THE FAILED SPINE

THE FAILED SPINE

Editors

SCOTT D. BODEN, M.D.

Professor of Orthopaedic Surgery,
Emory University School of Medicine, Atlanta, Georgia;
Director, The Emory Spine Center, Decatur, Georgia;
Chairman, National Spine Network, Marietta, Georgia

HENRY H. BOHLMAN, M.D.

Professor, Department of Orthopaedic Surgery,
Case Western Reserve University School of Medicine, Cleveland, Ohio;
Director, Spine Institute, University Hospitals of Cleveland, Cleveland, Ohio

LIPPINCOTT WILLIAMS & WILKINS
A **Wolters Kluwer** Company

Philadelphia • Baltimore • New York • London
Buenos Aires • Hong Kong • Sydney • Tokyo

Acquisitions Editor: Bob Hurley
Developmental Editor: Keith Donnellan
Supervising Editor: Mary Ann McLaughlin
Production Editor: Erica Broennle Nelson, Silverchair Science + Communications
Manufacturing Manager: Tim Reynolds
Cover Designer: Christine Jenny
Compositor: Silverchair Science + Communications
Printer: Edwards Brothers

©2003 by LIPPINCOTT WILLIAMS & WILKINS
530 Walnut Street
Philadelphia, PA 19106 USA
LWW.com

Printed in the USA

Library of Congress Cataloging-in-Publication Data

The failed spine / [edited by] Scott D. Boden and Henry H. Bohlman.
    p. ; cm.
  Includes bibliographical references and index.
  ISBN 0-7817-1760-4
  1. Cervical vertebrae--Pathophysiology. 2. Thoracic vertebrae--Pathophysiology. 3. Spine--Diseases--Treatment. I. Boden, Scott D. II. Bohlman, Henry H.
  [DNLM: 1. Cervical Vertebrae--pathology. 2. Lumbar Vertebrae--pathology. 3. Thoracic Vertebrae--pathology. WE 725 F161 2002]
  RD533 .F35 2002
  617.5'606--dc21

                                  2002069433

CONTENTS

CONTRIBUTING AUTHORS

William A. Abdu, M.D., M.S. Associate Professor, Department of Orthopaedic Surgery, Dartmouth Medical School, Hanover, New Hampshire; Dartmouth-Hitchcock Medical Center, Lebanon, New Hampshire

Todd J. Albert, M.D. Professor and Vice Chairman, Department of Orthopaedics, Jefferson Medical College of Thomas Jefferson University, Philadelphia, Pennsylvania; Rothman Institute, Philadelphia, Pennsylvania

Howard S. An, M.D. Morton International Professor of Orthopedic Surgery, Department of Orthopedic Surgery, Rush Medical College of Rush University, Chicago, Illinois; Rush-Presbyterian-St. Luke's Medical Center, Chicago, Illinois

Gunnar B.J. Andersson, M.D., Ph.D. Professor and Chairman, Department of Orthopedic Surgery, Rush Medical College of Rush University, Chicago, Illinois; Rush-Presbyterian-St. Luke's Medical Center, Chicago, Illinois

Perry A. Ball, M.D. Section of Neurosurgery, Dartmouth-Hitchcock Medical Center, Lebanon, New Hampshire

Oheneba Boachie-Adjei, M.D. Associate Professor of Surgery, Department of Orthopaedics, Weill Medical College of Cornell University, New York, New York

Scott D. Boden, M.D. Professor of Orthopaedic Surgery, Emory University School of Medicine, Atlanta, Georgia; Director, The Emory Spine Center, Decatur, Georgia; Chairman, National Spine Network, Marietta, Georgia

Henry H. Bohlman, M.D. Professor, Department of Orthopaedic Surgery, Case Western Reserve University School of Medicine, Cleveland, Ohio; Director, Spine Institute, University Hospitals of Cleveland, Cleveland, Ohio

Keith H. Bridwell, M.D. Asa C. and Dorothy W. Jones Professor of Orthopaedic Surgery, Department of Orthopaedic Surgery, Washington University School of Medicine, St. Louis, Missouri

Frank P. Cammisa, Jr., M.D. Associate Professor of Clinical Surgery, Weill Medical College of Cornell University, New York, New York; Chief, Spinal Surgical Service, Hospital for Special Surgery, New York, New York

Gregory D. Carlson, M.D. Assistant Clinical Professor, Department of Orthopaedic Surgery, University of California, Irvine, College of Medicine, Irvine, California

Christopher J. DeWald, M.D. Orthopaedics and Scoliosis, LLC, Chicago, Illinois

John R. Dimar II, M.D. University of Louisville, Louisville, Kentucky

Ashish D. Diwan, M.D., Ph.D. Lecturer, University of New South Wales, Sydney, Australia; Chief of Spine Service, Department of Orthopaedic Surgery, St. George Hospital, Sydney, Australia

Susan J. Dreyer, M.D. Assistant Professor, Departments of Orthopaedic Surgery and Physical Medicine and Rehabilitation, Emory University School of Medicine, Atlanta, Georgia

Sanford E. Emery, M.D. Associate Professor, Department of Orthopaedic Surgery, Case Western Reserve University School of Medicine, Cleveland, Ohio; University Hospitals of Cleveland, Cleveland, Ohio

Robert W. Gaines, Jr., M.D., F.A.C.S. Emeritus Professor of Orthopaedic Surgery, University of Missouri—Columbia School of Medicine, Columbia, Missouri; Columbia Spine Center, Columbia Orthopaedic Group, Columbia, Missouri

Steven D. Glassman, M.D. Associate Professor of Orthopaedic Surgery, Department of Orthopaedics, University of Louisville School of Medicine, Louisville, Kentucky

Michael E. Goldsmith, M.D. Clinical Instructor, Department of Orthopaedics, Georgetown University School of Medicine, Washington, D.C.

Carey D. Gorden, M.A. Assistant Clinical Professor of Medicine, Department of Medicine, University of California, Irvine, College of Medicine, Irvine, California

Eric J. Graham, M.D. Spine Fellow, Department of Orthopaedic Surgery, University of Pittsburgh School of Medicine, Pittsburgh, Pennsylvania; University of Pittsburgh Medical Center, Pittsburgh, Pennsylvania

John G. Heller, M.D. Professor of Orthopaedic Surgery and Spine Fellowship Director, Department of Orthopaedic Surgery, Emory University School of Medicine, Atlanta, Georgia; The Emory Spine Center, Decatur, Georgia

Alan S. Hilibrand, M.D. Assistant Professor of Orthopaedic Surgery, Department of Orthopaedic Surgery, Jefferson Medical College of Thomas Jefferson University, Philadelphia, Pennsylvania

Louis G. Jenis, M.D. Clinical Assistant Professor of Orthopaedic Surgery, Department of Orthopaedic Surgery, Tufts University School of Medicine, Boston, Massachusetts; New England Baptist Hospital, Boston, Massachusetts

Eldin E. Karaikovic, M.D., Ph.D. Department of Orthopaedic Surgery, University of Missouri—Columbia School of Medicine, Columbia, Missouri

Safdar N. Khan, M.D. Research Fellow, Spinal Surgical Service, Hospital for Special Surgery, New York, New York

William C. Lauerman, M.D. Professor and Chief of Spine Surgery, Department of Orthopaedics, Georgetown University School of Medicine, Washington, D.C.; Georgetown University Hospital, Washington, D.C.

Carl Lauryssen, M.D. Associate Professor, Department of Neurological Surgery, Washington University School of Medicine, St. Louis, Missouri

Richard D. Lazar, M.D. The Spine Center, Colorado Springs Orthopaedic Group, Colorado Springs, Colorado

Lawrence G. Lenke, M.D. Jerome J. Gilden Professor of Orthopaedic Surgery, Department of Orthopaedic Surgery, Washington University School of Medicine, St. Louis, Missouri

Howard I. Levy, M.D. Assistant Professor, Departments of Orthopaedics and Physical Medicine and Rehabilitation, Emory University School of Medicine, Atlanta, Georgia; The Emory Spine Center, Decatur, Georgia

Faiq Mahmud, M.D.* Spine Fellow, Spine Institute for Special Surgery, P.S.C., Louisville, Kentucky

John J. Oro, M.D. Professor, Department of Surgery, Division of Neurosurgery, University of Missouri—Columbia School of Medicine, Columbia, Missouri; University of Missouri Health Sciences Center, Columbia, Missouri

Hari K. Parvataneni, M.D. Orthopaedic Resident, Department of Orthopaedic Surgery, Lenox Hill Hospital, New York, New York

Nahshon Rand, M.D. Adjunct Professor of Orthopaedics, Department of Orthopaedics and Rehabilitation, Vanderbilt University School of Medicine, Nashville, Tennessee; Senior Surgeon, Israel Spine Center, Assuta Hospital, Tel Aviv, Israel

Mitchell F. Reiter, M.D. Assistant Professor of Orthopaedic Surgery, Department of Orthopaedic Surgery, UMDNJ—New Jersey Medical School, Newark, New Jersey

K. Daniel Riew, M.D. Associate Professor, Department of Orthopaedic Surgery, Washington University School of Medicine, St. Louis, Missouri; Barnes-Jewish Hospital, St. Louis, Missouri

Jonathan F. Rosenfeld, M.D., M.B.A. Resident in Orthopaedic Surgery, Department of Orthopaedic Surgery, Union Memorial Hospital, Baltimore, Maryland

Harvinder S. Sandhu, M.D. Associate Professor of Orthopaedic Surgery, Department of Orthopaedic Surgery, Weill Medical College of Cornell University, New York, New York; Hospital for Special Surgery, New York, New York

Gregory M. Sassmannshausen, M.D. Section of Orthopaedic Surgery, Dartmouth-Hitchcock Medical Center, Lebanon, New Hampshire

Farid F. Shafaie, M.D., M.S. Staff Neuroradiologist, Department of Radiology, MacNeal Hospital, Berwyn, Illinois

William O. Shaffer, M.D. Associate Professor, Department of Surgery, University of Kentucky College of Medicine, Lexington, Kentucky; Albert B. Chandler Medical Center, Lexington, Kentucky

Alexander R. Vaccaro, M.D. Professor of Orthopaedic Surgery, Department of Orthopaedics, Jefferson Medical College of Thomas Jefferson University, Philadelphia, Pennsylvania; Rothman Institute, Philadelphia, Pennsylvania

Thomas S. Whitecloud III, M.D. Professor and Chairman, Department of Orthopaedic Surgery, Tulane University School of Medicine, New Orleans, Louisiana; Tulane University Health Sciences Center, New Orleans, Louisiana

Scott C. Wilson, M.D. Assistant Professor and Chief, Department of Orthopaedic Surgery, Section of Orthopaedic Oncology, Tulane University School of Medicine, New Orleans, Louisiana; Tulane University Health Sciences Center, New Orleans, Louisiana

Neill M. Wright, M.D. Assistant Professor of Neurological Surgery, Department of Neurological Surgery, Washington University School of Medicine, St. Louis, Missouri

Wicharn Yingsakmongkol, M.D. Assistant Professor of Orthopaedic Surgery, Department of Orthopaedic Surgery, Faculty of Medicine, Chulalongkorn University, Bangkok, Thailand

*Deceased.

PREFACE

The last two decades have seen an explosion in our understanding of the pathophysiology of spinal problems and the technology available to diagnose and correct them. Unfortunately, not all spine surgery results in successful outcome. Careful selection of patients, an accurate diagnosis, and choice of an appropriate surgical procedure all increase, but do not guarantee, the likelihood of a good result. Once the first operation has failed, the chances for subsequent successful surgery diminish, and the medical and social costs to society increase exponentially. Although patients with one or more failed spine procedures are appearing more frequently at tertiary spine referral centers, little has been written to specifically help tackle the difficult problem of managing this unique group of patients.

The purpose of this book is to present an organized and rational approach to the clinical and radiographic evaluation of these complex patients with failed cervical, thoracic, and lumbar spine surgery after degenerative, traumatic, neoplastic, and infectious disorders. Particular emphasis is placed on new diagnostic techniques such as gadolinium-enhanced modalities, including myelography and computed tomography. Case illustrations are included to guide the reader through the pitfalls of diagnosis unique to the postoperative patient. After outlining how to select patients who can be helped with additional surgery, the remainder of the text concentrates on the specific surgical options and techniques. Revision spine surgery is quite a different animal from the first-time operation, and helpful technical hints are illustrated to minimize complications. In addition, immediate and delayed postoperative complications are discussed.

This book was written not only for the spine surgeon but also for the generalist, who frequently is faced with evaluation of these complicated patients. Although not all orthopedic surgeons and neurosurgeons actually perform revision spine surgery, an understanding of the consequences of failed spine operations is essential to prevent them. This understanding is also important for radiologists, who assist in outlining the most cost-effective diagnostic regimen and who must have a working knowledge of the most relevant radiographic findings in these patients. In addition, this text is intended to help physiatrists and neurologists, who often see these patients after unsuccessful surgery, to identify patients who may be candidates for further surgery and those who should be directed to a chronic pain management program. The authors hope the multidisciplinary audience of this text will help control the increasing magnitude of the problem of the failed spine surgery patient.

The National Spine Network (NSN) is a not-for-profit consortium of Spine Centers of Excellence throughout the United States. Founded in 1996, the organization focuses on collecting outcomes data for spinal patients and performing multicenter clinical trials to evaluate new and existing treatments. NSN has one of the largest outcomes databases on spine patients and has fostered a variety of educational programs to encourage informed decision making for patients with spinal disorders and improve the quality of spine care delivered. This textbook is one such educational effort, and all proceeds go to NSN to continue to study ways to improve the care of patients with spinal disorders. For more information about NSN, contact Harry Freedman at HafatNSN@aol.com.

Scott D. Boden, M.D.
Henry H. Bohlman, M.D.

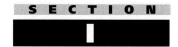

SECTION
1

CERVICAL SPINE

CERVICAL SPINE: EVALUATION

ALAN S. HILIBRAND AND NAHSHON RAND

It is estimated that over a recent 3-year period there were approximately 76,000 hospitalizations annually in the United States for the surgical treatment of disorders of the cervical spine (10). It is likely that most of these patients experienced relief of their preoperative symptoms and returned to normal activities. Indeed, long-term follow-up studies of posterior (14,17,18,25) and anterior (5–7,11,16,18,20,29–31,34,40) cervical spine procedures have shown that between 80% and 90% of patients experience these so-called satisfactory results. Unfortunately, this leaves 10% to 20% of patients with "unsatisfactory" results that may deteriorate over longer follow-up periods. Use of the term *failed neck* to describe these patients may be inappropriate, however, as new disease at an adjacent level develops in many patients long after surgery that is probably not due to a "failure" of the surgical technique. It is, therefore, imperative to identify elements in the clinical presentation, physical examination, and diagnostic workup that are suggestive of persistent, as opposed to new, pathology in the cervical spine.

CLINICAL PRESENTATION

The clinical evaluation of a patient following failed neck surgery begins with a thorough review of all prior surgical procedures. Usually, this requires a meticulous chronology of the disease process from the time of the initial onset of symptoms, documenting the exact surgical interventions. It is essential to understand the presenting symptoms before the previous procedure(s) and how they were affected by treatment. Important factors to consider are the presence or absence of a postoperative pain-free interval, the length of the interval, and any differences in the location or radiation, or both, of the present pain in comparison with prior symptoms.

It is also important to query the patient regarding recent trauma, which may have precipitated recurrence of symptoms. Major traumatic events, such as falling from a height or a motor vehicle accident, may result in a ligamentous or bony injury, a disk

herniation at an adjacent level, or "failure" of a stable fibrous nonunion. Furthermore, in patients who underwent a prior anterior or posterior fusion for a traumatic injury, late deformity or recurrence of neck pain, arm pain, or myelopathy may develop as a result of persistent instability (8,36,38).

The presenting complaint of the failed neck patient can now be considered in the context of the patient's history of cervical spinal pathology. The current symptoms should be compared with previous complaints with respect to location, radiation, quality, and precipitating factors. This should allow differentiation between recurrence of a previous problem and the development of a new disease process. Persistent pain in the same dermatomal distribution usually indicates an inadequate decompression at the index procedure. Initial pain relief, followed by the insidious recurrence of the same radicular complaints over the following 6 to 12 months, may suggest the development of a pseudarthrosis or failure of any internal fixation, or both. Late recurrence of pain in the *same* distribution is indicative of a recurrent disk herniation or foraminal stenosis at a level previously treated by foraminotomy or diskectomy, or both, but is very unusual in patients who underwent a complete decompression and successful arthrodesis at the index operation. In patients in whom new symptoms develop after a prolonged pain-free interval in a different radicular distribution, the development of symptomatic new disease at an adjacent segment should be considered. This occurrence has been reported in patients who have undergone cervical spine surgery at a rate of 3% per year, with adjacent segment disease developing in more than 25% of patients by 10 years following surgery (19).

As with patients who present with primary cervical complaints, evaluation of the failed neck patient must include localization of the patient's symptoms and his or her radiation, if any. Mechanical, or "diskogenic," neck pain is typically limited to the paracervical, supraclavicular, intrascapular, and infrascapular regions and may be difficult to localize (2) (Fig. 1). Neurologic symptoms, due to anatomic compression or chemical irritation of a spinal nerve root, usually extend beyond

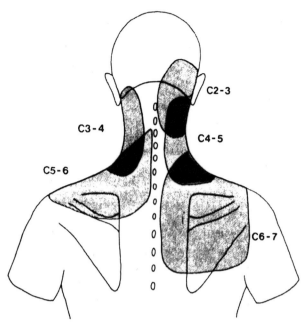

FIGURE 1. Patterns of referred pain from degenerative changes within the cervical spine. (From Aprill C, Dwyer A, Bogduk N. Cervical zygapophyseal joint pain patterns II: a clinical evaluation. *Spine* 1990;15:458–461, with permission.)

the edge of the acromion into the arm or the forearm, or both. The pattern of these symptoms is classically described by the dermatomal representation of the affected nerve root, although it should be remembered

that in the unusual circumstance of compression of the third or fourth cervical nerve root patients may present with only neck pain (Fig. 2).

Associated factors that increase or decrease symptoms may also be helpful in making the correct diagnosis. Patients who have compressive pathology in the neural foramina usually experience amplification of their symptoms with rotation toward the side of the symptoms (9). The symptoms may also be exacerbated with cervical flexion or extension. Similarly, these symptoms may be relieved with shoulder abduction, resting the affected hand on top of the head (9). In patients with mechanical neck pain due to adjacent disk degeneration or a pseudarthrosis, any significant motion or jarring of the axial skeleton may be painful but should be alleviated in a soft or hard cervical collar. For patients with myelopathy due to iatrogenic kyphosis or instability, extremes of flexion may result in electric shock–like sensations into the upper or lower extremities, while recurrent or persistent cervical spondylotic myelopathy related to cervical stenosis leads to these same symptoms in cervical extension.

Other exacerbating factors may suggest a nonspondylogenic source and should also be considered. Shoulder and arm pain that originates in the shoulder itself and is worsened with overhead activities is

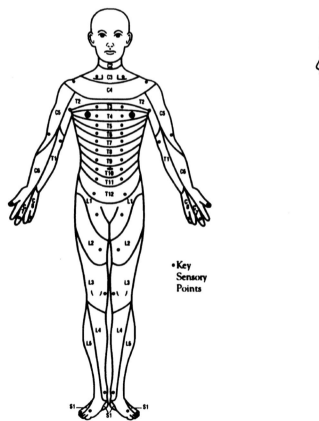

• Key Sensory Points

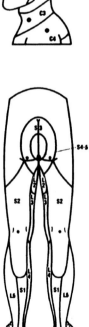

FIGURE 2. Dermatomal representation of the spinal nerve roots. (From *International standards for neurological and functional classification of spinal cord injury.* American Spinal Injury Association, rev 1996, with permission.)

suggestive of shoulder impingement or rotator cuff disease, or both. Pain in the hand and forearm that is exacerbated with repetitive motions of wrist flexion/extension may be due to compression of the median or ulnar nerves in the forearm or wrist. Other peripheral neuropathies may also produce arm pain that may radiate as far as the shoulder and are usually related to positional changes of the affected upper extremity.

The patient's response to previous treatment modalities should also be considered. Was there a response to antiinflammatory medications or a steroid taper? Did the patient respond to isometric cervical strengthening? Was cervical traction effective in "centralizing" the patient's radicular symptoms? Did a selective cervical root injection or epidural steroid injection provide at least temporary relief? Mechanical neck pain usually shows some improvement with antiinflammatory medications and isometric strengthening, whereas steroid preparations and cervical traction may be especially helpful in relieving radicular pain (32).

If the symptoms have been unresponsive to prior therapeutic interventions, or if the patients have been noncompliant with previous treatments, the existence of mitigating circumstances should be considered. Are the patients employed, and are they currently working? Are they able to perform their work duties, and is the workplace accommodating their difficulties? Although never specifically studied for patients with cervical spine complaints, it has been clearly identified that low job satisfaction and prior low back surgery are prognostic of a poor treatment outcome for a low back injury (3). The patient should also be asked whether the development or recurrence of symptoms is related to a compensable injury. Was the injury work related, and is there any ongoing litigation? Although never published for cervical disk disease, the outcome of lumbar diskectomy has been shown to correlate strongly with these factors (22).

The medical history of the patient with neck or arm pain, or both, following previous cervical spine surgery should also be carefully investigated. A history of malignancy and a family history of malignancies should be sought, keeping in mind solid neoplasms, which are most likely to metastasize to bone (prostate, breast, lung, kidney, and gastrointestinal) (23). The review of systems should include symptoms and conditions that are suspicious for an underlying infectious process, such as recent fevers, chills, or sweats, and a history of recent infections, immunosuppression, or intravenous drug abuse. Symptoms of unexplained weight loss, anorexia, malaise, or fatigue and system-specific complaints, such as hemoptysis, hematemesis/melena/hematochezia, hematuria, the appearance of a breast mass, or the development of a bleeding diathesis, should raise concerns of a malignant process and warrant further diagnostic evaluation. In patients who have undergone a previous grafting procedure, documentation of smoking status is important; a positive smoking history should raise concerns for a pseudarthrosis, as significantly lower rates of arthrodesis have been observed in smokers who are undergoing anterior cervical interbody grafting at more than one level (43).

PHYSICAL EXAMINATION

The physical examination of the failed neck begins with an overall inspection of posture and gait when the patient enters the room. At this time, a judgment can be made concerning the overall alignment of the cervical spine. Kyphosis may be present, especially after a destabilizing laminectomy, anterior cervical decompression without fusion, or graft failure after anterior cervical reconstruction. Rotatory abnormalities may be present as a result of muscle spasm or contracture, facet subluxation or dislocation, or malalignment following previous cervical spine arthrodesis.

The skin should be examined for scars from previous surgery on the cervical spine, thyroid, carotid arteries, or trachea. The location of these may influence the approach used in future cervical spine surgery. Special consideration should be given to the possibility of an asymptomatic unilateral vocal cord paralysis due to an injury to the recurrent laryngeal nerve, especially following a right-sided anterior approach to the cervical spine. In these cases, performing revision surgery through a contralateral approach places the patient at risk for bilateral vocal cord paralysis (39).

The patient's gait should be assessed and the use of any ambulatory assistive devices documented (see Neurologic Assessment). Upper extremity coordination may be inferred from the patient's ability to dress him- or herself in an office gown, legibly complete a questionnaire, and maintain personal hygiene. Fasciculations or muscle atrophy, or both, in the deltoid, biceps, or triceps muscles may provide a clue to the specific level of neurologic compression. Subtle muscle wasting can be documented by measuring the midbrachial and midantebrachial circumferences.

Palpation of the neck should be performed in search of any local tenderness or palpable deformity.

The general cervical anatomic landmarks should be identified, including the hyoid bone (C-3), thyroid cartilage (C4-5), cricoid ring (C-6), and carotid tubercle (C-6). Palpable soft tissue landmarks in the anterior neck are the sternocleidomastoid muscle, the thyroid gland, the lymph node chains, the carotid pulse, and the supraclavicular fossa. A cervical rib is sometimes palpable in this region. The presence of asymmetry, tenderness, or a lump in an identified structure may localize to underlying pathology.

Posterior bony landmarks include the occiput, the inion, the nuchal line, the mastoid processes, and the spinous processes of the second, sixth, and seventh cervical vertebrae. It is sometimes possible to palpate the facet joints, which are felt as small domes lateral to the spinous processes. Identifiable soft tissue landmarks include the trapezius muscle, the lymph node chains, and the superior nuchal ligament. If inflamed or affected by trauma or another process, the greater occipital nerves, located at the base of the skull near the inion, may be palpable and tender. The presence of tenderness, spasm, or deviation from the normal alignment should raise suspicion of underlying pathology.

The shoulders, arms, and hands should be assessed as part of the examination of the neck. Cervical spine disorders share some symptoms with extraspinal pathologies in the shoulder and entrapment syndromes of the peripheral nerves. Examining the range of motion of the shoulder or elbow and the relation of pain to motion can differentiate between symptoms that originate in the cervical spine and those related to impingement syndrome, shoulder instability, or lateral epicondylitis of the elbow.

The normal cervical range of motion includes flexion/extension, axial rotation, and lateral bending, although most day-to-day neck motion involves a coupled motion in all three planes. Restriction of a specific motion may be caused by abnormal articulations at one or more levels, although it should be remembered that almost any cervical spine disorder may cause reactive muscle spasm with limited range of motion. Voluntary restriction of motion may also occur as a result of guarding against the impinging effect of an osteophyte, a herniated disk, or other compressive pathology on the neural elements. The patient may also have general limitation of motion in all directions following a multilevel arthrodesis, especially when it involves the upper cervical spine.

Provocative maneuvers test for the presence of neural element compression within the cervical spine or upper extremities. They are very specific, as they are rarely present under normal conditions. The Valsalva maneuver raises intrathecal pressure due to the reduction of venous return caused by an increase in intrathoracic pressure. If a space-occupying lesion is present in the spinal canal (such as a herniated disk or a tumor), the increased intrathecal pressure caused by the Valsalva maneuver is likely to exacerbate the radicular symptoms. Spurling's maneuver (36) involves a combination of cervical extension, vertical compression, and axial rotation. When compressive pathology is present in the neural foramen, this maneuver should reproduce radicular symptoms with ipsilateral axial rotation. *Lhermitte's phenomenon* is defined as the production of electric shock–like sensations into the arms or legs, or both, with extremes of motion in the sagittal plane. In spondylotic myelopathy, these symptoms can be elicited with cervical extension, which usually narrows the sagittal canal diameter. In patients with posttraumatic or iatrogenic cervical kyphosis, however, extremes of flexion may exacerbate the "draping" of the spinal cord across posterior vertebral osteophytes, exacerbating the patient's symptoms.

Several "provocative" tests can also be used to differentiate a peripheral source of pain from spondylogenic pathology. Impingement test and Hawkins sign identify impingement of the rotator cuff muscles between the humeral head and the acromion. As the patient's arm is flexed from 60 to 120 degrees, the production of shoulder or arm pain, or both, is noted. Symptoms derived from cervical pathology may overlap, but usually cervical pathology should not be exacerbated within this specific range of motion. Hawkins test requires placement of the arm at 90 degrees' flexion with the elbow flexed. The reproduction of symptoms as the arm is internally rotated also suggests shoulder impingement.

The commonest site of peripheral compression of the ulnar nerve is in the groove between the olecranon and the medial epicondyle; the commonest site of peripheral compression of the median nerve is around the transverse carpal ligament (the carpal tunnel). *Tinel's sign* describes eliciting pain and paresthesias by tapping over an entrapped nerve. Phalen's test involves placement of the wrist in extreme flexion for up to 1 minute. This test, when positive, elicits pain, numbness, or tingling in the index, middle, and ring fingertips. Phalen's and Tinel's signs are useful in differentiating cervical versus peripheral sources of neural element compression.

Adson's test assesses possible compression of the subclavian artery and other structures in the thoracic outlet by a cervical rib or tight scalenus muscle. While the radial pulse is palpated, the patient's arm is abducted, extended, and externally rotated. The patient is then instructed to turn his or her head toward the examined arm while taking a deep breath. Diminution or elimination of the radial pulse is considered a positive test.

NEUROLOGIC ASSESSMENT

Clinical evaluation of the failed neck must include a comprehensive assessment of neurologic function. This evaluation begins with consideration of the patient's gait pattern and overall physical station. In particular, a wide-based gait in association with dizziness or unsteadiness may be caused by cervical spinal cord compression or cerebellar dysfunction. The presence of spinal cord compression may cause difficulties with tandem gait, which can be observed in the office.

Neurologic evaluation continues with a detailed level-by-level assessment of motor, sensory, and reflex functions to localize neural element compression within the cervical spine that is causing neural element compression (Table 1). Pathology at the C4-5 level may result in radicular findings in a C-5 distribution. This pathology may include motor weakness of the deltoid or biceps brachii muscles, sensory abnormalities (hyperesthesia, hypoesthesia, or, rarely, anesthesia) across the lateral arm in the distribution of the cutaneous branch of the axillary nerve, and/or a diminished biceps reflex. Radiculopathy in a C-6 distribution is usually caused by compressive pathology at the C5-6 level where the C-6 nerve root exits the spinal canal. However, pathology in a paracentral location at the C4-5 level can sometimes compress the sixth motor root anteriorly where it exits the spinal cord, resulting in C-6 weakness. Several muscles receive innervation from the C-6 level, including the biceps brachii, extensor carpi radialis longus/brevis, supinator, and pronator teres, although all of these groups also receive innervation from other levels. Sensation may be affected in the distribution of the musculocutaneous nerve, which includes the lateral forearm, thumb, and index finger. The primary C-6 reflex arc involves the brachioradialis reflex, although C-6 pathology may also attenuate the biceps reflex, which receives C-5 and C-6 input. Alternatively, spinal cord compression at or above the C4-5 level may result in hyperactivity of the brachioradialis reflex.

Compressive pathology at the C6-7 level (or, less commonly, at C5-6) usually results in a C-7 radiculopathy. The C-7 motor groups include the triceps brachii, flexor carpi radialis, and extensor digitorum muscles. The purest site of C-7 sensory representation is in the long finger, although there may be overlap with C-6 or C-8. C-7 pathology may attenuate the triceps reflex, whereas spinal cord compression above the C5-6 level may amplify the triceps reflex.

Radiculopathy in a C-8 distribution (due to pathology at the C-7 to T-1 or C6-7 levels) may be associated with finger flexion (grip strength) or altered sensation in the distribution of the ulnar nerve along the medial forearm and ring and little fingers. Pathology at T1-2 or C-7 to T-1 may cause a T-1 radiculopathy, with weakness of the intrinsic muscles of the hand or sensory changes across the medial arm. Neither the C-8 nor T-1 level has a reflex arc. Compressive pathology in this region of the spine is much less common than at the higher levels.

Patients who have spinal cord compression in the neck may have neurologic findings in the lower extremities. Motor or sensory changes may be present, although they are rarely dermatomal, and often present as "global" changes in an entire lower extremity. Deep tendon reflexes may be brisk in cases of cervical myelopathy, although they may be decreased if coexistent lumbar stenosis is present.

The neurologic evaluation should also include evaluation of proprioception and vibration sensation. Although most compressive pathology lies anterior to the spinal cord and nerve roots, posterior compression due to infolding, hypertrophy, or ossification of the ligamentum flavum may also occur. This compression can affect posterior column function, including vibration and proprioception, which can also be seen in gait pattern abnormalities. The neurologic evaluation then concludes with an assessment for any pathologic reflexes. These include Hoffmann's sign, Babinski's sign, and the presence of myoclonus. When

TABLE 1. NEUROLOGIC ASSESSMENT OF THE CERVICAL SPINE

Level	Motor Group	Sensory Distribution	Reflex
C-5	Deltoid biceps	Lateral arm	Biceps
C-6	Wrist extensors	Lateral forearm, thumb, and index fingers	Biceps, brachioradialis
C-7	Triceps, wrist flexors	Middle finger	Triceps
C-8	Finger flexors	Ring and little fingers, medial forearm	None
T-1	Hard intrinsics	Medial arm	None

present, these are suggestive of spinal cord compression, although other conditions, including hyperthyroidism, multiple sclerosis, stroke, closed head injury, and other intracranial processes, may also cause the appearance of pathologic reflexes.

DIAGNOSTIC TESTING

Diagnostic imaging of the postoperative cervical spine begins with comprehensive plain radiographs. Radiography usually includes the standard "five views" (anteroposterior, lateral, two oblique views, and the open mouth odontoid) as well as dynamic flexion/extension lateral views. Many patients cannot recall the exact technique or operated levels of the previous procedure, and the anteroposterior and lateral views can assist in identifying the prior surgical procedure. If a fusion was attempted, the dynamic lateral views can be used to identify the development of a pseudarthrosis. In the scientific literature, various criteria have been used to identify a nonunion, including the presence of greater than 1- to 3-mm motion between spinous processes or the absence of continuous bony trabeculae between vertebrae, or both (6,11,13,21) (Fig. 3). In patients who

have achieved successful fusion, dynamic views may demonstrate the development of degenerative instability above or below the solid fusion (Fig. 4). In individuals who underwent a posterior decompression without fusion, lateral radiographs should be used to screen for the development of a kyphotic deformity. When overall cervical kyphosis exceeds 20 degrees, anterior spinal cord compression may develop as the spinal cord is "draped" across osteophytes on the posterior margins of the vertebral bodies (41) (Fig. 5). In patients who have undergone spinal instrumentation, malposition of hardware may be identified between the anteroposterior and lateral views. Resorption of foraminal spurs on oblique radiographs is highly specific for a solid arthrodesis (30) but lacks sensitivity as a diagnostic sign. When the presence of a solid arthrodesis cannot be identified with dynamic lateral radiographs, plain or computer-assisted tomography should be used (Fig. 6).

The advent of magnetic resonance imaging (MRI) in the mid-1980s provided a valuable tool for the evaluation of the postoperative spine. The principal value of *postoperative* MRI has been in the differentiation of epidural scarring from residual neural element compression. In the postoperative spine, the injection

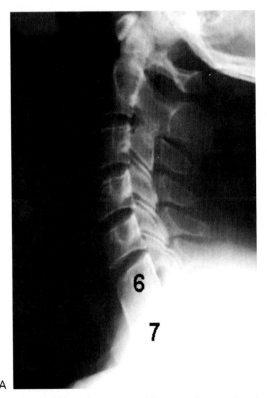
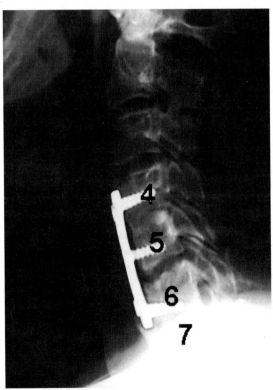

A   B

FIGURE 3. Patient with a previous arthrodesis at C6-7 **(A)** who underwent fusion of the adjacent levels C5-6 and C4-5 using iliac crest bone graft and an anterior cervical plate. At 1-year follow-up **(B)**, there is clear evidence of a nonunion at C5-6, with absence of bridging trabecular bone and loosening of the screws placed into the C-6 vertebral body.

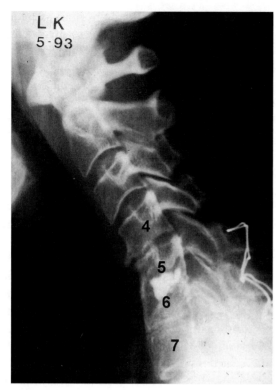

FIGURE 4. Degenerative instability at C4-5 above a solid anterior/posterior fusion at C5-6.

of the paramagnetic contrast agent gadolinium–diethylenetriamine pentaacetic acid enhances epidural scarring but does not enhance recurrent or residual disk herniations on early (within 10 minutes) T-1 images (12). MRI has been shown to be very sensitive

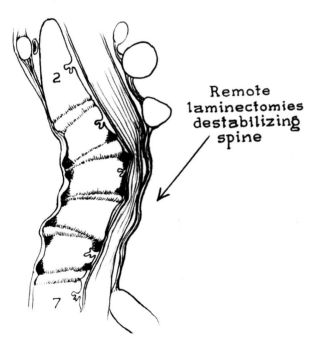

FIGURE 5. Destabilizing effects of a prior wide laminectomy in the cervical spine. Note the development of tethering and anterior spinal cord compression secondary to the deformity.

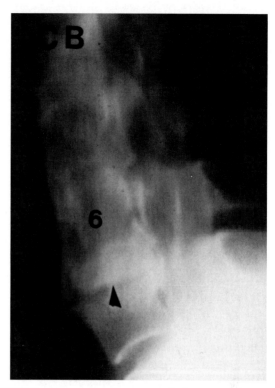

FIGURE 6. Conventional tomograph demonstrating a non-union at the C6-7 level after a three-level anterior cervical interbody grafting. Note solid arthrodesis and bony trabeculation across the interspaces at C4-5 and C5-6. The arrowhead indicates the site of the prior laminectomy.

at demonstrating neural compressive pathology, with accuracy similar to that of postmyelography computed axial tomography (27,28). It can also demonstrate the degree of disk hydration (so-called disk degeneration) at adjacent motion segments.

MRI offers some distinct advantages over computed tomography myelography (CTM). T2-weighted images can be used to evaluate patients who present with cervical myelopathy, myelomalacia (intrinsic spinal cord degeneration, which may be due to prior spinal cord compression), a traumatic or iatrogenic injury, or an intrinsic pathologic process (Fig. 7). The technique of magnetic resonance angiography has been used to identify the patency and function of the vertebral arteries, which may be damaged by trauma or prior surgical procedures (15,35). Unfortunately, although MRI is very sensitive for pathology, it has relatively low *specificity* (produces many false-positive findings); in one study, approximately 20% of asymptomatic persons were found to have compressive pathology on MRI of the cervical spine (4).

Although MRI is an excellent screening study, many surgeons still prefer CTM of the postoperative cervical spine in patients who demonstrate recurrent or new-onset radiculopathy or myelopathy. CTM provides sharper definition of spinal cord and nerve

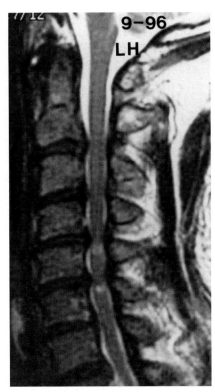

FIGURE 7. Sagittal T2-weighted magnetic resonance image demonstrating areas of increased signal within the spinal cord at C4-5 and C5-6 secondary to a spinal cord contusion with a "central cord" syndrome.

root dimensions than current MRI technology, and sagittal/coronal reconstructions can identify an established pseudarthrosis. Persistent posterior osteophytes are more clearly seen on CTM because of the better definition of bone versus soft tissue (Fig. 8).

Laboratory tests may provide supportive evidence for a diagnosis in complicated cases, although they generally have a minor role in diagnosing the source of neck pain after cervical spine surgery. Laboratory tests can confirm the diagnosis of inflammation or infection and should be considered for patients with severe or atypical mechanical neck pain. The most useful tests are white blood cell count (WBC), erythrocyte sedimentation rate (ESR), blood chemistry, urinalysis, and cultures.

The WBC and the ESR are quite sensitive but nonspecific means of searching for infectious or inflammatory disorders. Both are elevated with any acute-phase response of the body to injury. They can also be used for monitoring the activity level of the disease process as well as the response to treatment. The WBC usually responds rapidly to treatment, whereas a lag period may exist before changes in the ESR are observed. In spondyloarthropathies and malignancy, the ESR is generally elevated, although the WBC may still be in the upper range of normal.

The WBC and ESR are usually normal in patients with mechanical neck pain due to degenerative spondylosis. C-reactive protein is another acute-phase product that is elevated in the setting of inflammation, malignancy, or infection. It usually reaches a peak level within 3 to 4 days of an acute event and then recedes to normal over a few days. However, it may remain elevated in chronic situations.

Blood chemistries may be helpful in the setting of "red flags" identified in the history. Hypercalcemia is associated with primary and metastatic malignancies, although alterations in serum calcium and phosphorus may also reflect osteomalacia. Increased serum calcium and low serum phosphorus are typical of primary hyperthyroidism. Elevated alkaline phosphatase may be detected in osteomalacia, healing fracture, bony metastases of carcinoma, or Paget's disease. The total protein and serum albumin levels may reflect chronic inflammation and nutritional depletion situations. Marked hyperproteinemia or proteinuria, determined by a serum or urine electrophoresis test, may be associated with multiple myeloma. Otherwise, no specific electrolyte changes are associated with degenerative osteoarthritis or mechanical neck problems.

Technetium bone scans are sensitive to bone activity and may be helpful when imaging findings are lagging behind the bone activity, as in cases of acute infection or pathologic stress fracture. They enable early detection of infection, inflammation, trauma, or neoplasm and may help localize the process. One important exception is multiple myeloma. In myeloma, the neoplastic plasma cells may cause large bone defects, which can clearly be seen on a radiograph, although the bone scan may be negative. In contrast to their high sensitivity, technetium scans are nonspecific and cannot differentiate between inflammation, trauma, and degenerative change. Gallium or indium radionuclide scans are more specific for the presence or absence of infection. In the era of high-resolution, high-sensitivity contrast-enhanced MRI, a patient often has an MRI performed before a radionuclide scan, and the MRI findings may, therefore, render such a scan unnecessary in many cases.

Electrodiagnostic studies (EDS) can provide objective data regarding nerve damage. They can demonstrate the integrity of the nerve-muscle unit and different spinal cord tracts. EDS can confirm existing damage objectively and define severity and distribution of damage. However, they cannot diagnose the etiology of the damage. EDS may serve to identify the level of a cervical injury as well as to differentiate central versus spinal nerve versus truncal (brachial plexus)

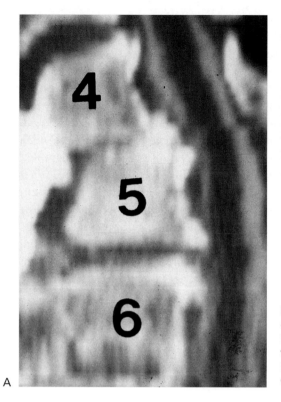

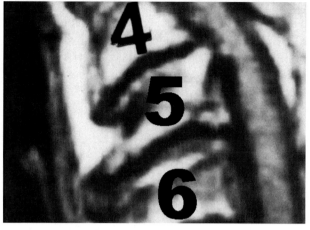

FIGURE 8. Sagittal images of C-4 through C-6 from a postmyelogram computed tomogram **(A)** and a magnetic resonance image **(B)** from a patient with cervical spondylosis and kyphosis with myelopathy. Anterior spinal cord compression due to draping of the spinal cord across chondroosseous spurs is present at C4-5 and C5-6.

versus peripheral disease. The studies may assist in identifying symptomatic pathology when multiple abnormalities are present on imaging studies. EDS can also be used in the failed neck patient to document the patient's status before any surgical intervention.

EDS can also be used to differentiate between myopathy and neural damage and between peripheral neuropathy, radiculopathy, and myelopathy. The commonly used studies include electromyography (EMG), nerve conduction velocity (NCV), and somatosensory evoked potentials (SSEPs). EMG measures the action potentials of muscle fibers. NCV measures the conduction velocity through a nerve and its latency. Because both tests require direct or indirect access to the nerve or muscle, they are primarily used to diagnose a peripheral neuropathy. Motor and sensory nerve conduction velocities may be normal in patients with radiculopathy or myelopathy, because they measure only the conduction velocity in the peripheral, uninjured nerve. The H-reflex (the electrical analogue of a tendon reflex) should also be evaluated. It is affected almost immediately after nerve root compression or damage, and it can detect a lesion in the sensory and the motor parts of the reflex arc. It is generally useful in diagnosing cervical radiculopathy, especially of C-7. A comparison must be done between right and left, and it should be remembered that, once damaged, the H-reflex never recovers, which limits its usefulness in chronic cases. In addition, the H-reflex cannot diagnose between damage to the spinal cord, sensory roots, motor roots, brachial plexus, or peripheral nerve. Furthermore, EMG/NCV studies are considered specific but have poor sensitivity; a normal EMG and NCV cannot exclude spinal or radicular pathology, although significant findings on EMG/NCV indicate an organic source to the patient's symptoms (26). EDS may be helpful in differentiating cervical spondylotic myelopathy from anterior motor horn cell disease and in differentiating between shoulder-neck symptoms that arise in peripheral entrapment syndromes and those arising in cervical radiculopathy (37).

SSEPs evaluate the conduction of peripheral neural stimuli along the spinal cord to the cerebral cortex. The small potentials that arise from peripheral stimulation are averaged together to determine the latency. They can detect abnormalities in peripheral sensory and mixed nerves and assess the integrity of the sensory tracts of the spinal cord. One advantage of SSEPs over EMG/NCV is the ability to evaluate spinal cord integrity. However, because peripheral nerves usually carry fibers that originate in several cervical levels, conventional SSEPs cannot be reliably used to diagnose the specific level of the pathology. SSEPs that are read at a spinal rather than a cortical level may improve the accuracy, however. Mixed nerve SSEPs are mainly useful for detecting spinal cord abnormalities, such as spinal tumors, demyelinating diseases, and compressive myelopathy (24). This test, like the

EMG and NCV, is specific but not sensitive. Another method for reading SSEPs is by directly stimulating the specific dermatome of interest (dermatomal SEP). In the cervical spine, stimulating a relatively limited and well-defined skin area should correspond to a specific dermatome of interest (C-6: thumb, C-7: middle finger, C-8: little finger), although it is a technically demanding examination.

DIFFERENTIAL DIAGNOSIS (ALGORITHM)

Persistence or recurrence of neck or arm pain, or both, may occur for many reasons after cervical spinal surgery. The previous operation may have been done for the wrong diagnosis, or the wrong operation may have been done for the correct diagnosis. In other instances, the correct operation may have been performed for the appropriate diagnosis but in a patient with secondary factors that mitigate against a successful outcome. When the previous surgery involved an inadequate decompression, stabilization, or alignment, revision surgery is usually required due to failure of the prior surgical technique (14,29,41,42). In patients in whom new symptoms develop after a prolonged pain-free interval in a different distribution due to new disease at an adjacent level, nonoperative treatments may be effective (19). When these patients require another procedure, it usually involves surgery on an unoperated segment and is not the result of technical "failure." Finally, there is a subset of patients who may not achieve a satisfactory outcome from the previous surgery because of persistent mechanical neck pain or factors that are unrelated to the cervical spondylotic disease.

We propose a stepwise algorithm for the differential diagnosis of the failed neck patient as outlined in Figure 9. The evaluation begins by ruling out the presence of a serious underlying medical or neurologic condition that may be responsible for the patient's complaints. An infectious or pathologic process (primary or metastatic cancer) may be suspected based on the presence of certain constitutional symptoms or organ system–specific complaints. If suspected, further medical evaluation should be sought immediately; the patient "leaves" the differential diagnostic algorithm of the "failed neck" until the medical workup is completed and any urgent treatment is delivered. Consultation with a neurologist may be appropriate in the patient who has progressive "myelopathy" symptoms in spite of a complete anterior decompression for cervical spondylotic myelopathy to rule out demyelinating disease or an intracranial process.

After ruling out any "red flags," the next diagnostic step is the evaluation by plain radiographs, including dynamic views. These films may identify an underlying structural problem, such as a fracture or deformity, or the presence of a pseudarthrosis, which usually requires flexion/extension lateral radiographs for diagnosis in the absence of hardware failure. When a cervical spine fracture is identified, the patient should be given the appropriate orthopedic management, although the possibility of an underlying pathologic process should be considered. If the plain films demonstrate a deformity such as postlaminectomy kyphosis and the patient is symptomatic, he or she should be sent for CTM to evaluate the possibility of spinal cord compression and should be treated appropriately.

In patients with initial pain relief followed by recurrent axial symptoms during the first year after surgery, the possibility of pseudarthrosis should be considered. In some cases, these patients may note recurrence of radicular complaints in the preoperative distribution. Usually, the diagnosis of a pseudarthrosis can be made using dynamic plain film criteria. If pseudarthrosis is suspected but dynamic plain films are inconclusive, further evaluation by conventional tomography can confirm the diagnosis. If the patient with a symptomatic pseudarthrosis of the cervical spine requires surgical treatment, preoperative CTM should be performed to identify any residual compressive pathology or symptomatic adjacent segment disease that may affect the surgical treatment plan (see Chapter 3).

In the "failed neck" patient with unremarkable plain radiographs, the remainder of the diagnostic algorithm is driven by the patient's radicular symptoms, if any. If the patient's radicular complaints are the same as they were before the previous procedure(s), an inadequate decompression should be suspected. Either MRI with gadolinium contrast (preferred for failed posterior decompression without fusion) or CTM (preferred for failed anterior procedures) should be used to confirm the diagnosis and to assist in presurgical planning. If the advanced imaging study is negative for residual compressive pathology, electrodiagnostic testing is appropriate to evaluate for a peripheral neuropathy or an underlying neurologic disorder. If the electrodiagnostic workup is negative and the patient underwent an arthrodesis, conventional tomograms should be obtained to rule out pseudarthrosis.

If the patient's radicular symptoms are different from what they were before the previous operation, the possibility of symptomatic disease at an adjacent

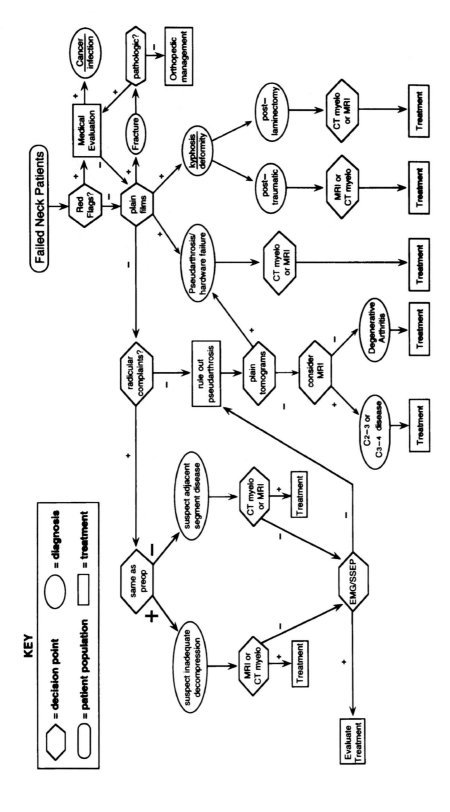

FIGURE 9. Algorithm developed by the authors for the evaluation of the patient with new or recurrent symptoms following previous surgical treatment of the cervical spine. CT myelo, computed tomography myelography; EMG/SSEP, electromyography/somatosensory evoked potential; MRI, magnetic resonance imaging.

motion segment should be considered. Once again, the diagnosis can be confirmed by either MRI or CTM, which can also be used for presurgical planning. If imaging studies are negative or inconclusive, electrodiagnostics may be helpful in ruling out the possibility of a peripheral neuropathy. If these are negative, the possibility of pseudarthrosis should be evaluated with conventional tomography.

If the patient has negative plain films and no radicular complaints but continues to complain of neck, paracervical, or periscapular pain, a pseudarthrosis should be ruled out with conventional tomography. If this study confirms a solid arthrodesis, it is most likely that the patient has degenerative changes elsewhere in the cervical spine that are causing nonspecific mechanical neck pain, which usually cannot be helped by surgical treatment. However, less common syndromes of third or fourth cervical nerve root compression may also result in neck pain only. Consequently, MRI evaluation of patients with a solid arthrodesis and no radicular complaints should be considered, especially if the cephalad end of a prior fusion extends to the fourth or third cervical vertebrae.

In some cases, large spurs may remain symptomatic even with a solid arthrodesis, especially if there has been significant collapse of the graft material with healing. In general, these findings are most easily identified on CTM, and are usually amenable to surgical management, as is discussed in Chapter 3.

In spite of a thorough surgical decompression, some patients may experience persistence of their preoperative symptoms as a result of an inadequate surgical stabilization, resulting in a pseudarthrosis. When graft material fails to consolidate into a solid fusion mass, foraminal spurs will continue to cause nerve root irritation with persistent motion. In other cases, an inadequate stabilization may be due to extrusion or collapse of graft material, leading to segmental kyphosis and further narrowing of the neural foramina with recurrence of the preoperative symptoms. Common risk factors for inadequate stabilization include a history of smoking (43) and the use of allogeneic bone graft materials [both have been shown to result in a higher pseudarthrosis rate (1)] and the use of onlay grafting techniques (Fig. 10). Although an inadequate stabilization may result in the same preoperative radicular symptoms, there is usually proportionally more mechanical neck pain and less radicular pain.

When previous neck surgery fails because of "inadequate alignment," the commonest finding is kyphosis. Kyphosis may occur in patients who undergo cervical laminectomy and is usually the result of an aggressive posterior decompression without a con-

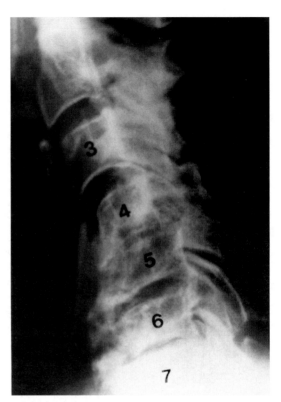

FIGURE 10. Example of onlay fibular grafting from C-4 to C-6. Note listhesis and collapse of C-4 on C-5 and lack of any structural support provided by the anterior fibular graft, which is partially reabsorbed.

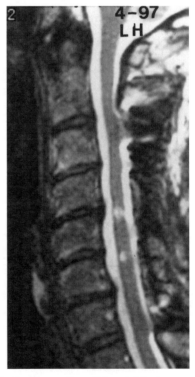

FIGURE 11. Postoperative T2-weighted magnetic resonance image of the same patient shown in Figure 7 following five-level cervical laminoplasty. In spite of complete spinal cord decompression, the two foci of increased signal intensity at C4-5 and C5-6 persist.

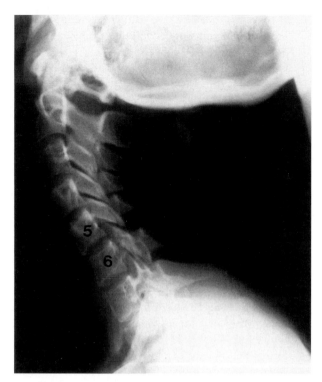

FIGURE 12. Lateral radiograph demonstrating interspinous widening between C-5 and C-6 four weeks after a cervical injury that was treated nonoperatively.

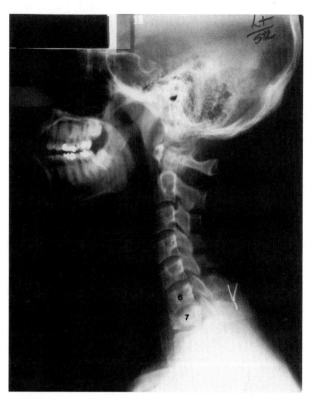

FIGURE 13. Lateral radiograph of a patient with a C6-7 flexion-compression injury treated with a posterior interspinous wiring only. Note collapse of the C-7 vertebral body and recurrence of kyphosis at the C6-7 segment.

comitant stabilization procedure, especially in the patient with a preoperative loss of cervical lordosis (41). These changes may also develop in the patient who has a well-maintained disk space height and undergoes anterior cervical diskectomy without interbody grafting. Other causes are extrusion or collapse of graft material after anterior interbody or strut grafting, with concomitant shortening of the anterior column of the cervical spine (Fig. 10). Patients in whom cervical kyphosis develops may experience persistent mechanical pain related to chronic muscle strain from attempting to maintain forward vision (21). More significant kyphosis may result in draping of the spinal cord across any residual chondroosseous spurs along the posterior vertebral margin, with persistence or recurrence of cervical myelopathy requiring more aggressive surgical management (see Chapter 3). The spinal cord deformity caused by draping across the posterior aspect of the vertebral body is well delineated by CTM or MRI, although MRI can also identify signal change within the spinal cord itself, suggestive of neuronal damage (Fig. 11).

Inadequate alignment may develop after treatment of fractures and dislocations of the cervical spine in cases in which normal anatomic alignment was not restored with the initial treatment. Progressive cervical kyphosis may develop after a posterior ligamentous disruption treated nonoperatively (Fig. 12). In

addition, patients with an injury to the anterior and posterior portions of the vertebral column who were not adequately stabilized may develop future instability and deformity (Fig. 13).

Symptomatic adjacent segment disease is usually the result of progressive cervical spondylosis at motion segments adjacent to a previous anterior or posterior surgical procedure. Like cervical spondylosis, this process is commonest when the adjacent open interspaces lie at C5-6 or C6-7. In younger patients, this usually results from the herniation of disk material at the adjacent level. In older patients, this condition is more likely to be due to spondylotic compression of the neural elements. In some cases, the adjacent segment may become symptomatic due to the development of a degenerative listhesis long after the initial procedure. The authors consider this new disease at the adjacent segment rather than "inadequate alignment," because it does not reflect failure of the previous surgical technique.

In the absence of inadequate decompression, inadequate stabilization, inadequate alignment, adjacent segment disease, or upper cervical pathology, persistent symptoms after prior cervical spine surgery are most likely related to degenerative arthritis. This pain may originate in a desiccated intervertebral disk, zygapophyseal (posterior facet) joints, or a paraspinal ligamentous structure. Schellhas et al. (33) have shown the technique of cervical diskography to be superior to MRI in identifying "painful" disk degeneration, although they did not describe the outcomes of any operative treatment that was based on cervical diskography. At the present time, the technique remains controversial.

CONCLUSION

Focusing on the patient's symptoms, treatment, and recovery following the previous treatment of cervical spine pathology can facilitate the diagnostic evaluation of the postoperative cervical spine patient. Neurologic changes, including evidence of progressive spinal cord compression since the previous operation, should be sought. Many causes of failed cervical spine surgery, such as pseudarthrosis, graft dislodgment, and cervical kyphosis, are easily recognized on plain radiographs. For patients with radicular symptoms, advanced imaging (CTM) can provide the best definition of any nerve root or spinal cord compression. On the other hand, MRI remains the most useful technique for identifying neural compression due to a retained disk herniation and can demonstrate signal changes within the spinal cord that are suggestive of myelomalacia. Once the cause of the failed neck is identified, options for nonoperative and operative treatment can be considered, as is discussed in Chapters 2 and 3.

REFERENCES

1. An HS, Simpson JM, Glover JM, et al. Comparison between allograft plus demineralized bone matrix versus autograft in anterior cervical fusion. A prospective multicenter study. *Spine* 1995;20(20):2211–2216.
2. Aprill C, Dwyer A, Bogduk N. Cervical zygapophyseal joint pain patterns II: a clinical evaluation. *Spine* 1990;15:458–461.
3. Bigos SJ, Battie MC, Spengler DM, et al. A longitudinal, prospective study of industrial back injury reporting. *Clin Orthop* 1972;279:21–34.
4. Boden SC, McCowin PR, Davis DO, et al. Abnormal magnetic-resonance scans of the cervical spine in asymptomatic subjects. *J Bone Joint Surg Am* 1990;72A:1178–1184.
5. Bohlman HH, Emery SE, Goodfellow DB, et al. Robinson anterior cervical discectomy and arthrodesis for cervical radiculopathy. Long-term follow-up of one hundred and twenty-two patients. *J Bone Joint Surg Am* 1993;75:1298–1307.
6. Brodke DS, Zdeblick TA. Modified Smith-Robinson procedure for anterior cervical discectomy and fusion. *Spine* 1992;17:2427–2430.
7. Clements DH, O'Leary PF. Anterior cervical discectomy and fusion. *Spine* 1990;15:1023–1025.
8. Cybulski GR, Douglas RA, Meyer PR, et al. Complications in three-column cervical spine injuries requiring anterior-posterior stabilization. *Spine* 1992;17:253–256.
9. Davidson R, Dunn E, Metzmaker J. The shoulder abduction test in the diagnosis of radicular pain in cervical extradural compressive monoradiculopathies. *Spine* 1982;6:441–446.
10. Davis H. Increasing rates of cervical and lumbar spine surgery in the United States, 1979–1990. *Spine* 1994;19:1117–1124.
11. DePalma AF, Rothman RH, Lewinnek GE, et al. Anterior interbody fusion for severe cervical disc degeneration. *Surg Gynecol Obstet* 1972;134:755–758.
12. Djukic S, Lang P, Morris J, et al. The postoperative spine. Magnetic resonance imaging. *Orthop Clin North Am* 1990;21:603–624.
13. Emery SE, Bolesta MJ, Banks MA, et al. Robinson anterior cervical fusion. Comparison of the standard and modified techniques. *Spine* 1994;19:660–663.
14. Farey ID, McAfee PC, Davis RF, et al. Pseudarthrosis of the cervical spine after anterior arthrodesis. Treatment by posterior nerve root decompression, stabilization, and arthrodesis. *J Bone Joint Surg Am* 1990;72A:1171–1177.
15. Giacobetti FB, Vaccaro AR, Bos-Giacobetti MA, et al. Vertebral artery occlusion associated with cervical spine trauma. A prospective analysis. *Spine* 1997;22:188–192.
16. Gore DR, Sepic SB. Anterior cervical fusion for degenerated or protruded discs. *Spine* 1984;9:667–671.
17. Henderson CM, Hennessey RG, Shuey HM. Posterior-lateral foraminotomy as an exclusive operative technique for cervical radiculopathy: a review of 846 consecutively operated cases. *Neurosurgery* 1983;13:504–511.
18. Herkowitz HN, Kurz LT, Overholt DP. Surgical management of cervical soft disc herniation. A comparison between the anterior and posterior approach. *Spine* 1990;15:1026–1030.
19. Hilibrand AS, Carlson GD, Palumbo MA, et al. Radiculopathy and myelopathy at segments adjacent to an anterior cervical arthrodesis. *J Bone Joint Surg Am* 1999;81:519–528.
20. Hilibrand AS, Tannenbaum DA, Graziano GP, et al. The sagittal alignment of the cervical spine in adolescent idiopathic scoliosis. *J Pediatr Orthop* 1995;15:627–632.
21. Hilibrand AS, Yoo JU, Carlson GD, et al. The success of anterior cervical arthrodesis adjacent to a prior fusion. *Spine* 1997;22:1574–1579.
22. Klekamp J, McCarty E, Spengler DM. Results of elective lumbar discectomy for patients involved in the worker's compensation system. *J Spinal Disord* 1998;11:277–282.
23. Kostuik JP. Differential diagnosis and surgical treatment of metastatic spinal tumors. In: Frymoyer JW, ed. *The*

adult spine: principles and practice, 2nd ed. Philadelphia: Lippincott–Raven Publishers, 1997:989–1014.

24. LaBan MM, Tamler MS, Wang AM, et al. Electromyographic detection of paraspinal muscle metastasis: correlation with magnetic resonance imaging. *Spine* 1992;17:1144–1147.

25. Lunsford LD, Bissonette JD, Jannetta PJ, et al. Anterior surgery for cervical disc disease. Part 1: Treatment of lateral cervical disc herniation in 253 cases. *J Neurosurg* 1980;53:1–11.

26. Massey EW, Riley TL, Pleet AB. Coexistent carpal tunnel syndrome and cervical radiculopathy (double crush syndrome). *South Med J* 1981;74:957–959.

27. Modic MT, Masaryk T, Boumphrey F, et al. Lumbar herniated disc disease and canal stenosis: prospective evaluation by surface coil MR, CT, and myelography. *AJR Am J Roentgenol* 1986;147:757–765.

28. Modic MT, Masaryk T, Mulopulos GP, et al. Cervical radiculopathy: prospective evaluation by surface coil MR imaging, CT with metrizamide, and metrizamide myelography. *Radiology* 1986;161:753–759.

29. Phillips FM, Carlson GD, Emery SE, et al. Anterior cervical pseudarthrosis. Natural history and treatment. *Spine* 1997;22:1585–1589.

30. Riley LH, Robinson RA, Johnson KA, et al. The results of anterior interbody fusion of the cervical spine: review of 93 consecutive cases. *J Neurosurg* 1969;30:127–133.

31. Robinson RA, Walker AE, Ferlick DC, et al. The results of anterior interbody fusion of the cervical spine. *J Bone Joint Surg Am* 1962;44A:1569–1587.

32. Saal JS, Saal JA. Nonoperative management of herniated cervical intervertebral disc with radiculopathy. *Spine* 1996;21:1877–1883.

33. Schellhas KP, Smith MD, Gundry CR, et al. Cervical discogenic pain. Prospective correlation of magnetic resonance imaging and discography in asymptomatic subjects and pain sufferers. *Spine* 1996;21:300–312.

34. Simmons EH, Bhalla SK. Anterior cervical discectomy and fusion. A clinical and biomechanical study with eight-year follow-up. *J Bone Joint Surg Br* 1969;51B:225–237.

35. Smith MD, Emery SE, Dudley A, et al. Vertebral artery injury during anterior decompression of the cervical spine. A retrospective review of ten patients. *J Bone Joint Surg Br* 1993;75B:410–415.

36. Spurling RG. *Lesions of the intervertebral disc.* Springfield, IL: Charles C Thomas Publisher, 1956.

37. Stark RJ, Kennard C, Swash M. Hand wasting in spondylotic high cord compression: an electromyographic study. *Ann Neurol* 1981;9:58–62.

38. Stauffer ES, Kelly EG. Fracture-dislocations of the cervical spine: instability and recurrent deformity following treatment by anterior interbody fusion. *J Bone Joint Surg Am* 1977;59A:45–48.

39. Weisberg NK, Spengler DM, Netterville JL. Stretch-induced nerve injury as a cause of paralysis secondary to the anterior cervical approach. *Otolaryngol Head Neck Surg* 1997;116:317–326.

40. White AA, Southwick WO, Deponte RJ, et al. Relief of pain by anterior cervical-spine fusion for spondylosis. *J Bone Joint Surg Am* 1973;55A:525–534.

41. Zdeblick TA, Bohlman HH. Cervical kyphosis and myelopathy: treatment by anterior corpectomy and strut-grafting. *J Bone Joint Surg Am* 1989;71A:170–182.

42. Zdeblick TA, Hughes SS, Riew KD, et al. Failed anterior cervical discectomy and arthrodesis. Analysis and treatment of thirty-five patients. *J Bone Joint Surg Am* 1997; 79A:523–532.

43. Hilibrand AS, Fye MS, Emery SE, et al. Impact of smoking on the outcome of anterior cervical arthrodesis with interbody or strut-grafting. *J Bone Joint Surg Am* 2001;83A:668–673.

2

CERVICAL SPINE: NONOPERATIVE TREATMENT

SUSAN J. DREYER AND SCOTT D. BODEN

Neck and shoulder pain are common in the general population and in postoperative patients. Surveys of the general population have found a 1-year prevalence rate of 16% to 18% (58,62). The prevalence of postoperative axial pain is as high as 60% when laminoplasty is performed for cervical myelopathy (29). Patients with successful surgical outcomes may have persistent pain or a recurrence of neck or arm pain, or both; they may develop pain as a result of cervical sprain, repetitive strain, disk herniation, or painful progression of spondylosis, including facet joint arthropathy. Optimally, patients have been educated regarding these possibilities preoperatively. Recurrence of neck pain in the postoperative patient is often frightening for the patient and frequently prompts concern that the surgery was not performed properly even when the patient had previously enjoyed a period of relief from a painful cervical condition. Many musculoskeletal conditions respond quickly to treatment and heal without sequelae. Patients who are familiar with positive, long-term results from orthopedic intervention for a sprained ankle or acutely torn knee meniscus often expect that spine surgery will provide a similar long-term solution to their problem and prevent future deterioration or injury. Although the aging cervical spine is ubiquitous and may be accompanied by pain, the process of spondylosis is often unexpected by patients. The finding of degenerative changes on radiographs is often misconstrued as pathology. Radiographic evidence of cervical degeneration is observed in some 30-year-olds and is present in more than 90% of persons older than 60 years of age (25,55). Unfortunately, spine surgery treats the presenting problem and is not prophylactic for future cervical degeneration or injuries. Thus, the treatment of patients with musculoskeletal neck and upper extremity pain that begins years after their original surgery must include reeducation regarding the natural history of neck pain.

The reasons for neck, shoulder, and, occasionally, arm pain after cervical spine surgery are numerous. The differential diagnosis and workup for surgically treatable causes, such as pseudarthrosis, and late insta-

bility or kyphosis, are reviewed in Chapter 1. Epidural hematoma and dural tears are typically identified in the immediate postoperative period. This chapter focuses on those patients whose surgery was technically successful but who present with either persistent neck and upper extremity complaints or recurrence of pain after a period of pain relief. After these patients have been evaluated to exclude extrinsic causes of their pain and determine that no further operative intervention is warranted, the challenge remains how to best help these patients. The first step involves determining their most likely pain generator. Potentially painful musculoskeletal structures include bone, muscles, ligaments, zygapophyseal (facet) joints, and intervertebral disks. Neural structures, including the dorsal root ganglia and nerve roots, may also mediate pain. Based on a presumptive diagnosis, treatment is initiated and may include enforced inactivity including orthoses, enforced activity often under the direction of a physical therapist, topical agents, oral medications, psychological support and counseling, fluoroscopically guided spinal injections, transcutaneous interventions, or the multidisciplinary approach used in treating chronic pain.

GENERAL CONSIDERATIONS

Little published research is available on the treatment of neck pain after spine surgery. Many of the following recommendations are based on the authors' experience and extrapolation of data from the nonoperative population and from applications of principles used in treating persistent lumbar pain after spine surgery. Evaluation of neck pain after cervical surgery should proceed in an orderly fashion. As in preoperative evaluation, a focused history and careful neurologic examination provide the basis of clinical decision making. Specific diagnoses are then confirmed or refuted using selective imaging and, if necessary, provocative tests. The details of such evaluation are outlined in Chapter 1. It is assumed that appropriate diagnostic workup has excluded medical causes of persistent neck and upper extremity symptoms such as Pancoast's tumor as well as surgical problems such as postlaminectomy instability. This chapter addresses those patients in whom no surgical lesions or medical causes are identified. These individuals can be broadly subdivided into three main groups: those with axial or nonradicular pain, those with radicular symptoms, and those with painful myelopathy.

Patients with neck and extremity pain must be evaluated and treated comprehensively. Pain is not a primary sense like sight, hearing, and smell but rather an unpleasant emotional state. It is the result of abnormal activity within the nociceptor system after it has been subjected to varying degrees of facilitation and inhibition (65). By its nature, pain is a subjective experience. This individual variability must be recalled as one approaches patients. Furthermore, pain is often accompanied by depression. Up to 10% of the general population is clinically depressed (51). Most likely the rate of clinical depression is at least that high in postoperative patients who experience persistent or recurrent neck or upper extremity pain, or both. Clinical depression should be identified and aggressively treated. Often a combination of psychotherapy and medications is needed. The newer serotonin reuptake–inhibiting drugs (e.g., paroxetine, sertraline) are generally well tolerated but require monitoring of liver function tests due to recent reports of hepatotoxicity. Tricyclic antidepressants (e.g., amitriptyline) have been used for decades but are limited by their sedating and anticholinergic side effects in some patients. The potentiation of multiple neurotransmitter activity, including serotonin, norepinephrine, and dopamine, by venlafaxine offers another class of antidepressants to be tried. The authors have found that starting with very low doses of the antidepressants and slowly titrating them to more therapeutic levels improves patient tolerance while minimizing side effects. The sedating aspect of the tricyclic antidepressant medications can be used for the benefit of patients with depression and sleep disturbance. The anorexic effect of the serotonin reuptake inhibitors can be a beneficial side effect in patients who are trying to lose weight.

Antidepressant medication is not addicting; however, the potential exists for serious morbidity and mortality with overdoses of the tricyclic antidepressants. Patients with major depression or suicidal ideation, or both, should be evaluated for appropriate psychiatric intervention.

Analgesic medications can be divided into two main classes: narcotic and nonnarcotic agents. The use of potentially addicting medications in patients with chronic neck and arm pain remains somewhat contro-versial. Substance abuse affects the doctor-patient relationship in addition to affecting pain perception. It is estimated that 8% of the general population engages in substance abuse. Alcoholics are predisposed to painful peripheral neuropathies, and their metabolic status may impair nerve healing in the presence of chronic compression and inflammation. Identifying those patients who are substance abusers allows physicians to adjust their prescribing habits and consider seeking consultation with the pain service for more comprehensive management.

Prescription of nonnarcotic analgesics such as acetaminophen, aspirin, and nonsteroidal antiinflammatory agents for pain control is common practice. One must recall that these agents have analgesic and, in the case of aspirin and nonsteroidal antiinflammatory products, antiinflammatory effects. Pain may be due to mechanical, chemical, or combined mechanical and chemical factors. When sufficient forces act on the nociceptors to stress, deform, or damage them, mechanical pain results. On other occasions, chemical mediators such as lactic acid or phospholipase A_2 stimulate the nociceptors and cause chemical pain. In general, mechanical pain is significantly influenced by motion and often relieved by rest or certain positions. It is imperative that physicians query patients as to the amount of rest relief they obtain. This information provides an important clue to guide the physician in the treatment plan. On the other hand, chemical pain is more constant and less influenced by motion but is generally more responsive to medications, including nonsteroidal antiinflammatory agents and corticosteroids. Although acute inflammatory pain is best treated with rest and immobilization, more chronic inflammatory conditions are often accompanied by mechanical pain associated with the formation of adhesions and scarring as the healing process occurs. Active or passive range of motion treatments are typically more effective for the mechanical component of pain. Aerobic exercise increases the general sense of well-being and should be a part of all exercise programs.

The goals of treating neck pain in postoperative patients are to decrease pain, restore motion within the available range, and improve strength and function. Treatment of perioperative pain is not addressed in this chapter.

AXIAL NECK PAIN

The neck is designed to allow maximum flexibility while still providing stability and protection of vital neural and vascular structures passing between the head and body. Examination of the patient who complains of neck, interscapular, and shoulder pain without radicular pain or paresthesias begins as the physician enters the room. The patient's body habitus and behavior provide important clues. A head-forward, rounded shoulder posture chronically strains the posterior cervical muscles and ligaments. Evaluation of cervical active range of motion can be quickly accomplished by noting if the patient can touch the chin to the chest, gaze upward while positioning the face nearly horizontal to the ground, touch the ears to the neutral shoulders, and rotate to each side so that the chin contacts each shoulder (8). Patients who can accomplish these motions typically enjoy full range of motion of the cervical spine, including 60 degrees of flexion, 75 degrees of extension, 45 degrees of side bending, and 80 degrees of bilateral rotation.

Repetitive Strains

Cervical pain often arises from poor posture, which in turn results in abnormal forces and strain on the musculature that must balance and control the head. Persistent pain postoperatively is often due to inadequately addressed compensatory posture. Typically, a head-forward posture is acquired when the patient learns that slumping the thoracic spine requires no energy expenditure. Flexion of the thoracic spine disrupts spinal balance and often drives a patient to attempt to compensate by thrusting the head further forward, thus exacerbating the condition. This posture can be summarized as increased kyphosis of the thoracic spine, secondary increased lordosis of the cervical spine initially, and increased capital extension. This forward-head posture results in muscle length adaptations that alter normal spinal biomechanics. Later, a decrease in midcervical lordosis results, along with adaptive soft tissue changes as capital extension is maintained. Over time, the body attempts to keep the eyes horizontal using greater capital extension (24,37,57). Normal motion undertaken in this poor postural environment produces abnormal muscular strain, particularly of the levator scapulae, upper trapezius, sternocleidomastoid, scalene, and suboccipital muscles. Other adaptations associated with this posture include a retruded mandible, rounded shoulders, and protracted scapulae with tight anterior muscles and stretched posterior muscles (34,54,57). Patients often present with these postural abnormalities after surgery, especially after posterior approaches in which there has been greater dissection of the muscles. The

traumatized muscles may cause pain, which in turn causes patients to restrict their motion. In patients with these postural abnormalities, secondary myofascial pain may develop that can cause referral zone pain (59).

Treatment of chronic cervical strain must include postural reeducation. A skilled physical therapist works with the patient to teach proper body mechanics and posture. Taping across the shoulder blades can serve as a postural cue for a patient not to return to a rounded shoulder, head-forward position. Use of a full-length mirror also allows patients to cue in on their alignment and make corrections to their posture. Workstation ergonomics should be addressed. A chair that provides adequate support and encourages the patient to maintain lumbar lordosis provides a stable platform for the cervical spine. Feet should easily touch the floor, and the thighs should be horizontal to the ground. Adjustable-height chairs allow patients to correct sitting posture for their height. Computer monitors should be positioned to allow a slight, 20-degree downward slope of the eyes. Patients who wear bifocals and work extensively on the computer may benefit from a specially manufactured pair of bifocals that places the bifocal lens superiorly or from a second pair of glasses that they use exclusively for their monitor work. These changes prevent hyperextension to view the screen through the lower portion of the glasses. For patients who spend a significant portion of their workday on the telephone, use of a headset encourages proper posture by eliminating the need to cradle the phone between an ear and a shoulder to free both hands. Patients who work without a headset often cradle the phone between an ear and a shoulder, and chronic muscular stress develops.

In addition to instruction in body mechanics and ergonomics, a physical therapy prescription typically includes a stretching regimen and myofascial release techniques to help normalize tissue tone and range of motion. A brief period of use of modalities such as heat, cold, and electrical stimulation over 1 to 3 weeks can facilitate stretching of the muscles and provide some analgesia. After physiologic range of motion has been returned, posture corrected, and tender points addressed, strengthening becomes the main focus. Strengthening often begins with isometric contractions against manual resistance applied by the patient. Patients are taught to hold their hand against the side, front, back, or opposite side of the head and push against their own manual resistance.

Neck pain that arises from repetitive strain is best addressed by correcting the underlying mechanics.

Medications play only a minor role. Occasionally, acetaminophen, aspirin, or nonsteroidal antiinflammatory agents are used for several weeks to help control pain. Used in isolation, they rarely allow for resolution of symptoms. Narcotic analgesics and muscle relaxants are not part of the usual treatment plan. For neck pain that persists despite correction of biomechanical stresses, patients should be reevaluated for other causes of their pain.

Acute Cervical Strains and Sprains

Muscular strain and ligamentous sprains are common noncatastrophic injuries that occur regardless of a patient's previous operative status. Almost 85% of neck pain results from acute or repetitive neck injuries or chronic stresses and strain (32). Neck strain is more of a clinical syndrome describing nonradiating neck pain associated with acute or static stresses. Cervical strains and sprains are often associated with local muscular tenderness and restriction of vertebral motion. A cervical strain is produced by an overload injury to the muscle-tendon unit due to excessive forces on the cervical spine. The etiology is believed to be due to elongation and tearing of muscles or ligaments. Secondary edema, hemorrhage, and inflammation may occur. Many cervical muscles do not terminate in tendons but instead attach directly to bone by myofascial tissue that blends into the periosteum (50). The response of the muscles to injury is contraction with recruitment of surrounding muscles in an attempt to splint the injured muscle.

A strain typically involves stretching or tearing of muscle fiber. With greater injury forces, vertebral motion restriction may develop. The levels of restriction are determined by palpating over the junction of two adjoining vertebral levels and determining their relative motion. This skill is akin to that developed when palpating other deep structures such as the liver, spleen, or ovaries. The pathomechanics of these restrictions are not known. Possible explanations include entrapment of synovial material or a meniscoid (7), hypertonic contracted musculature (33), changes in nervous reflex activity such as sympathicotonia (41) or gamma bias (40), or abnormal stresses on an unguarded spine (12). With more extreme forces, fracture, dislocation, and neurologic injury may occur. Treatment of these acute injuries is well delineated in other sources.

Patients with cervical strains present with complaints of neck pain, headache, and occasional extremity or chest pain. Typically, the pain has a dull and aching quality and is aggravated by any motion. Guarding and limitation of motion may be present due to the pain. Palpation nearly always reveals tenderness but no true spasm. The most commonly involved muscles are the upper trapezius and sternocleidomastoid. Neurologic examination is normal. Radiographs typically reveal only the previous surgical intervention and perhaps additional nonspecific straightening of the spine due to muscle contraction.

Treatment of neck sprain varies with the degree of pain. Physical modalities such as heat, electrical stimulation, and ultrasound can be used to relax the muscles in the acute period (less than 4 weeks). Acetaminophen and nonsteroidal antiinflammatory medications aid in controlling the pain. Muscle relaxants have a sedative effect that can be useful in inducing sleep. Light cervical traction may reduce pain and diminish spasm. A cervical collar, especially if worn at night, when the patient is most at risk of inadvertently placing the neck in a position of further strain, is often beneficial. Graduated return to activities should begin 2 to 4 weeks after the injury, and the patient's exercise program should include strengthening. Physical therapy can be beneficial in reducing neck pain and improving mobility (38). In more refractory cases judicious use of trigger point injections of local anesthetic may be helpful in breaking reflex spasm and relieving pain, thus allowing the patient to participate more fully in stretching and strengthening to restore normal range of motion and function. Treatment of cervical strains is nonsurgical. Many patients improve within 8 weeks. If pain persists for many months, one should suspect that more severe ligamentous, disk, or associated facet injuries have occurred. If significant pain persists past 4 to 8 weeks, flexion and extension radiographs may be useful to exclude late instability. Occasionally, a cervical strain can persist for months or years. A posttraumatic myofascial pain may result from an acute cervical strain.

Myofascial Pain

Myofascial pain syndrome involves pain and autonomic responses referred from active myofascial trigger points in the muscle (30). Myofascial trigger points are hyperirritable areas within a taut band of skeletal muscle or in the muscle's fascia that are painful on compression. Typically, palpation of these trigger points causes pain in a predictable referral pattern. Normal muscle tissue does not exhibit these characteristics. Pressure over a trigger point may produce a pathognomonic twitch response, a visible contraction of the muscle.

TABLE 1. LOCATION OF THE TENDER POINTS IN FIBROMYALGIA

Name	Description of Location
Posterior	
Bilateral occipital	Suboccipital muscle insertions
Bilateral trapezius	Midpoint of the upper border
Bilateral supraspinatus	Above the medial border of the scapular spine
Bilateral gluteal	Upper outer quadrants of buttocks
Bilateral greater trochanter	Posterior to the trochanteric prominence
Anterior	
Bilateral medial knees	Medial fat pad proximal to the joint line
Bilateral lateral epicondyle	2 cm distal to the epicondyles
Bilateral second rib	Second costochondral junctions
Bilateral low cervical	Anterior aspects of the intertransverse spaces at C5-7

Myofascial pain may be either primary, as discussed in this section, or a secondary tissue response to disk or facet injuries. Primary myofascial trigger points are thought to begin after a muscular strain that becomes a site of sensitized nerves with altered metabolism. Active trigger points cause pain, whereas latent trigger points restrict range of motion and produce weakness of the affected muscle, with the patient being unaware of the tender area until the examination. Latent trigger points may persist for years after a patient recovers from an injury and may become active and create acute pain in response to minor overstretching, overuse, or chilling of the muscle (57,59). Primary myofascial pain is distinguished from secondary myofascial pain via careful examination for underlying pathology.

Primary fibromyalgia remains a poorly understood complex of generalized body aches and is probably the musculoskeletal system's response to stress. Pain should be present in at least 11 of 18 tender point sites (Table 1) for at least 3 months (22). Sleep is usually poor, and sleep studies show that stage IV sleep is the most interrupted. Patients may also complain of numbness into the upper extremities (60%) in a nonradicular pattern. Others have swelling in the hands and feet. Hot baths, local application of heat, and warm weather often provide temporary relief. An association depression should be sought and treated when present. Even in patients without clinical depression, the use of tricyclic antidepressants is often useful. An evening dose of amitriptyline, nortriptyline, or doxepin aids sleep and decreases alpha wave intrusion patterns, resulting in improvement of the rapid eye movement and restorative sleep patterns. Occasionally, a bedtime dose of alprazolam, 0.5 to 1.0 mg, can be used to control concomitant restless leg syndrome that interferes with sleep. Other studies document improvement in fibromyalgia patients with the use of cyclobenzaprine, 10 to 40 mg per day. Acetaminophen or nonsteroidal antiinflammatory medications used for brief periods of activity-related flares can be beneficial. Opioids are usually not effective.

Stretching is the key to treatment of myofascial pain; it can be facilitated through the use of ice massage, a vapor coolant spray, ischemic compression, and/or trigger point injections. Superficial cooling with ice massage or vapor coolant fluormethane spray appears to decrease muscle spasm and tenderness temporarily; used in conjunction with stretching, this technique offers a noninvasive treatment of trigger points. Patients can be taught the circular motions of ice massage using water frozen in a Styrofoam cup. The upper edge of the cup can easily be peeled back, allowing for a convenient exposure of the ice while maintaining an insulated grip on the ice. Ischemic compression is achieved by sustaining direct pressure over the trigger point for 60 to 180 seconds. Most commonly the thumb is used to apply pressure. To facilitate self-treatment for inaccessible regions such as the rhomboid muscles, lying on a tennis ball or using the handle of a cane can be substituted for direct manual compression. Dry needling or injections with local anesthetic only have been shown to be equally efficacious to injections of corticosteroids in myofascial pain (28). Some authors strongly prefer the injection of local anesthetic over dry needling (20). The theory of local anesthetic injections into a trigger point is to stabilize the muscle membrane physically as well as to interrupt the involved muscle fibers. Typically, either bupivacaine or lidocaine without epinephrine is used in volumes of 2 to 3 mL per trigger point. All of these methods of inactivating the trigger points must be followed by stretching and joint range of motion. Stretches should be performed slowly and smoothly for 30 to 60 seconds. Initially, patients benefit from frequent stretching four to five times a day. After 2 to 4 weeks, a maintenance stretching program of only one to two times a day is often adequate. Oral medications are typically ineffective in treating isolated trigger points (31).

Cervical Facet Joint Pain

The cervical facet (zygapophyseal) joints are responsible for a significant portion of chronic neck pain in patients who have had cervical spine surgery as well as those who have not had surgery. The first report on the prevalence of cervical facet pain in patients with chronic neck pain documented that 26% of the sample population achieved relief with zygapophyscal joint blocks and estimated that up to 63% of the population has experienced painful cervical facet joints (if the joints had been investigated in all cases; that is, if the joints had been evaluated despite known painful disk pathology). Such an investigative process should identify the cases of mixed pathology in which the disk and joint both contributed to the pain (1). A more recent study found the prevalence of chronic cervical facet pain after motor vehicle accident whiplash injuries to be 54% (4). More than one million whiplash injuries occur each year in the United States (19); 20% to 40% of these patients experience symptoms that persist for years. Halo immobilization is also associated with the development of facet joint arthritis. One study reported that degenerative changes in the cervical facet joints subsequently developed in 47 of 100 patients who were immobilized with a halo (60). Facet joint degeneration was positively correlated with age and length of time in the halo. Age-matched control patients were not studied to determine the relative increase over normal progression of spondylosis with age. It quickly becomes apparent that the cervical facet joint is a significant source of chronic neck pain. Established referral zones for the cervical facet joint (2,16) overlap myofascial and diskogenic pain patterns (Fig. 1).

Cervical facet pain typically presents as unilateral, dull, aching neck pain with occasional referral into the occiput or interscapular regions, depending on the cervical facet joint that was injured. Neurologic examination should be intact or unchanged if permanent neurologic deficits exist from previous injury. Palpation laterally often reveals regional soft tissue changes in response to the underlying facet injury, and motion testing reveals altered mechanics corresponding to the injured facet (35). Traditional imaging studies [x-ray, magnetic resonance imaging (MRI), computed tomog-

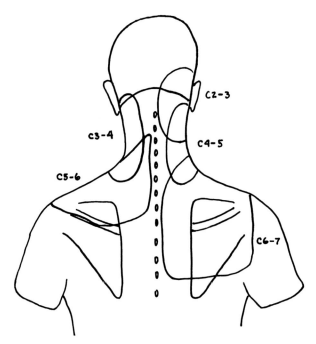

FIGURE 1. Referral zones for cervical facet joint overlapping myofascial and diskogenic pain patterns.

raphy scans] are typically unremarkable, although incidental or painful disk pathology may be noted. Presently, clinical suspicion of facet injuries is best confirmed by diagnostic intraarticular facet injections or blockade of the facet's nerve supply, also known as the medial branch of the dorsal ramus, at the vertebral level below and the level above (3,4). For example, the C5-6 facet joint is blocked by interrupting the medial branches located at the articular "waist" of C-5 and C-6 as seen on anteroposterior imaging.

Treatment for pain arising from the cervical facet joints remains controversial. The only controlled study on intraarticular corticosteroid injections for the treatment of whiplash facet pain has found these injections to be ineffective (44). Their potential use in more degenerative/inflammatory conditions of the spine has not been studied in a blinded and controlled fashion and needs to be determined through the use of well-designed studies on carefully selected patient populations.

Typical conservative care of cervical facet joint injuries without dislocation includes nonsteroidal antiinflammatory drugs, postural exercises and education, cervical pillow, active and passive stretching, positional releases and manual therapy, specific strengthening, and short-term judicious use of modalities to facilitate these interventions. Unfortunately, as in other cervical injuries, no studies on documented, isolated cervical facet pain exist to guide the practitioner through the most cost-effective/efficacious algorithm.

In patients with recalcitrant, disabling neck pain due to documented facet nociception, radiofrequency neurotomies of the medial branches may be an effective long-term pain control measure (45). Radiofrequency heat can be used to interrupt the innervation of the facet joint and thereby halt the noxious stimuli. Because of the possibility of neural regeneration of the small medial branches of the dorsal rami, pain relief from radiofrequency lesioning may decrease after 9 to 12 months. The procedure can be repeated in such cases.

Cervical Spondylosis

Cervical spondylosis occurs gradually and as a result of aging. Eventually, all persons exhibit degenerative changes on their radiographs or autopsies. The degeneration is noticed earlier in men than in women. Postoperative spines are not spared this degenerative cascade. Not all cervical spondylosis is painful, but the degenerative changes may result in painful lesions in some individuals. The C5-6 segment is most commonly and severely involved. Over time, the cervical intervertebral disk degenerates as a result of loss of water content of the nucleus pulposus and loss of anulus fibrosis elasticity. These changes result in loss of the disk space height and narrowing of the foramen. If degeneration of the disk is accompanied by posterior disk protrusion, further compromise of the canal and roots may occur. The vascular supply also diminishes. Over time, these changes result in irregular transmission of forces through that segment and secondary injury to the ligaments and facet joint complex. Instability of the segment stimulates osteophyte growth as the body tries to fuse or autostabilize the injured area. Changes associated with cervical spondylosis include posterior vertebral body osteophytes and bony bars, osteophytes of the lateral joints of Luschka, thickening of the ligamentum flavum, and degenerative changes in the facet joints.

Cervical spondylosis typically presents in patients older than 40 years of age with neck or referred pain without known antecedent trauma. Headaches commonly accompany the neck pain if the upper cervical segments are involved. Approximately 15% of subjects may present with tinnitus or vertigo, and 5% may give a history of syncope due to vertebrobasilar insufficiency from the narrowing of the foramen transversaria (14).

Physical examination is typically fairly normal. At times, a restriction in cervical range of motion is noted. Palpation usually reveals midline tenderness.

Radiographs are positive for cervical spondylosis in 70% of persons older than 70 years of age (26), but there is no correlation between radiographic abnormalities and symptoms (10,18,66). MRI is usually not indicated, partially because of its high false-positive rates. One study found degenerative cervical disks in 62% of asymptomatic persons older than 40 years old. However, no degenerative disks were noted in persons younger than 30 years old (49). The diagnosis of cervical spondylosis is one of exclusion.

Treatment for cervical spondylosis is needed only when significant pain is present. Painful cervical spondylosis is subdivided into three main categories: patients with neck pain alone, those with spondylitic radiculopathy, and those with primarily myelopathic features. Unless rapid neurologic progression is noted, patients with cervical spondylosis should be treated nonoperatively (11). Treatment of patients with primarily myelopathic or radicular symptoms is discussed in the following sections. This section focuses on treatment for neck pain secondary to cervical spondylosis. Gore et al. (23) followed patients with spondylotic neck pain for 10 years and found that 79% improved with 43% pain free at the end of the follow-up period. Often, rest of the neck joints, musculature, and disks provides substantial relief and can be readily accomplished by using a cervical orthosis for a few days. Activity modifications such as limiting overhead work also help to reduce the mechanical stresses to the inflamed region. Oral nonsteroidal antiinflammatory drugs are another method of achieving an antiinflammatory effect. Ergonomic evaluation of daily activities and work often leads to small but effective changes, such as stepping back to look at elevated objects, wearing special reading glasses or glasses with bifocals at the top instead of bottom of the lens for computer work, or using a headset for telephone work.

Isometric exercise, strengthening against resistance without joint motion, is recommended to improve stability and strength without overstressing the joints. Application of moist heat at home is easily accomplished and may provide temporary relief, as may other modalities, such as electrical stimulation, ultrasound, and neuroprobe. Physical therapy modalities are effective in temporizing acute painful flares and are best reserved for such cases (11). Some try epidural steroid injections for particularly severe flares of cervical spondylotic pain, especially when radiating symptoms are present. Facet joint injections for focal lateral tenderness over a specific facet joint in combination with an exercise program may also temporize the pain (63). These forms of treatment await validation in randomized, controlled clinical trials.

In a double-blind, controlled study evaluating the role of manipulation in chronic neck pain, no difference was found between the control group and the group that received a single manipulation for chronic neck pain (56). Conservative care of painful cervical spondylosis must also include longitudinal follow-up of neurologic examinations to monitor for insidious progression of myelopathy. For patients with more severe or recalcitrant pain, pain centers with their multidisciplinary teams can provide relief. Techniques such as behavioral modification, acupuncture, biofeedback, and guided imagery are often used to augment more traditional approaches of medications, exercise, and injections.

Cervical Disk Injuries

Cervical disks may become painful as part of the degenerative cascade described above, from repetitive microtrauma, or from an excessive single load. When the anulus fails without nuclear extrusion, an annular fissure results. At times these annular tears trigger an intense inflammatory response and may be noted as high-intensity zones on an MRI. When nucleus pulposus extrudes through a defect in the anulus, a herniated nucleus pulposus (HNP) results. Depending on the size and location of the lesion, pain from the disk injury may result from inflammation (21,53) or compression of local nervous or vascular tissue. The pain may be radicular or axial, or both. Patients with an HNP without radiculopathy usually complain of neck and interscapular pain aggravated by cervical flexion or extension and relieved with traction (13,57,61). Cervical disk herniations can often be treated successfully without surgery. The incidence of recurrent disk herniations is 10% to 15%. Patients who have had a previous anterior cervical diskectomy and fusion and experience a new disk herniation should be evaluated and given the benefit of nonoperative treatment provided that there is no progressive neurologic compromise. Treatment of cervical diskogenic pain includes oral medications, cervical traction, soft cervical collar, and physical therapy. Patients without neurologic deficit or significant arm pain have not proved to benefit from surgical intervention over the long run (15).

Oral medications include primarily the antiinflammatory agents but may also include a limited course of narcotic agents and muscle relaxants. Cervical traction can be applied manually by the physician, thera-

pist, or appropriately trained family member and can be quite effective. Devices are also available to apply cervical traction using a hand-held pneumatic pump in the supine position, over-the-door weights, and over-the-bed pulley weights. Contraindications to cervical traction include an unstable spine, tumor, infection, significant osteoporosis, extreme anxiety, temporomandibular joint disease, vertebrobasilar arterial disease, carotid artery disease, large midline disk herniations, and acute neck injuries. Traction provides a stretch to the muscles and may thereby relieve spasm; heavier weights (greater than 20 lb) begin to result in vertebral body distraction, which may produce a negative pressure within the disk and allow decompression. The separation also allows for effective enlargement of the foramina.

Soft collars are fit with the wide portion anteriorly. A small elliptical cutout is usually made to allow for appropriate positioning of the mandible. A properly fit soft collar holds the neck in a neutral position with the chin horizontal to the ground. Cervical collars provide support and rest for the neck musculature. Exercise programs are individualized; however, most patients obtain analgesia using cervical retraction or posterior gliding of the lower cervical spine in combination with extension of the lower cervical spine and flexion of the upper cervical spine. The net result is a motion similar to tucking the chin. For patients who have difficulty in mastering this motion, overpressure by the hand pressing on the mandible or maxilla can be of benefit. Adding lateral flexion or sidebending to the neck in the retracted position helps to reduce pain further and to improve physiologic range of motion. Exercise may also improve the diskal nutrition and collagen alignment, strength, and flexibility. Improvements in muscular strength and flexibility may provide protection from further injury by improving resistance to applied forces. Ultimately, exercises must address both flexibility and strength.

Radicular Pain

Pain, numbness, and occasionally weakness in the upper extremity are often due to compression of a spinal nerve by either a cervical disk herniation or stenosis from spurs. Other causes of pain radiating into the upper extremity, such as idiopathic brachial plexitis, are not included in the following discussion. The paresthesias associated with radiculopathy should be in a dermatomal pattern and the weakness in the appropriate myotome. Any changes in the reflexes should correspond to the suspected root involvement. Radicular pain becomes worse with positional foraminal compression maneuvers and with cervical extension and rotation, that is, Spurling's maneuver. The annual incidence of cervical HNP with radiculopathy is 5.5 per 100,000 in Rochester, Minnesota (39). Peak incidence for cervical HNP is 45 to 54 years old, and it is only slightly less common in the 35- to 44-year-old group. C5-6 is the most commonly affected level, followed by C6-7 and C4-5. The combined prevalence of C5-6 and C6-7 HNPs accounts for 75% of cervical disk herniations (36). Of these disk herniations, 23% were attributed to a motor vehicle accident. Cigarette smoking and frequent lifting were both shown to be associated with a higher risk of HNP.

Patients with cervical disk herniations often report a history of neck pain for days to weeks before the onset of their arm pain. As time passes, radicular complaints overshadow axial ones. Physical examination typically reveals a loss of range of motion and occasional torticollis, with the head tilted toward the side of the disk herniation. Abnormalities on manual muscle testing have greater specificity than reflex or sensory abnormalities. Radicular pain is often exacerbated by compression of the neural foramen (Spurling's maneuver) and relieved by abduction of the affected arm (5). Electromyography (EMG) may be useful in assessing for radiculopathy in patients with deficits of questionable neurologic origin. Accuracy of EMG examination is 80% to 90% and improves with the more classic presentation and findings on physical examination. False-negative EMG may occur if there is selective involvement of only the sensory fibers of the root, if the electromyographer fails to study the cervical paraspinal muscles and an adequate sampling of the peripheral muscles, or if the test is performed within the first 3 weeks after presentation. When the physical examination alone is not conclusive, EMG and nerve conduction studies can be helpful in distinguishing ulnar nerve entrapments from C-8 radiculopathies and C-6 radiculopathies from high median neuropathies, evaluating for possible brachial plexitis and carpal tunnel syndrome.

Treatment of cervical radiculopathy due to disk herniations is primarily nonoperative. Treatment of persistent radicular pain despite appropriate decompression is also nonoperative. In acute radiculopathy, whether due to an adjacent level disk herniation or first-time disk herniation, rest and immobilization are important, usually requiring a few days of bed rest with bathroom privileges. The pain of radiculopathy is often relieved with cervical traction (13,57,61). Typically, the pain begins to ease within 2 weeks of restricted activities. At that point it is important to taper the use of the cervical orthotic and begin gentle reactivation. Most patients are able to return to restricted-duty work. Medication includes nonsteroidal antiinflammatory drugs as well as muscle relaxants for their soporific effects. Occasionally, corticosteroids or a short course of oral narcotics, or both, are required (17). The need for narcotics can be minimized by adequate rest and patient education. Cervical traction can provide dramatic relief, and consideration should be given to training the patient in the use of a home unit. Patients can use a unit at home two to three times a day for 15-minute sessions. The efficacy of traction has not been scientifically proven with a randomized controlled trial, but it is commonly used and thought to be of benefit (13,17,57,61). Therapeutic modalities may also provide temporary analgesia but should only be used acutely. Exercises begin with isometrics to prevent atrophy and progress to gentle stretching and finally strengthening. The use of a cervical pillow, a soft pillow tied in the middle with a ribbon to allow cradling of the neck, or a cervical collar at night often improves sleep. A patient's posture should be corrected, and he or she should be taught to avoid prolonged static postures, especially those that involve cervical extension. Selective cervical epidural steroid injections may allow for further pain control and reduction of inflammatory mediators (17,46,47,64).

Despite appropriate conservative care, a small percentage of patients who present with acute cervical radiculopathy will continue to have significant and debilitating arm pain and possibly persistent neurologic deficits. These patients should be referred for surgical consultation after a minimum of 6 weeks to 3 months of conservative care.

Patients with persistent radicular pain without a compressive lesion may have an inflammatory radiculitis, residual nerve dysfunctions from the now decompressed area, or operative neural injury. Neurologic complications range from 0.64% to 2.18% depending on the route of surgery (57). Medications to treat neuropathic pain include nonsteroidal antiinflammatory agents, antidepressants that block norepinephrine (e.g., amitriptyline, nortriptyline, desipramine, doxepin), cortisone, and anticonvulsants. Gabapentin is commonly used for neuropathic pain. Other anticonvulsants, including carbazepam, clonazepam, phenytoin, and valproate, have been used for the lancinating or shooting pains of chronic radiculopathy. These latter drugs require monitoring of blood levels and have relatively narrow therapeutic windows. They are believed to exert their effect through their membrane-stabilizing properties. Mexiletine, an antiarrhythmic agent, is occasionally beneficial in reducing neuropathic pain. Long-term opioid therapy may also have a role in cases in which there is known nociceptive input, such as a damaged nerve with pain that interferes and limits function.

Cervical Myelopathy

Posterior disk herniations, often in combination with degenerative osteophytes, may lead to compression of the spinal cord and result in cervical myelopathy. Patients with cervical myelopathy frequently have difficulties with balance and a stooped, wide-based jerky gait. Spasticity is nearly uniformly present, and radicular pain is present in approximately one-third of patients (14). Patients may experience loss of dexterity, nonspecific weakness, numbness, and paresthesias of the upper extremities. Bladder incontinence is uncommon. Lhermitte's sign may be present. Lower motor neuron deficits at the level of the cervical lesion and upper motor neuron signs below the lesion may be found on physical examination.

Lower extremity symptoms may occur before upper extremity difficulties. Patients often have trouble describing their symptoms but frequently report difficulty in walking, peculiar sensations, spontaneous leg movement, shuffling of the feet, and fear of falling. The clinical presentation is often variable, depending on the number and location of levels involved (6). The five cervical spondylotic myelopathic clinical syndromes are (a) lateral, causing radicular arm pain, often unilateral; (b) medial, presenting with bilateral lower extremity involvement but no pain; (c) combined medial and lateral syndromes, upper extremity radicular pain with lower extremity clumsiness; (d) anterior, causing painless unilateral upper extremity weakness; and (e) vascular, the least common. Symptoms generally begin insidiously in patients older than 55 years of age.

Cervical spinal cord neurapraxia may occur, particularly given certain predisposing factors that may cause the anteroposterior diameter of the spinal canal to narrow. These factors include developmental spinal stenosis, instability, HNP, and spondylosis. Hyperflexion or hyperextension injuries of the cervical spine may further decrease the size of an already stenotic central canal. These forced injuries may result in brief but abrupt mechanical compression of the spinal cord, causing transient interruption of

motor or sensory function, or both, distal to the lesion. Both arms, both legs, or all four extremities may be involved. These bilateral findings help differentiate spinal cord neurapraxia from radiculopathy or from brachial plexus injury, both of which are almost always unilateral. By definition, the neurologic deficit associated with cervical spinal cord neurapraxia is transient and completely reversible (27).

Physical examination in myelopathy typically reveals hyperreflexia and may include positive Babinski's and Hoffmann's signs, gait abnormalities of a stooped, wide-based shuffling pattern. Sensory changes usually involve the spinothalamic tract (pain temperature) or posterior columns (vibration and proprioception).

Radiographs often demonstrate advanced degenerative changes. Congenital stenosis should be assessed. Pavlov's ratio is the anteroposterior diameter of the canal divided by the anteroposterior diameter of the corresponding vertebral body. Values of less than 0.8 suggest stenosis. If Pavlov's ratio is less than 0.8, stenosis should be excluded using more advanced imaging techniques such as computed tomography myelography or MRI.

Cervical myelopathy should be treated conservatively unless rapid onset of symptoms or clear progression has occurred (11). The natural history of cervical myelopathy is that the majority of patients remain stable (9,43,48,52). Surgical decompression aims to halt the progression of the disease; recovery of neural function is variable (42,52).

Conservative therapy for cervical myelopathy includes immobilization in a rigid orthosis, rest, nonsteroidal antiinflammatory medication, physical therapy avoiding aggressive stretching or manipulation, and occasionally epidural steroid injections. Epidural steroid injections can be administered in a generalized fashion with the entry point between the lamina, or they can be performed laterally, localized to the sight of the radiculopathy. Interlaminar epidural corticosteroid injections should not be performed at the level(s) of stenosis because of the obliteration of the epidural space at this (these) level(s) and the resultant risk of further neurologic damage from the pressure of the injectant. Also, it is best to avoid interlaminar injections at the level of previous posterior cervical surgery because of the possibility of scarring and adhesion of the dura to the ligamentum flavum. For these reasons, a transforaminal epidural approach for radicular pain in the postoperative patient is recommended.

Surgical intervention achieves better outcomes in the early stages of the disease, as it aims to halt progression rather than restore neurologic function. Anterior cervical diskectomies, anterior corpectomies and arthrodesis, and posterior laminoplasty are all methods of decompressing the cervical spine. Cervical myelopathy is generally a slowly progressive disease with long quiescent periods following bouts of worsening signs or symptoms. Occasionally (approximately 20%), slow progression without remissions is encountered.

CONCLUSION

Neck pain is a complex, subjective experience with a variety of musculoskeletal causes that can generally be treated nonoperatively. Accurate diagnosis rests heavily on a careful history and physical examination. Imaging studies are important tools that are used to support or refute a suspected diagnosis. Treatment of musculoskeletal neck pain generally follows rehabilitative principles: Functional deficits are identified, realistic goals are set, and a multifaceted treatment program is initiated to control pain and to restore range of motion, strength, and function.

REFERENCES

1. Aprill C, Bogduk N. The prevalence of cervical zygapophyseal joint pain: a first approximation. *Spine* 1992; 17:744–747.
2. Aprill C, Dwyer A, Bogduk N. Cervical zygapophyseal joint pain patterns II: a clinical evaluation. *Spine* 1990; 15:458.
3. Barnsley L, Bogduk N. Medial branch blocks are specific for the diagnosis of cervical zygapophyseal joint pain. *Reg Anesth* 1993;18:343–350.
4. Barnsley L, Lord SM, Wallis BJ, et al. The prevalence of chronic cervical zygapophyseal joint pain after whiplash. *Spine* 1995;20:20–25.
5. Beatty RM, Fowler FD, Hanson EJ Jr. The abducted arm as a sign of ruptured cervical disc. *Neurosurgery* 1987;21:731.
6. Bernhardt M, Hynes R, Blume H, et al. Cervical spondylotic myelopathy. *J Bone Joint Surg Am* 1993;75:119–128.
7. Bogduk N, Engle R. The menisci of the lumbar zygapophyseal joints: a review of their anatomy and clinical significance. *Spine* 1984;9:454–460.
8. Braddon RL. Management of common cervical pain syndromes. In: Delisa JA, ed. *Rehabilitation medicine: principles and practice*, 2nd ed. Philadelphia: JB Lippincott Co, 1993:1037.
9. Bradshaw P. Some aspects of cervical spondylosis. *QJM* 1957;26:177–208.
10. Clark CR. Cervical spondylotic myelopathy: history and physical findings. *Spine* 1988;13:847–849.
11. Clark CR. Differential diagnosis and nonoperative management. In: Frymoyer JW, ed. *The adult spine: principles and practice*, 2nd ed. Philadelphia: Lippincott–Raven Publishers, 1997:1145.
12. Clarke K. An epidemiologic view. In: Torg JS, ed. *Athletic injuries to the head, neck, and face*. St. Louis: Mosby–Year Book, 1991:15–27.
13. Colachis S, Strohm B. Cervical traction: relationship of traction time to varied tractive force with constant angle of pull. *Arch Phys Med Rehabil* 1965;46:815–819.
14. Crandall PH, Batzdorf U. Cervical spondylotic myelopathy. *J Neurosurg* 1966;25:57–66.
15. Dillin W, Booth R, Cuckeler J, et al. Cervical radiculopathy: a review. *Spine* 1986;11:988–991.
16. Dwyer A, Aprill C, Bogduk N. Cervical zygapophyseal joint pain patterns I: study in normal volunteers. *Spine* 1990;15:453–457.
17. Ellenberg MR, Honet JC, Treanor WJ. Cervical radiculopathy. *Arch Phys Med Rehabil* 1994;75:342–352.
18. Epstein NE, Epstein JA, Carras R, et al. Coexisting cervical and lumbar spinal stenosis: diagnosis and management. *Neurosurgery* 1984;15:489–496.
19. Evans RW. Some observations on whiplash injuries. *Neurol Clin* 1992;10:975–997.
20. Fischer AA. Trigger point injection. In: Lennard TA, ed. *Physiatric procedures in clinical practice*. Philadelphia: Hanley & Belfus, 1995:28–35.
21. Franson R, Saal J. Human disc phospholipase A_2 is inflammatory. *Spine* 1992;17:S129–S132.
22. Freundlich B, Leventhal L. The fibromyalgia syndrome. In: Schumacher HR, Klippel JH, Koopman WJ, eds. *Primer on the rheumatic diseases*, 10th ed. Atlanta: Arthritis Foundation, 1993.
23. Gore DR, Sepic SB, Gardner GM, et al. Neck pain: a long-term follow-up of 205 patients. *Spine* 1987;12:1–5.
24. Grieve G. Common patterns of clinical presentation. In Grieve G, ed. *Common vertebral joint problems*, 2nd ed. London: Churchill Livingstone, 1988.
25. Heine J. Uber die arthritis deformans. *Virchows Arch Pathol Anat* 1926;260:521–663.
26. Heller JG. The syndromes of degenerative cervical disease. *Orthop Clin North Am* 1992;23:381–394.
27. Herzog RJ, Wiens JJ, Dillingham MF, et al. Normal cervical spine morphometry and cervical spinal stenosis in asymptomatic professional football players: plain film radiography, multiplanar computed tomography, and magnetic resonance imaging. *Spine* 1991;16:S178–S188.
28. Hong C. Lidocaine injection versus dry needling to myofascial trigger point. The importance of the local twitch response. *Am J Phys Med Rehabil* 1994;73:256–263.
29. Honsono N, Yonenobu K, Ono K. Neck and shoulder pain after laminoplasty: a noticeable complication. *Spine* 1996;21:1969–1973.

30. Hubbard DR, Berkhoff GM. Myofascial trigger points show spontaneous needle EMG activity. *Spine* 1993; 18:1803–1807.

31. Irving GA, Wallace MS. Myofascial pain. In: Irving GA, Wallace MS, eds. *Pain management for the practicing physician.* New York: Churchill Livingstone, 1997:159.

32. Jackson R. Cervical trauma: not just another pain in the neck. *Geriatrics* 1982;37:123–126.

33. Janda V. Muscles, central nervous regulation and back problems. In: Korr IM, ed. *Neurobiologic mechanisms in manipulative therapy.* New York: Plenum Publishing, 1978:27–41.

34. Janda V. *Muscle function testing.* London: Butterworth, 1983.

35. Jull G, Bogduk N, Marsland A. The accuracy of manual diagnosis for cervical zygapophyseal joint pain syndromes. *Med J Aust* 1988;148:233–236.

36. Kelsey J, Githens P, Walter S, et al. An epidemiological study of acute prolapsed cervical intervertebral disc. *J Bone Joint Surg Am* 1984;66-A:907–914.

37. Kendall FP, Kendall-McCreary E. *Muscles: testing and function,* 3rd ed. Baltimore: Williams & Wilkins, 1983.

38. Koes BW, Bouter LM, van Mameren H, et al. The effectiveness of manual therapy, physiotherapy and treatment by the general practitioner for nonspecific back and neck complaints: a randomized clinical trial. *Spine* 1992;17:28–35.

39. Kondo K, Molgaard C, Kurland L, et al. Protruded intervertebral cervical disc. *Minn Med* 1981;64:751–753.

40. Korr I. Proprioceptors and somatic dysfunction. *J Am Osteopath Assoc* 1975;74:638–650.

41. Korr I. Sustained sympathicotonia as a factor in disease. In: Korr IM, ed. *Neurobiologic mechanisms in manipulative therapy.* New York: Plenum Publishing, 1978:229–268.

42. LaRocca H. Cervical spondylotic myelopathy: natural history. *Spine* 1988;13:854–855.

43. Lee F, Turner JW. Natural history and prognosis of cervical spondylosis. *BMJ* 1963;2:1607–1610.

44. Lord SM, Barnsley L, Bogduk N. The utility of comparative local anesthetic blocks versus placebo-controlled blocks for the diagnosis of cervical zygapophyseal joint pain. *Clin J Pain* 1995;11:208–213.

45. Lord SM, Barnsley L, Wallis BJ, et al. Percutaneous radio-frequency neurotomy for chronic cervical zygapophyseal-joint pain. *N Engl J Med* 1996;335:1721–1726.

46. Malanga GA. The diagnosis and treatment of cervical radiculopathy. *Med Sci Sports Exerc* 1997;S236–S243.

47. Mimura M, Moriya H, Watanabe T, et al. Three-dimensional motion analysis of the cervical spine with special reference to the axial rotation. *Spine* 1989;14:1135–1139.

48. Nurick S. The natural history and the results of surgical treatment of the spinal cord disorder associated with cervical spondylosis. *Brain* 1972;95:101–108.

49. Pavlov H, Torg JS, Robie B, et al. Cervical spinal stenosis: determination with vertebral body ratio method. *Radiology* 1987;164:771–775.

50. Press JM, Herring SA, Kibler WB. *Rehabilitation of musculoskeletal disorders. The textbook of military medicine.* Washington, DC: Borden Institute, Office of the Surgeon General, 1996.

51. Ransford AO, Cairns D, Mooney V. The pain drawing as an aid to the psychologic evaluation of patients with low-back pain. *Spine* 1976;1:127–134.

52. Roberts AH. Myelopathy due to cervical spondylosis treated by collar immobilization. *Neurology* 1966;16:951–954.

53. Saal J, Franson R, Dobrow R, et al. High levels of inflammatory phospholipase A_2 activity in lumbar disc herniations. *Spine* 1990;15:674–678.

54. Saunders H. *Evaluation, treatment and prevention of musculoskeletal disorders,* 2nd ed. Minneapolis: Viking Press, 1985.

55. Schmorl G, Junghanns H. *The human spine in health and disease.* New York: Grune & Stratton, 1971.

56. Sloop PR, Smith DS, Goldenberg E, et al. Manipulation for chronic neck pain: a double-blind controlled study. *Spine* 1982;7:532–535.

57. Stratton SA, Bryan JM. *Dysfunction, evaluation, and treatment of the cervical spine and thoracic inlet. Orthopaedic physical therapy,* 2nd ed. New York: Churchill Livingstone, 1993:77–122.

58. Takala J, Sievers K, Klaukka T. Rheumatic symptoms in the middle-aged population in southwestern Finland. *Scand J Rheumatol* 1982;47:15–29, 59.

59. Travell JG, Simons DG. *Myofascial pain and dysfunction: the trigger point manual.* Baltimore: Williams & Wilkins, 1992.

60. Tredwell SJ, O'Brien JP. Apophyseal joint degeneration in the cervical spine following halo-pelvic distraction. *Spine* 1980;5:497–501.

61. Valtonen E, Kiurn E. Cervical traction as a therapeutic tool: a clinical analysis based on 212 patients. *Scand J Rehabil Med* 1970;2:29–36.

62. Westerling D, Jonsson BG. Pain from the neck-shoulder region and sick leave. *Scand J Soc Med* 1980;8:131–136.

63. Wilson SP, Iacobo C, Rocco AG, et al. Cervical epidural steroid injection (CESI): clinical classification as predictor of therapeutic outcome. Presented at the Annual Meeting of the Cervical Spine Research Society, New Orleans, 1989.

64. Woodard JL, Herring SA, Windsor RE, et al. Epidural procedures in spine pain management: cervical and thoracic. In: Lennard TA, ed. *Physiatric procedures in clinical practice.* Philadelphia: Hanley & Belfus, 1995:260–291.

65. Wyke B. The neurology of low back pain. In: Jayson M, ed. *The lumbar spine and back pain,* 3rd ed. New York: Churchill Livingstone, 1987:56.

66. Yiannikas C, Shahani BT, Young RR. Short-latency somatosensory–evoked potentials from radial, median, ulnar, and peroneal nerve stimulation in the assessment of cervical spondylosis: comparison with conventional electromyography. *Arch Neurol* 1986;43:1264–1271.

3

CERVICAL SPINE: DEGENERATIVE DISEASE

HENRY H. BOHLMAN

Over the past 20 years, there has been a tremendous evolution of newer techniques of the anterior approach applied to various problems of the patient with cervical spine degenerative disease, trauma, tumors, and infections. Since the advent of Dr. Robert A. Robinson's report of the first anterior cervical diskectomy and fusion in 1955, this approach has been widely applied to solve many of the problems of cervical spine disease. In the past we have witnessed the use of laminectomy for degenerative disease, herniated disk, primary tumors, and trauma of the cervical spine, with the attendant short-term, as well as long-term, risks of increased neurologic deficit, deformity, and further incapacitation (10–12,18,20). Long-term follow-up outcome studies have proved the superiority of anterior decompression and arthrodesis over laminectomy for the above pathologic states (1,4,5).

Through the 1980s, newer diagnostic techniques completely revolutionized our diagnostic ability of the failed spine surgery patient. Specifically, water-soluble myelographic dye in conjunction with computed tomography (CT) scanning has allowed us to see the neurologic structures in association with the bony architecture as well as tumors and trauma in a much more accurate way. Gadolinium-enhanced magnetic resonance imaging (MRI) has also been a major advance in our diagnostic ability. All of these newer techniques have made preoperative planning much more accurate and have enhanced our ability to diagnose the etiology of failure in the postoperative spine patient.

The clinical evaluation of the postoperative failed cervical spine patient must include a careful history and physical as well as neurologic examination. The treating physician must delve back into the preoperative symptoms and neurologic findings before the index procedure and determine whether any immediate or delayed neurologic deficit occurred. A thorough review of the initial preoperative examination as well as the diagnostic studies performed gives many clues as to the cause for the failed spine surgery. For instance, if the patient originally presented with a herniated disk and radiculopathy with weakness and an anterior or posterior procedure was per-

formed, following which the patient had no relief of arm pain or paralysis, one would strongly consider inadequate decompression of the nerve roots for a variety of reasons. If, on the other hand, the patient had initial relief of arm and neck pain and then, over a period of months, increasing neck pain and finally recurring arm pain slowly developed, one would consider a pseudarthrosis of an anterior cervical diskectomy and fusion or pathology at a new level, which would be very unusual (13).

Almost all of the patients who present with cervical spondylosis and myelopathy have a combination of radiculopathy and spinal cord signs, that is, upper as well as lower motor neuron signs. If an operative procedure is performed and the patient wakes up with an increased neurologic deficit, one would consider iatrogenic damage to the spinal cord (8). However, if the patient does not have relief of the neurologic deficit over a period of time and has increasing difficulties in walking with or without neck pain, one would consider inadequate decompression of the spinal cord and possibly inadequate stabilization of the spine. Further diagnostic studies should point to those facts.

Physical examination should demonstrate the patient's walking ability as to whether any wide-based gait or staggering or evidence of spasticity is present. Notation should be made of the patient's pain pattern, whether it be purely cervical or radiating into the shoulder and arm and into any particular fingers. Radiating paresthesias may be a clue to a specific nerve root compression. Palpation of the cervical spine posteriorly and anteriorly may give clues to a level of pathology if pain is elicited at a very specific level. Range of motion of the cervical spine is critically important and may demonstrate loss of extension of the cervical spine in the patient with marked cervical cord or nerve root compression. In addition, loss of extension with lateral rotation that then reproduces a Lhermitte's sign indicates continued nerve root compression. On occasion, pure extension producing a Lhermitte's sign into the arms and legs indicates a cause of spinal cord compression that has not been decompressed.

The examining physician should assess the posture of the head and neck because a patient with residual spinal cord compression may hold the head and neck in flexion or in a kyphotic way or a fixed kyphotic deformity may be present. Neurologic examination should include a thorough motor examination as well as testing of reflexes to determine if any reflexes have been lost or if any reflexes are pathologic in the upper and lower extremities. Sensation should be tested for pin prick, position, and vibratory sense in all four extremities. The neurologic findings should then be compared to the preoperative findings of the original surgeon or other surgeons before the index procedure. Careful documentation of a graded motor examination is critically important in determining the progression of neurologic disease, either for the worse or an improvement.

Diagnostic evaluation of the failed postoperative cervical spine patient should include plain radiographs with anteroposterior, lateral, and flexion/extension laterals and obliques of the cervical spine. These should specifically help to identify any abnormal motion or subluxation that was not present before the surgery, the congenitally narrow cervical spinal canal or stenosis, other associated levels of cervical spondylosis, and solid arthrodesis, if present. CT scan reconstruction is often helpful if one suspects pseudarthrosis or wants to prove a solid arthrodesis. By and large, the trabeculation across the disk space in an anterior fusion should be quite apparent on the postoperative films, as should resorption of bony spurs by the process of normal bone remodeling.

In the author's experience, it is almost unheard of for a postoperative infection to develop from an anterior cervical diskectomy and fusion. If this does occur, however, a bone scan and MRI, as well as sedimentation rate, can further help in the diagnosis.

The MRI, with or without gadolinium enhancement, is a major addition to our armamentarium in diagnosing the etiology of the failed postoperative cervical spine patient unless metal artifact is present either from using a power burr or an implant. We are able to diagnose pseudarthroses with MRI, sometimes more accurately than with bending films, and the rare cervical infection may be well demonstrated on the MRI. The presence of residual herniated disk or retained osteophytes compressing the neural structures can be outlined and adequate decompression of the nerve roots and spinal cord demonstrated by MRI. Ultimately, if bone or disk compression of the spinal cord or nerve roots is suspected, a myelogram with enhanced CT scan is the test of choice, which in our hands is much more sensitive and specific in demonstrating residual osseous and disk compression of the neural structures in the central canal and intraforaminally.

Electrodiagnostic studies may be useful in the patient with persistent radiculopathy or myelopathy or if an associated disease is suspected. Amyotrophic lateral sclerosis can be differentiated from cervical spondylosis or occur in conjunction with it and be defined by electromyographic (EMG) studies. Diabetic neuropathy may be associated with cervical spondylosis and radiculopathy and can be differentiated by EMG studies. Various forms of myopathy can be differentiated from cervical spondylosis and radiculopathy by EMG or may occur in conjunction with radiculopathy. Muscle biopsies and enzyme studies may be very helpful in this situation as well. It is not uncommon that persistent median hand pain and paresthesias secondary to an associated carpal tunnel syndrome can be diagnosed by nerve conduction studies.

ETIOLOGY AND UNCOMMON REASONS FOR FAILURE

Initially, the wrong diagnosis may have been entertained in view of how commonly spondylosis is seen on x-ray at the fourth decade and in older patients. We have seen patients operated on for cervical radiculopathy when, in fact, they have a tumor that is producing the neck and arm pain. This may be a primary tumor of the cervical spine that has been overlooked initially or a lung tumor, such as a Pancoast's tumor, that is producing shoulder and upper arm pain similar to that of C-5 nerve root compression (Fig. 1). Various neurologic diseases may mimic cervical radiculopathy or myelopathy in symptoms and in findings on examination. Amyotrophic lateral sclerosis may produce a combination of upper and lower motor neuron signs and be progressive either in association with cervical spondylosis or as a separate entity. Multiple sclerosis may produce intermittent myelopathy and gait disturbances, and Guillain-Barré disease may at onset present with paresthesias and weakness that is very mild. Occasionally, the wrong level may have been operated on, either by misinterpretation of diagnostic radiologic studies or diagnostic neurologic examination, and for that reason pain persists.

Another problem is selection of patients in whom the operative procedure was not indicated in the first place and in whom a conservative approach should be the primary mode of treatment. In general, patients

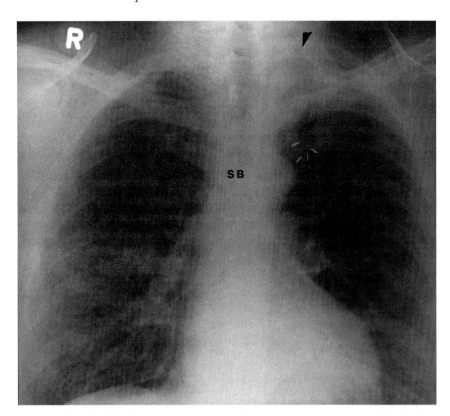

FIGURE 1. This 55-year-old man presented with a history of previous bypass surgery and more recent onset of neck and left shoulder pain. He had evidence of a Pancoast's tumor in the left apex of the lung, which was later resected, with the cure of his carcinoma.

with degenerative disk disease, especially at more than one level, with axial pain and no neural compression are treated conservatively with immobilization in a collar, physical therapy, and antiinflammatory agents. It is very rare that we operate on these patients unless radiculopathy develops manifested by arm pain and paresthesias as well as neurologic deficit.

In general, the commonest cause of failed spine surgery that we see today is secondary to inadequate decompression of the neural structures and, therefore, persistent radicular pain and nerve root or spinal cord compression. Failed arthrodesis may in turn produce persistent pain or recurring pain and is another cause that is more frequent than misdiagnosis.

DIFFERENTIAL DIAGNOSIS ALGORITHM FOR THE FAILED CERVICAL SPINE PATIENT

We have developed an algorithm for the diagnosis and treatment of failed cervical spine surgery patients. This includes patients who generally present with neck pain alone, neck and arm pain, or paralysis, which may occur immediately after the index operation or has increased in the postoperative period. By and large, all patients should have routine cervical spine radiographs, which should include dynamic flexion/extension views to determine the integrity of an arthrodesis or to dis-

cern whether any pathologic subluxations may occur. If a pseudarthrosis or subluxation is discovered after the dynamic cervical spine radiographs are performed, we occasionally proceed with CT scan reconstruction to determine in more osseous detail the presence of the pseudarthrosis. In addition, more recently, gadolinium-enhanced MRIs more accurately identified pseudarthroses and vascular fibrous tissue making up these entities. If the above studies are negative for pseudarthrosis and neural compression and the patient continues to have chronic pain, he or she is sent to the pain center for further nonoperative treatment. On the other hand, if the CT scan and MRI are positive for a pseudarthrosis and the patient has persistent neck or arm pain, or both, a repeat arthrodesis is carried out. In the case of an anterior fusion, a repeat anterior resection of the pathologic material and autogenous fusion are usually performed. In some situations, a posterior arthrodesis may be necessary.

FAILED DECOMPRESSION FOR DEGENERATIVE DISK DISEASE AND ARTHRITIS

Anterior Operations

As previously mentioned, one of the commonest causes of failed cervical spine surgery is secondary to inadequate decompression of the neural structures, and a common cause of the latter is the microscopic decompression, usually without fusion. We have seen a large number of patients who have had micro-diskectomies for radiculopathy and myelopathy and have persistent neural deficit as well as neck and arm pain. The problem with the micro approach is that a very limited exposure of the disk space is carried out, and, although the decompression may appear to be adequate through the microscope, in fact, it not uncommonly may leave a residual herniated disk or neural compression secondary to bony osteophytes. In addition, in the patient with a congenital cervical spinal stenosis, the microscopic approach is usually inadequate to decompress the entire spinal canal, which is necessary in the patient with myelopathy. Not infrequently in the patient who has had a dis-kectomy without fusion, the arm pain may subside after the nerve root is decompressed, but the neck pain persists, and on repeated studies the disk space collapses and frequently a soft tissue outpouching posteriorly of fibrous tissue continues to compress the nerve root. In addition, spontaneous fusion does not always occur, and motion continues at that seg-ment, which adds to the irritation and compression of the nerve root or spinal cord (Fig. 2).

Another cause of failed anterior operations is the anterior cervical diskectomy and fusion for spondylo-sis in which the decompression itself may be inade-quate with or without a failure of arthrodesis (7). This situation usually occurs with the inexperienced sur-geon. In some patients, a soft herniated disk can be extruded posterior to the vertebral body and migrated superiorly or inferiorly, and if the anterior diskectomy is performed without removing a portion of the verte-bral body, a retained disk fragment will result, with persistent pain or neurologic deficit, or both. Cer-tainly today, with our sophisticated diagnostic tools such as an MRI and myelography with CT scanning, one should be able to identify accurately the exact position of an extruded disk fragment and be prepared to perform a hemicorpectomy to retrieve the soft disk.

Inadequate decompression of cervical osteophytes may result in persistent neurologic deficit or pain, or both. The usual cause of this technical problem is not removing enough of the vertebrae above and below to visualize the osteophyte adequately to remove it safely from the posterior longitudinal liga-ment. This may occur if only a diskectomy is per-formed without removing part of the vertebrae. On the other hand, if the osteophyte is small and the patient only has radiculopathy, it is not necessary to remove the osteophyte because it will remodel with

the process of arthrodesis, and in our experience this occurs over 9 to 18 months.

Inadequate decompression with neural structures may occur even with a cervical corpectomy if the midline trough is not wide enough and if the sur-geon fails to burr away the osteophytes posterolater-ally in the joints of Luschka. Technical causes for inadequate decompression in cervical corpectomies are inexperience of the surgeon and use of the micro-scope, which may lead to the false impression of an adequate decompression because of the magnifica-tion and also may result in further decompression on the side opposite where the surgeon is standing. The latter may occur even with use of magnifying loupes, because it is much more difficult to decompress the left side of the spinal canal if the surgeon is standing to the left of the patient unless the surgeon switches sides of the table, which is preferable to perform an adequate decompression bilaterally (Fig. 3).

It has been our general principle to decompress all levels of neural compression that appear to be signif-icant on the diagnostic studies, even though one level may be worse than the other. In our experience, this principle has stood the test of time, and the results of neurologic recovery are excellent in radicu-lopathy as well as myelopathy patients.

An additional complication that can occur to pro-duce a failed cervical spine patient (which, fortunately, is less common today than previously) is an overly vig-orous removal of osteophytes with large instruments using the Cloward technique in a patient with cervical stenosis, spondylosis, and myelopathy. We have seen approximately ten patients in 20 years in whom quad-riparesis or quadriplegia developed secondary to this technique in whom iatrogenic damage occurred to the spinal cord itself. This results from removal of osteo-phytes through a small hole with inadequate exposure of the spinal canal (Fig. 4). It is in reality much safer to perform multiple-level corpectomies to totally visu-alize the chondroosseous masses that are compressing the spinal cord and directly remove them by peeling them back from the posterior longitudinal ligament.

By the same token, decompression may be totally inadequate if all of the compressive pathology is unrecognized, especially in cervical myelopathy, and the exposure is a very limited small hole through the disk space. Although in this situation the neurologic deficit may not become worse, it will not improve either if residual cord compression remains.

On rare occasions, new pathology may develop after an adequate anterior decompression. We had two patients with adequate anterior decompression and arthrodeses in whom ossification of the posterior lon-

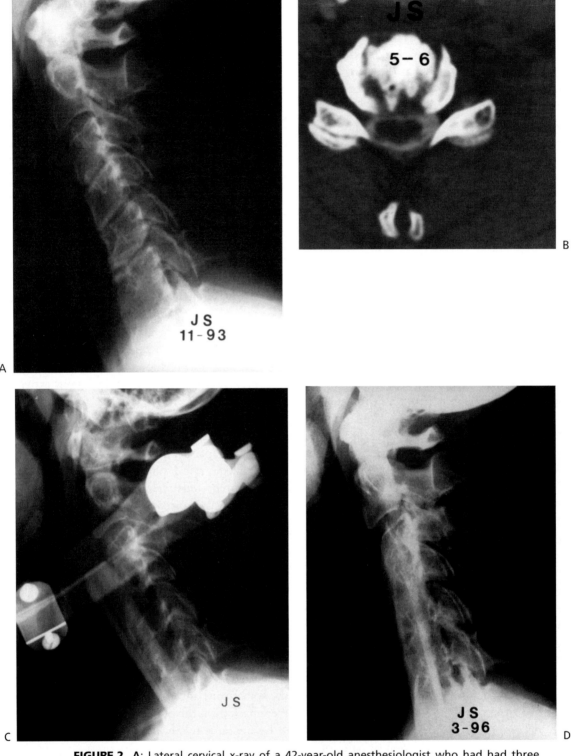

FIGURE 2. A: Lateral cervical x-ray of a 42-year-old anesthesiologist who had had three previous anterior microdiskectomies without fusion for cervical myelopathy with continued myelopathy and neck pain. The C6-7 level is spontaneously fused. **B**: Enhanced computed tomography scan at the C5-6 level showing continued spinal cord compression in a congenitally narrow spinal canal. **C**: Lateral x-ray of the cervical spine in a brace immediately following surgery revealing superior extrusion of the fibular graft. **D**: Lateral x-ray of the cervical spine revealing complete incorporation of the replaced fibular graft 2 years and 8 months following the anterior corpectomies and fusion surgery.

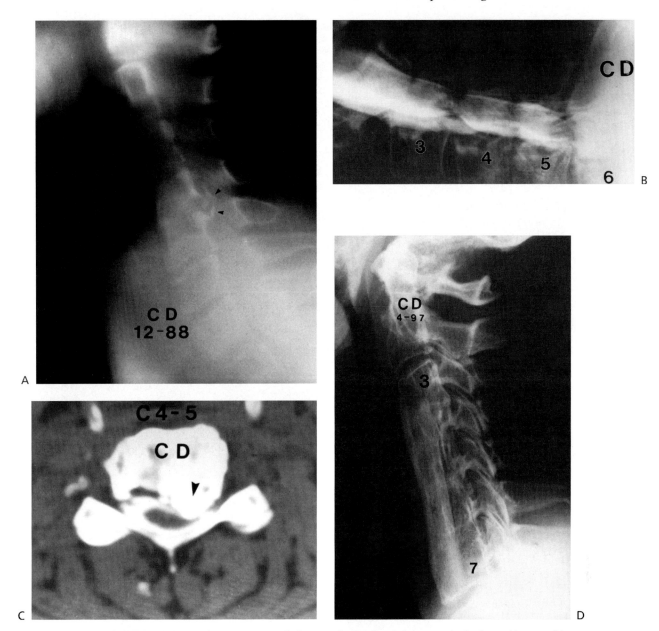

FIGURE 3. A: Lateral tomogram of the cervical spine postoperatively in a 49-year-old woman with Brown-Séquard's syndrome and cervical myelopathy who had had a previous anterior diskectomy and fusion without relief of her hemiparesis. Note the persistent ossification at the C4-5 level protruding into the spinal canal (*arrows*). **B**: Postoperative myelogram revealing persistent C3-4 and C4-5 spinal cord compression. **C**: Enhanced computed tomography scan revealing a unilateral persistent, severe bony compression of the spinal cord at the C4-5 level where the previous surgery had been performed (*arrow*). **D**: Lateral cervical spine film revealing total incorporation of the fibular graft after an anterior cervical corpectomy at C-4, C-5, and C-6 performed in 1988. With a 9-year follow-up, the patient recovered all of her neurologic deficit. [**B** and **C** from Zdeblick TA, Hughes SS, Riew KD, et al. Failed anterior cervical diskectomy and arthrodesis. Analysis and treatment of thirty-five patients. *J Bone Joint Surg Am* 1997;79A:523–532, with permission.]

gitudinal ligament (OPLL) developed with progressive cord compression and myelopathy or radiculopathy that has required further decompression and arthrodesis. Additionally, an adjacent level may develop spondylosis and new neural compression (14).

A rare complication of anterior cervical corpectomy is injury to the vertebral artery, which may have to be ligated to control bleeding. This usually occurs when there is an anomalous tortuosity of the artery that can be identified on preoperative CT scan. The incidence of these anomalies is approximately 2.8% (3,23).

Posterior Operations

Posterior decompressive operations may also result in failed spine patients. A posterior foraminotomy for

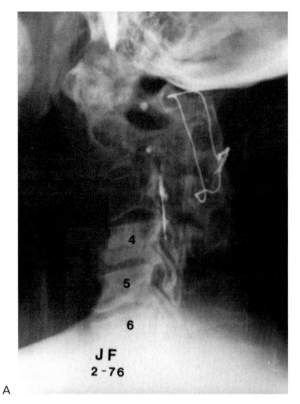

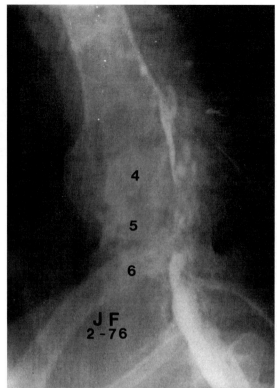

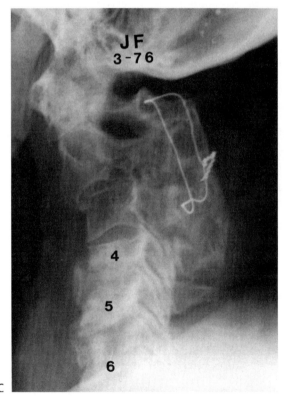

FIGURE 4. A: Lateral cervical spine x-ray revealing a remote posterior cervical fusion at C2-3 for a traumatic subluxation; however, this patient presented with cervical myelopathy and spondylosis with posterior osteophyte formation at C4-5 and C5-6. **B:** Lateral myelogram revealing severe spinal cord compression at C4-5 and C5-6. **C:** The patient underwent an anterior Cloward decompression and fusion at C4-5 and C5-6 and was immediately quadriplegic postoperatively secondary to removal of osteophytes with instrumentation used within a narrow spinal canal. This technique produces iatrogenic cord injury.

anterior nerve root compression may not relieve osteophytic compression of the nerve root anteriorly or even adequately remove disk material. The radicular pain persists with or without neurologic deficit, which then has to be resolved by an anterior decompression and fusion. In addition, total facetectomy posteriorly may produce instability and recurring radiculopathy and pain secondary to the instability, which requires posterior stabilization (16).

More significantly, the complete laminectomy at multiple levels has proved to be a poor operation during long-term follow-up for radiculopathy as well as myelopathy. It can produce a progressive kyphotic deformity, does not relieve anterior cord compres-

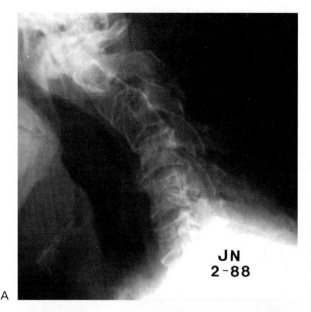

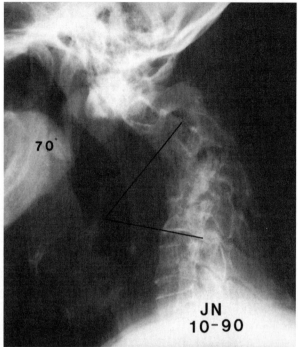

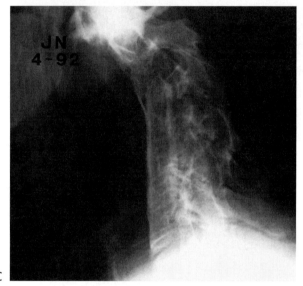

FIGURE 5. A: This 57-year-old man had a remote cervical laminectomy for spastic torticollis 17 years previously. He presented with progressive cervical kyphosis and myelopathy. This lateral x-ray demonstrates the previous laminectomy at C-1, C-2, C-3, and the kyphotic deformity. **B:** The patient underwent an anterior cervical corpectomy and iliac strut fusion, which, because of his osteoporosis, collapsed into an increased kyphosis of 70 degrees. **C:** The patient then had a reconstructive procedure with intraoperative skeletal traction and a repeat anterior cervical corpectomy and autogenous fibular strut fusion; ultimately, his spine was stabilized. This lateral radiograph reveals an incorporated fibular graft 4 years following his surgery, with partial recovery from his myelopathy.

sion, and may produce iatrogenic cord damage during the procedure. Even though the facets are spared, kyphosis or swan neck deformity frequently develops over a long follow-up period (21,25).

Most importantly, if a laminectomy is carried out in a teenager or child, the kyphotic deformity that ensues is almost universal. In addition, if the erector spinae muscles are not reattached to the C-2 spinous process properly following the laminectomy, the muscles become splayed laterally, and this increases the deformity and loss of muscle control of the cervical spine (Fig. 5).

Once the kyphotic deformity occurs after a laminectomy, it becomes more or less fixed with the cervical spondylosis, and in the patient with myelopathy the anterior cord compression persists. The patient may become worse neurologically with time, develop increasing neck and arm pain, and have difficulty with the deformity itself, with neck muscle fatigue, pain,

and difficulty in looking forward or drinking a glass of water. This situation can ordinarily be rectified by carrying out multiple anterior cervical corpectomies at the pathologic levels with intraoperative spinal cord monitoring and skeletal traction; the patient's deformity is corrected once the decompression is carried out and there is no longer any danger to the spinal cord. After the skeletal traction is increased and the cervical spine is extended, a fibular strut graft is used. These patients are always placed in a halo vest postoperatively for 6 weeks, following which a soft collar is worn for another 2 weeks for protection.

Even in the patient who has undergone anterior arthrodesis as well as posterior laminectomy, a kyphotic deformity can develop, which may require a multiple level osteotomy and anterior corpectomy to correct the deformity (Fig. 6). An additional posterior fusion may be necessary in this situation and can be performed under the same anesthesia (12,19).

With regard to posterior decompressive operations, laminoplasty has been used by the Japanese for OPLL for many years and has more recently gained favor in the United States. Technical difficulties are presented with laminoplasty in that the opening may shut down if a graft technique that has been used collapses. It probably should not be recommended for segmental OPLL or multiple level cord compression except when the solid OPLL produces cord compression over many segments, which would be very diffi-

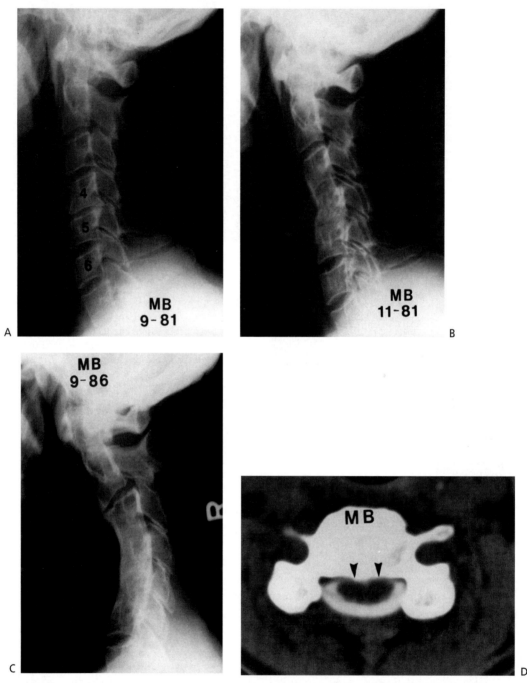

FIGURE 6. A: Lateral cervical spine film in a 50-year-old woman who presented initially with cervical myelopathy. Her lateral radiograph reveals osteophyte formation at C4-5 and C5-6. **B**: The patient underwent an anterior cervical Cloward procedure at two levels that produced the initiation of her cervical kyphotic deformity. When two large dowel-type grafts are used at adjacent levels, very little vertebral body is left in between, and the cervical spine drifts into kyphosis. **C**: The patient presented in 1986 with recurring cervical myelopathy, having undergone another anterior cervical Cloward procedure and then a posterior cervical laminectomy. Note the increased kyphotic deformity even though the anterior cervical spine is solidly fused. In this situation, the bone remodels in the kyphotic position. **D**: The enhanced computed tomography scan reveals flattening of the spinal cord at the kyphotic level (*arrowheads*). (*continued*)

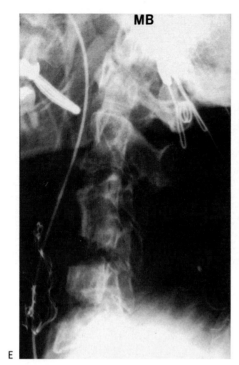

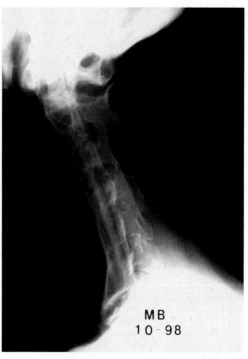

FIGURE 6. (*continued*) **E**: The lateral cervical spine x-ray intraoperatively demonstrating a three-level anterior cervical osteotomy to correct the kyphotic deformity using intraoperative skeletal traction. **F**: The patient underwent a multilevel anterior cervical corpectomy correction of her kyphotic deformity and an autogenous fibular strut graft. This lateral radiograph was taken 12 years after her surgery. She had completely recovered from her cervical myelopathy, and the fibular graft is well incorporated.

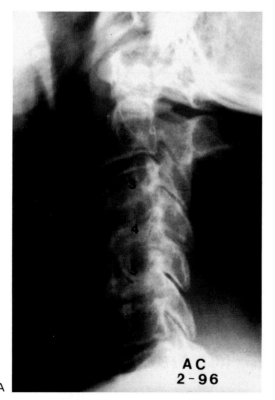

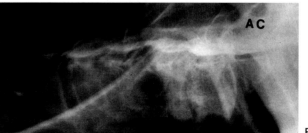

FIGURE 7. **A**: Lateral radiograph of a 66-year-old man presenting with recurring cervical myelopathy and radiculopathy. This x-ray revealed that he has had a cervical laminectomy from C-3 through C-6 and anterior cervical diskectomy and fusion at C3-4 and C4-5. After the two procedures were performed, the patient's neurologic deficit did not resolve. **B**: Lateral cervical myelogram revealing multiple level spinal cord compression anteriorly. (*continued*)

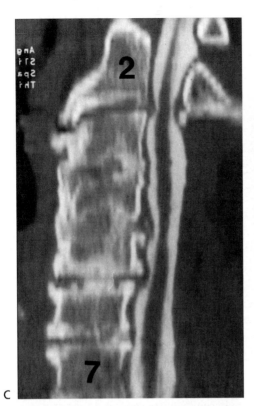

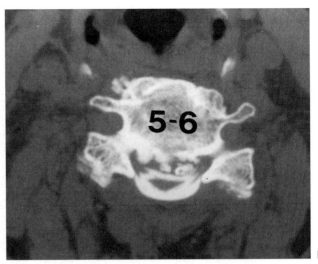

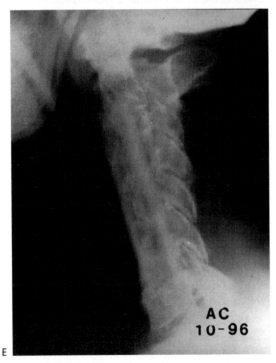

FIGURE 7. (*continued*) **C**: Sagittal computed tomography (CT) scan reconstruction reveals ossification of the posterior longitudinal ligament (OPLL) and multiple levels of cord compression. **D**: Enhanced CT scan at the C5-6 level reveals a persistent OPLL and spinal cord compression. **E**: The patient underwent an anterior cervical corpectomy of C-3, C-4, C-5, and C-6 with an autogenous fibular strut graft. The postoperative lateral cervical spine film reveals excellent incorporation of the fibular strut. The patient recovered from his cervical myelopathy and radiculopathy.

cult to resect from the anterior approach (17). Another technical problem with laminoplasty is that it is very difficult to carry out foraminotomies and it is designed to give a posterior central widening of the spinal canal. Reports have also indicated that patients have a high incidence of neck pain after laminoplasty (15). Laminectomy may also fail to decompress anterior cord compression (Fig. 7).

FAILED ARTHRODESIS FOR DEGENERATIVE DISK DISEASE AND ARTHRITIS

Anterior Arthrodesis

In general, an anterior arthrodesis may fail by graft extrusion, collapse, or pseudarthrosis. However, a pseudarthrosis is not necessarily painful and, in fact, may be totally asymptomatic. Currently, banked bone is being used by some surgeons, but we believe that this has a higher pseudarthrosis and collapse rate and is only justified in circumstances in which the patient is osteopenic and elderly or has poor bone stock. Plates are being widely used to fix the anterior cervical spine, but they do not prevent pseudarthroses, especially in the patient who smokes.

Pseudarthrosis is probably the commonest cause of failure in anterior cervical spine surgery. In a published paper on the results of Robinson anterior cervical diskectomy and arthrodesis for cervical radiculopathy with long-term follow-up in 122 patients, we demonstrated an overall pseudarthrosis incidence of 24 of 195 operatively treated segments (1). Of those, 16 of the patients were symptomatic but only four had sufficient pain to warrant revision surgery. The risk of pseudarthrosis was significantly greater in smokers and after multiple-level arthrodesis than after a single level arthrodesis. We have abandoned performing three-level arthrodeses (6). We have improved the healing rate in one- or two-level anterior diskectomy and fusions by burring off the vertebral endplates before insertion of the bone graft (5). Repair of the painful pseudarthrosis is usually necessary in cases of persistent and incapacitating neck pain or recurring radiculopathy. If the arthrodesis fails and the foraminal osteophytes were not removed, they do not resorb with the normal process of bone remodeling and they persistently irritate the nerve roots. By the same token, a ventral posterior osteophyte may enlarge if a pseudarthrosis occurs, producing spinal cord compression. The patient with cervical spinal stenosis and spondylosis is much more prone to having recurring problems with a pseudarthrosis and neural compression than is someone with a wide 18-mm spinal canal. Based on our own experience, we have seen very poor results from bank or bovine bone with collapse and pseudarthrosis.

We have published an analysis of treatment of 35 patients who had failed anterior cervical diskectomy and arthrodesis (26). Twenty-three patients had failure of arthrodesis without deformity but with neck or arm pain with radiculopathy or myelopathy. Four patients had migration of the grafts, two Robinson-type grafts anteriorly and two Cloward grafts posteriorly displaced. Six had received allograft bone. Eight patients had graft failure with kyphosis, of whom five had a Cloward procedure, one a diskectomy alone, and two a Robinson procedure. Treatment of these patients consisted of an anterior resection of the area of failed arthrodesis, decompression of the nerve roots or spinal cord, and arthrodesis with autogenous bone. The results were excellent in 29 patients, good in 1, fair in 4, and poor in 1. We concluded that repeat anterior arthrodesis can produce excellent results in the majority of patients with persistent symptoms.

The surgical repair of a pseudarthrosis after an anterior cervical diskectomy and fusion can be carried out by the anterior or posterior approach. In general, we restudy the patient with a gadolinium-enhanced MRI or myelogram and CT to determine if any significant anterior spinal cord or root compression is present. If it is, we proceed with a resection of the pseudarthrosis anteriorly and a repeat arthrodesis with or without plate fixation. If little or no anterior neural compression is present, a posterior arthrodesis with the triple wire technique or lateral mass plate fixation can be performed (9). Ultimately, when the posterior fusion consolidates, the anterior pseudarthrosis does also.

In our review of all of our anterior cervical arthrodeses with either iliac or autogenous bone, we found that the grafts may collapse if they are osteopenic and are associated with an osteoporotic cervical spine. This is true of iliac as well as fibular grafts. If the above situation is appreciated before the surgery, we occasionally use bank bone if the graft site is osteopenic. If the patient has an osteopenic cervical spine and a multilevel decompression and fibular graft is to be used, consideration for the use of a halo vest would be an important part of the procedure to stabilize the spine further until healing occurs. In addition, if an anterior decompression is going to be done in an osteopenic spine, a supplemental posterior arthrodesis should be considered. When a surgeon encounters a patient with a collapsed anterior graft that produces a kyphotic deformity and may be associated with pseudarthrosis, repeat diagnostic studies should be carried out by myelography and CT scan to determine the amount of neural compression. Even if the bone is solidly fused following the collapse of the graft, this usually requires an anterior cervical corpectomy at one or more levels, resection of the old graft, and use of a fibular graft. The kyphotic deformity can be corrected intraoperatively after the decompression is performed and before the new graft is inserted.

Extrusion of a fibular or iliac graft usually requires replacement with a longer graft. However, this may be a significant problem if the fibular graft was inserted over multiple segments such as from C-2 to C-7, in which case putting in a long, straight fibular graft may be difficult if the cervical spine is lordotic. The higher risk for graft extrusion is in the postlami-

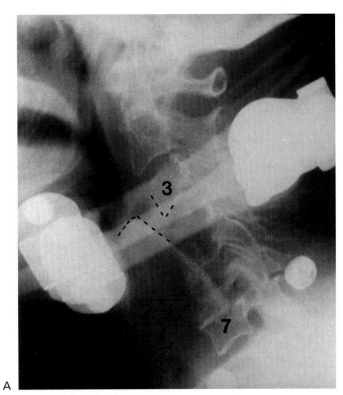
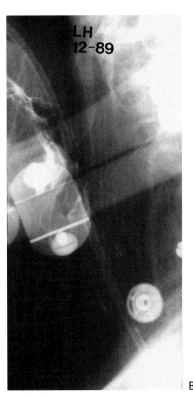

FIGURE 8. A: Lateral x-ray of an 80-year-old woman who had undergone an anterior cervical corpectomy and fusion from C-3 to C-7 for cervical myelopathy. Postoperatively, she extruded her superior iliac graft, which ultimately perforated her esophagus. The latter problem was initially unrecognized, and subsequently a fibular graft was inserted. **B**: After the second operation, fever and a pharyngeal abscess developed that extended down to the mediastinum. On barium swallow, one notes the extraneous barium anterior to the nasogastric tube. The patient had her cervical abscess drained, and the esophagus was repaired with recovery.

nectomy patient, in whom we now use the halo vest. If the graft extrudes inferiorly and is not producing dysphagia, replacement is not necessary, a supplemental posterior arthrodesis can be performed, and the patient can remain in a halo vest until healing occurs. The commonest location of a fibular graft extrusion in our experience is inferiorly where the vertebrae fracture at the seating hole, usually the anterior lip. An additional problem that we have had has been superior graft extrusion where the upper cervical vertebrae are quite small in diameter and seating is difficult. One problem that can occur in this situation is that the inferior part of the graft may angulate inward and produce osteophyte protrusion into the spinal canal and recurring radiculopathy. Repeat decompression and reinsertion of a graft may be necessary in this situation (Fig. 2). If at the time of surgery the surgeon perceives a problem with graft seating, a small buttress plate can be used.

We have had experience with one patient who extruded an iliac graft when coughing vigorously in the recovery room; the graft had a sharp edge that perforated the esophagus. This went unrecognized for approximately 3 days. The iliac graft was then replaced with a fibular graft, but it was not appreciated that the esophagus had been perforated and an abscess formed, resulting in repeat surgery to drain the abscess to prevent mediastinal spread and generalized sepsis. Finally, the esophagus was repaired, and the patient healed uneventfully (Fig. 8).

Anterior bone grafts may displace into the spinal canal, an occurrence that we find to be extremely rare, if the posterior longitudinal ligament is spared, which is our policy. The graft may be placed there inadvertently and not be recognized until the postoperative state. This situation may produce paralysis with spinal cord and nerve root compression. It has to be identified by appropriate diagnostic studies, such as repeat myelography, CT scanning, or MRI. The graft is then removed and replaced in its proper position (Fig. 9). We recommend spinal cord monitoring with evoked potentials in all spinal cord decompression operations.

We believe that Cloward dowel-type grafts are inadequate for a number of reasons. They are not as strong as block-type grafts; by this technique they may extrude into the spine, producing paralysis, especially when the posterior longitudinal ligament is

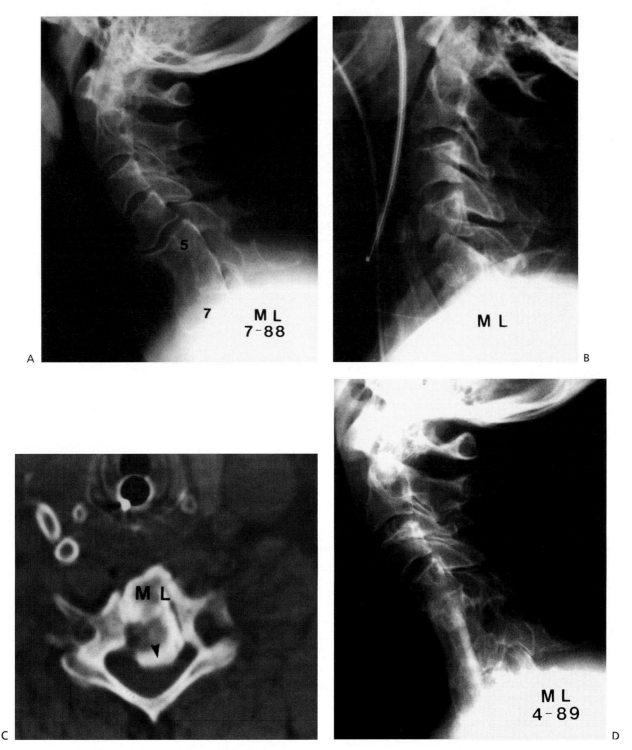

FIGURE 9. **A**: This 48-year-old man presented with progressive cervical myelopathy and neck pain. He had had anterior cervical diskectomy and fusions by the Cloward procedure 25 years previously with progressive kyphotic deformity. This lateral x-ray reveals a kyphosis and original tearing of the posterior interspinous ligaments at C5-6. **B**: The patient underwent an anterior cervical corpectomy of C-5 and C-6 and an iliac strut fusion. An hour after the patient's awakening and moving all extremities, a right hemiparesis developed. After a review of the lateral cervical radiograph, it appeared as though the bone graft had cocked back into the spinal canal inferiorly. Note the lateral radiograph and the angular placement of the bone graft. **C**: The immediate postoperative computed tomography scan that was carried out with the patient still intubated revealed the graft extrusion into the spinal canal (*arrowhead*). **D**: The patient was returned to the operating room immediately, where the iliac graft was removed and a longer fibular graft was replaced. Postoperatively, the patient recovered, although with neurologic deficit. This lateral radiograph reveals the incorporated fibular graft more than a year after the surgery.

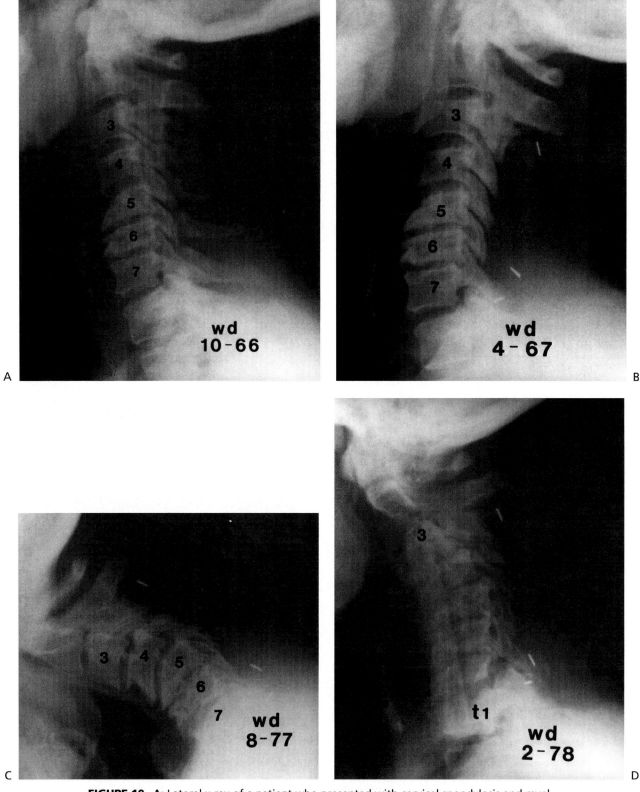

FIGURE 10. A: Lateral x-ray of a patient who presented with cervical spondylosis and myelopathy. Note the multiple levels of osteophyte formation at C5-6 and C6-7. **B**: The patient underwent a cervical laminectomy of C-3, C-4, C-5, and C-6, with initial improvement of the cervical myelopathy. Initially, he was Nurick grade 4 and then became ambulatory. This lateral radiograph was taken shortly after the operation was performed. **C**: Within 1 year, severe cervical kyphosis and subluxations developed, as noted on this lateral radiograph. **D**: The patient underwent an anterior cervical partial corpectomy at multiple levels with a fibular strut fusion, ultimately recovering from his myelopathy, attaining ambulatory status and walking without aid.

taken down, which is inadvisable. In addition, the dowel-type graft, when applied at multiple adjacent segments, leaves very little structure of the vertebral body in between, and kyphosis may occur, which can be progressive. This situation can be compounded when a laminectomy is additionally performed following the multiple-level Cloward procedure. The cervical spine remodels into kyphosis even though it may be solidly fused. This situation can only be rectified by a cervical corrective osteotomy and additional fusion, which is a rather complex procedure (Fig. 6).

In general, we have not used anterior plate fixation for routine reconstructive anterior cervical spine surgery. It is our contention that by using skilled techniques with autogenous bone grafting, the fusion rate is extraordinarily high. Certainly, for the Robinson Smith type of block fusions, graft extrusion is almost unheard of in our experience. We believe that the anterior plate is more applicable to the traumatic cervical spine injury. Anterior plates may fail for a variety of reasons. Screws may break or back out and perforate the esophagus. In addition, with the Caspar technique, the posterior cortex of the vertebral body is tapped and the screws are purposely placed through that into the spinal canal, which we believe to be dangerous.

Posterior Arthrodesis

Failure of a subaxial posterior cervical arthrodesis is an extremely uncommon problem. The commonest type of posterior fusion that has stood the test of time in our 25 years of experience has been the Bohlman triple-wire technique, using autogenous iliac crest graft. This is a safe, almost universally successful procedure in all types of degenerative cervical spine problems, including rheumatoid arthritis. We have never seen a failure of arthrodesis with this technique for degenerative disease, and we do not decorticate the subaxial cervical spine for a posterior arthrodesis. Plate fixation is an alternative to wiring but usually is not necessary. Another good technique with limited application is lateral facet fusion and wiring in patients who have had previous cervical laminectomies, although in that situation a lateral plate and lateral mass screw fixation can be used; there is very little bone surface exposed following plate insertion to allow bone-to-bone contact, however.

It is well known that banked bone fusions have a lower arthrodesis rate, and, therefore, except in extenuating circumstances, we use autogenous bone. We have seen pseudarthrosis with onlay grafts, which are not fixed to the spinous processes. These can be repaired with a repeat procedure posteriorly using grafts wired in place or an anterior arthrodesis. Posterior arthrodesis may fail if a flexible cable system is used and the bone graft resorbs somewhat in the healing process, in which case the cable system becomes loose and a pseudarthrosis will ensue. Once the pseudarthrosis is established, the cable system should be removed, and we believe that it is preferable to use more rigid monofilament wire to anchor the bone grafts or to use a lateral mass plate.

Although methylmethacrylate is rarely used to attempt a posterior stabilization of the spine today, it should be condemned for various reasons that have been published. Most importantly, the cement does not adhere to cortical bone and eventually loosens, and the fixation will fail. In addition, bone cement affects mobilization of white blood cells, and the infection rate is extremely high. In the past when we have treated the failures of cement fixation, the material, including the wires, had been removed and the standard arthrodesis was performed using the triple-wire technique.

POSTLAMINECTOMY INSTABILITY

In patients who have undergone a cervical laminectomy for tumor or degenerative disease who have had the facets removed, marked instability of the cervical spine, as well as kyphosis, has developed. Cervical kyphoses following laminectomy can be rectified with an anterior decompression and intraoperative correction of the deformity with strut fusion (Fig. 10). If the anterior approach is not feasible and the cervical kyphosis is flexible and correctable with traction, a posterior facet fusion and wiring or lateral mass plating can be performed with arthrodesis after the patient has been placed in skeletal traction and corrected. Fortunately, this is a very uncommon problem today.

POSTOPERATIVE PARALYSIS

Postoperative paralysis following anterior decompression and fusion fortunately is uncommon and occurs in fewer than 1% of these procedures (8). Immediate postoperative paralysis has many causes, including iatrogenic injury to the spinal cord during decompressive surgery, overextension and positioning on the operating table in the presence of severe spinal cord compression, excessive tension on the shoulders pulling them down for intraoperative lateral cervical spine x-rays, intraoperative ischemia of the spinal cord secondary to hypotension, and, as previously mentioned, graft extrusion posteriorly into the spinal canal (24).

We routinely use intraoperative spinal cord monitoring in patients with cervical myelopathy who require anterior cervical corpectomies and spinal cord decompression or in most of the other cervical corpectomies. We find somatosensory evoked potentials to be quite sensitive to spinal cord insults during positioning of the patient, before surgery on the operating table, and intraoperatively (2).

If the patient awakens with an increased neurologic deficit immediately, we may suggest carrying out radiographs and an emergency cervical MRI, but if the patient is recovering function over a number of hours, suggesting avascular insult, we might merely observe that individual if the postoperative x-rays reveal no graft extrusion and the procedure went uneventfully. In this situation, there is no scientific proof that steroids have any effect on recovery of the deficit unless direct trauma to the spinal cord occurred. We have never seen a postoperative hematoma that caused paralysis from anterior cervical surgery. If graft extrusion has occurred into the spinal canal, the graft should be removed immediately and replaced with another, usually longer graft.

SPINAL FLUID FISTULA

Although quite unusual, spinal fluid cutaneous fistula or spinal fluid leak may occur when the dura is absent, specifically in patients with OPLL with long-standing dural compression (22). In addition, an iatrogenic tear of the dura may be present, which, if inadequately repaired, can produce a spinal fluid leak. We have reported on the treatment of such cases with absence of the dura. If absence of the dura is encountered interoperatively, it is our policy to ask the anesthesiologist to respire the patient manually with less volume to decrease the subarachnoid pressure and, therefore, the loss of spinal fluid while a repair is carried out. Ordinarily, this situation occurs in anterior decompressions of the spinal cord with large osteophytes or in long-standing large segments of OPLL, which leave the arachnoid or spinal cord exposed after resection. An attempt is made to suture a muscle fascia patch down to the posterior longitudinal ligament or edge of the dura, which can be done with fine silk sutures and microinstruments in some situations. If no remaining posterior ligament or dura is available

to which to suture, an onlay muscle fasciae graft is placed. Once the wound is dry, the patch is covered with fibrin glue, following which the anterior graft is inserted. Before the patient is awakened, we place a lumbar drain to drain the spinal fluid distally while the cervical wound is sealing off. This requires approximately 3 days of drainage, during which time the patient remains semirecumbent.

If absence of the dura is suspected preoperatively and can be predicted in patients with a very large herniated disk or OPLL of long-standing duration, we place a lumbar subarachnoid drain before carrying out the anterior decompressive procedure. When the absent dura is encountered, the drainage is started and allows a dry field in which to carry out the dural repair.

Avoidance of the failed cervical spine surgery patient requires careful preoperative assessment of the pathologic problem and meticulous operative technique as well as postoperative care.

REFERENCES

1. Bohlman HH, Emery SE, Goodfellow DB, et al. Robinson anterior cervical discectomy and arthrodesis for cervical radiculopathy: long-term follow-up of one hundred and twenty-two patients. *J Bone Joint Surg Am* 1993;75A:1298–1307.
2. Bouchard JA, Bohlman HH, Biro C. Intraoperative improvements of somatosensory evoked potentials: correlation to clinical outcome in surgery for cervical spondylitic myelopathy. *Spine* 1996;21:589–594.
3. Curylo LJ, Mason HC, Bohlman HH, et al. Tortuous course of the vertebral artery and anterior cervical decompression: a cadaveric and clinical case study. *Spine* 2000;25:2860–2864.
4. Emery SE, Bohlman HH, Bolesta MJ, et al. Anterior cervical decompression and arthrodesis for the treatment of cervical spondylotic myelopathy. Two to seventeen-year follow-up. *J Bone Joint Surg Am* 1998;80A:941–951.
5. Emery SE, Bolesta MJ, Banks MA, et al. Robinson anterior cervical fusion: comparison of the standard and modified techniques. *Spine* 1994;19:660–663.
6. Emery SE, Fisher RS, Bohlman HH. Three-level anterior cervical discectomy and fusion: radiographic and clinical results. *Spine* 1997;22:2622–2624.
7. Farey ID, McAfee PC, Davis RF, et al. Pseudarthrosis of the cervical spine after anterior arthrodesis. Treatment by posterior nerve-root decompression, stabilization, and arthrodesis. *J Bone Joint Surg Am* 1990;72A:1171–1177.
8. Flynn TB. Neurologic complications of anterior cervical interbody fusion. *Spine* 1982;7:536–539.
9. Fuji T, Yonenobu K, Fujiwara K, et al. Interspinous wiring without bone grafting for nonunion or delayed

union following anterior spinal fusion of the cervical spine. *Spine* 1986;11:982–987.

10. Gregorius FK, Estrin T, Crandall PH. Cervical spondylotic radiculopathy and myelopathy. A long-term follow-up study. *Arch Neurol* 1976;33:618–625.

11. Heller JG, Silcox DH III. Postlaminectomy instability of the cervical spine. Etiology and stabilization technique. In: Frymoyer JW, Ducker TB, Hadler NM, et al., eds. *The adult spine—principles and practice*, 2nd ed. Philadelphia: Lippincott–Raven Publishers, 1997:1413–1434.

12. Hennan JM, Sonntag VK. Cervical corpectomy and plate fixation for postlaminectomy kyphosis. *J Neurosurg* 1994;80:963–970.

13. Hilibrand AS, Carlson GD, Palumbo MA, et al. Radiculopathy and myelopathy at segments adjacent to the site of a previous anterior cervical arthrodesis. *J Bone Joint Surg Am* 1999;81A:519–528.

14. Hilibrand AS, Yoo JU, Carlson GD, et al. The success of anterior cervical arthrodesis adjacent to a previous fusion. *Spine* 1997;22:1574–1579.

15. Hosono N, Yonenobu K, Ono K. Neck and shoulder pain after laminoplasty. A noticeable complication. *Spine* 1996;21:1969–1973.

16. McAfee PC, Bohlman HH, Ducker TB, et al. One-stage anterior cervical decompression and posterior stabilization: a study of one hundred patients with a minimum of two years of follow-up. *J Bone Joint Surg Am* 1995;77A:1791–1800.

17. McAfee PC, Regan JJ, Bohlman HH. Cervical cord compression from ossification of the posterior longitudinal ligament (OPLL) in non-orientals. *J Bone Joint Surg Am* 1987;69B:569–575.

18. Mikawa Y, Shikata J, Yamamuro T. Spinal deformity and instability after multilevel cervical laminectomy. *Spine* 1987;12:6–11.

19. Riew KD, Hilibrand AS, Palumbo MA, et al. Anterior cervical corpectomy in patients previously managed with a laminectomy: short-term complications. *J Bone Joint Surg Am* 1999;81A:950–957.

20. Saito T, Yamamuro T, Shikata J, et al. Analysis and prevention of spinal column deformity following cervical laminectomy. 1. Pathogenetic analysis of postlaminectomy deformities. *Spine* 1991;16:494–502.

21. Sim FH, Svien HJ, Bickel WH, et al. Swan-neck deformity following extensive cervical laminectomy. A review of twenty-one cases. *J Bone Joint Surg Am* 1974;56A:564–580.

22. Smith MD, Bolesta MJ, Leventhal M, et al. Postoperative cerebrospinal-fluid fistula associated with erosion of the dura: findings after anterior resection of ossification of the posterior longitudinal ligament in the cervical spine. *J Bone Joint Surg Am* 1992;74A:270–277.

23. Smith MD, Emery SE, Dudley A, et al. Vertebral artery injury during anterior decompression of the cervical spine. A retrospective review of ten patients. *J Bone Joint Surg Br* 1993;75B:410–415.

24. Yonenobu K, Hosono N, Iwasaki M, et al. Neurologic complications of surgery for cervical compression myelopathy. *Spine* 1991;16:1277–1282.

25. Zdeblick TA, Bohlman HH. Cervical kyphosis and myelopathy. Treatment by anterior corpectomy and strut-grafting. *J Bone Joint Surg Am* 1989;71A:170–182.

26. Zdeblick TA, Hughes SS, Riew KD, et al. Failed anterior cervical discectomy and arthrodesis: analysis and treatment of thirty-five patients. *J Bone Joint Surg Am* 1997;79A:523–532.

4

CERVICAL SPINE: DEFORMITY

RICHARD D. LAZAR AND TODD J. ALBERT

Cervical deformity is an unusual and potentially difficult problem for spine surgeons. The care and treatment of each patient must be individualized with regard to the etiology of the deformity, the extent of neural involvement, and the presence of associated medical problems or congenital anomalies. Surgical treatment must be approached with caution due to the inherent high risk of neurologic compromise. Surgical efforts should focus on improvement of function, pain relief, and cosmetic appearance. The etiology of failures of deformity surgery involving the cervical spine is similar to failures of deformity surgery involving the thoracic and lumbar spine. Common mechanisms of surgical failure include inadequate correction of sagittal or coronal balance, pseudarthrosis, instrumentation failure, adjacent segment disease, and neurologic injury.

Causes of cervical deformity include posttraumatic pyogenic infection, cervical scoliosis, Klippel-Feil syndrome, metastatic tumor, spondylosis, and iatrogenic causes. The latter is the commonest etiology for cervical deformity and clinically is most frequently seen as postlaminectomy kyphosis. All of these presentations are relatively rare and difficult to treat. The combination of limited clinical experience and difficult deformity creates a setting of risk for surgical failures. These failures may be due to loss of correction, graft collapse, nonunion, instrumentation failure, neurologic injury, or continued pain. This chapter explores the various etiologies of cervical deformity, mechanisms of treatment, and the treatment of postlaminectomy kyphotic deformity with revision surgery.

BIOMECHANICS OF CERVICAL KYPHOSIS

The majority of cervical deformities present as kyphosis. The etiology of kyphotic deformity in the cervical spine and its propensity for progression can be better understood by examining the biomechanics of cervical sagittal alignment. The average range of normal sagittal lordosis in the cervical spine from C-2 to C-7 was reported by Bridwell (5) to be 14.4 degrees. Normally, the weight-bearing axis of the cranium lies posterior to the vertebral bodies of C2-7. This helps to maintain normal lordotic sagittal contour and minimizes posterior cervical musculature tension to maintain balance of the weight-bearing forces. Pal and Sherk (34) tested load transmission in the anterior (vertebral bodies) and posterior cervical columns (facet joints) in cadavers. They found that 36% of the total load applied to the top of the specimen is transmitted through the anterior column and 64% through the posterior columns formed by the articular processes of the facets.

Because the neural arch in the cervical region transmits more load than the anterior column, extensive loss of facet integrity can produce cervical instability. Once the normal alignment of the cervical spine is lost in the sagittal plane, the weight-bearing axis of the cranium becomes aligned anteriorly with respect to the vertebral bodies. This loss of balance in the sagittal plane results in the posterior spinal musculature constantly contracting to maintain normal upright head position. Eventually, fatigue and pain occur and the kyphotic deformity progresses. As weight-bearing forces shift to the anterior column, the vertebral bodies and disks are responsible for the entire weight-bearing force. In the skeletally immature, Yasouka et al. (54) postulated that the wedging of the anterior vertebrae is due to increased compression of the cartilaginous endplates and at least partly responsible for the postlaminectomy kyphosis seen in such patients.

As kyphosis increases, the spinal cord becomes draped over the posterior aspect of the vertebral bodies. Breig (6) studied the microvascular supply to the spinal cord and found that cervical flexion produced flattening of the small feeder vessels to the cord. He additionally postulated an increase in cord tension longitudinally with flexion due to tethering of the cord by the dentate ligaments and cervical roots. This combination of spinal cord tension and ischemia may lead to direct neuronal injury as deformity progresses. Often, severe spinal cord changes such as myelomalacia and cord atrophy are seen as spinal cord signal changes on magnetic resonance imaging (MRI) in these patients.

POSTTRAUMATIC DEFORMITY

Posttraumatic deformity is usually secondary to late instability after acute injuries or progressive deformity of neglected injuries. Significant ligamentous injury of the cervical spine may result in chronic instability, deformity, and pain. Herkowitz and Rothman (21) demonstrated this phenomenon of late instability and deformity in their clinical series.

Kyphosis after cervical injury is the most frequently encountered posttraumatic deformity. This deformity is thought to be secondary to the elastic deformation of the posterior ligaments seen with flexion and axial loading. Other traumatic injuries that can produce cervical kyphosis following injury include unrecognized facet subluxation, facet fracture, or progressive anterior vertebral body collapse due to occult fracture (2). These unrecognized injuries often occur at or near the cervicothoracic junction as a result of poor plain radiographic resolution at this level (Figs. 1 and 2).

Prevention of posttraumatic deformity requires recognition of unstable injury patterns and subse-

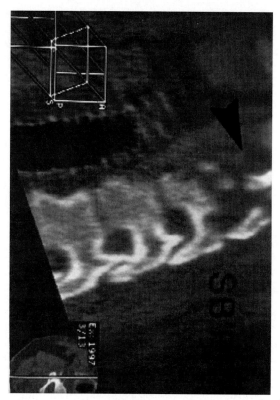

FIGURE 2. Sagittal reformatted tomogram of the same patient seen in Figure 1. This scan shows the extent of the T-1 vertebral body fracture and the perched facet.

quent treatment that ensures stabilization. Cervical kyphosis following decompressive laminectomy for cervical trauma is a well-recognized complication, and, therefore, laminectomy should be avoided as an isolated treatment. Morgan et al. (33) reported that 68% of patients treated with laminectomy for cervical trauma required a secondary arthrodesis.

Bohlman's retrospective review (3) of 300 cervical spine injuries demonstrated that posterior ligamentous injuries in combination with compression or wedge fractures of the vertebral bodies cannot be treated with halo immobilization (Fig. 3). This injury pattern was found to have a high incidence of late displacement and painful deformity.

A Cloward arthrodesis for treatment of anterior column disruptions in combination with posterior ligamentous injury may also result in late kyphotic deformity and pain. Stauffer and Kelly (47) described 16 patients with interbody fusions in whom late kyphotic deformity developed. In a retrospective review of the radiographs, all 16 patients had widening of one or more interspinous spaces.

McAfee and Bohlman (30) reported on 24 patients with anterior cervical column injuries in combination with posterior ligamentous disruption using simultaneous anterior and posterior arthrodesis. They believed that this approach ensures stabilization, arthrodesis, and

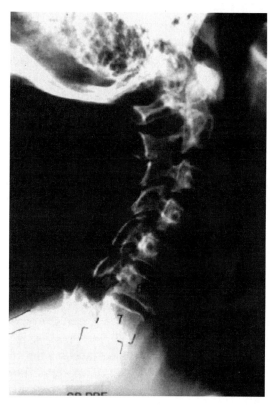

FIGURE 1. Lateral radiograph for neck pain evaluation following trauma showing traumatic spondylolisthesis at C7 to T1.

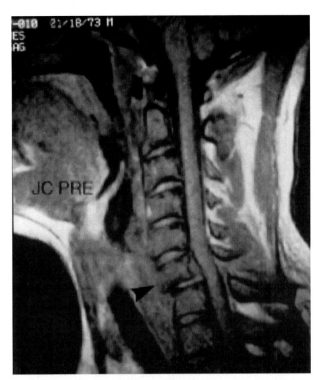

FIGURE 3. Sagittal T1-weighted magnetic resonance image clearly shows the anterior displacement of C-6, the retropulsed C-7, and the large prevertebral hematoma anteriorly *(arrow)*.

control of sagittal alignment. The prevention of post-traumatic cervical spine deformity depends on recognition of the injury pattern and the extent of posterior ligamentous injury. Once cervical kyphosis develops, reduction and stabilization become more difficult.

SPINAL INFECTIONS

Tuberculosis remains the leading cause worldwide of nontraumatic paraplegia (42). Several mechanisms are believed responsible for neurologic deficit in tuberculous spondylitis. Direct compression of the spinal cord can occur by abscess formation, displaced bone or disk, or the development of kyphotic deformity (16,22). The indications for operative intervention are the same as with pyogenic infections of the spine: the presence of severe bone loss and deformity, neurologic deficit with spinal cord compression, failure of antibiotic therapy, and presence of a paraspinal abscess (13). Cervical spine involvement with tuberculosis is rare but, when present, is associated with a greater than 40% incidence of cord compression and neurologic deficit (24). MRI is the radiographic study of choice due to its delineation of bone and soft tissue involvement. This is critical for preoperative planning when considering the extent of radical débridement that is

necessary, site of abscesses, and involvement of the epidural space.

The described Hong Kong procedure for the surgical treatment of tuberculous kyphosis consists of radical anterior resection and strut graft fusion. Ten-year follow-up of this technique demonstrated a 97% successful fusion rate and mean thoracic kyphosis decrease of 1.4 degrees (31). Débridement of the lower cervical spine (C3-7) can best be approached through the posterior triangle in cases of abscess formation, as purulence often tracks into the posterior triangle (23). After drainage and débridement of the paravertebral abscess, débridement of infected bone and disk is not complete until adjacent bleeding bone is seen. The anterior débridement should extend to the posterior longitudinal ligament in cases of kyphotic deformity and to the dura if the posterior longitudinal ligament is pathologically related to the spinal cord compression.

Kyphotic deformity is then corrected with anterior distraction and insertion of a strut graft. The Hong Kong study demonstrated a greater than 95% fusion rate with autogenous iliac crest strut graft and excellent maintenance of deformity correction (31). For long constructs in the cervical spine, we prefer autogenous fibular graft.

VERTEBRAL OSTEOMYELITIS

Pyogenic vertebral osteomyelitis represents 2% to 8% of all cases of osteomyelitis (50). The incidence of cervical spine osteomyelitis is approximately 6% for all cases of vertebral osteomyelitis (29). The primary routes of infection appear to be hematogenous. Identifiable sources of bacteria include the genitourinary tract (29%) (38), soft tissue infections (13%) (40), upper respiratory tract (11%) (40), and intravenous drug abuse (2%) (27). However, Sapico and Montgomerie (40) found that 27% of cases of cervical osteomyelitis involved intravenous drug abusers. Endress et al. (14) postulated that the increased incidence of cervical involvement could be due to the use of central venous injection sites, particularly the jugular veins.

Infections by hematogenous spread typically involve the vertebral metaphysis first because of the rich vascular supply along the anterior body. The upper cervical spine has a distinct venous plexus around the odontoid called the *pharyngeal vertebral vein*. This plexus is thought to be responsible for hematogenous infectious spread to the upper cervical spine (35). Once established within the meta-

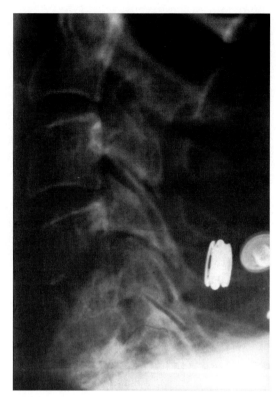

FIGURE 4. Lateral radiograph of healthy male who presented with neck pain, fever, and upper extremity weakness. Note the destruction of the C4-5 disk space accompanied by vertebral collapse and localized kyphosis.

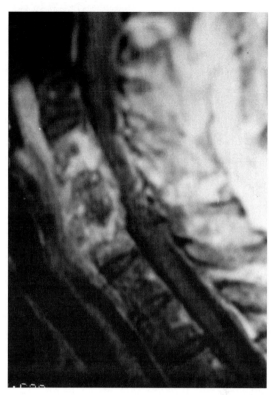

FIGURE 5. Sagittal T1-weighted magnetic resonance image of the same patient shown in Figure 4 demonstrates intervertebral diskitis at C4-5 and C5-6 with epidural abscess formation.

physis, the infection may spread into the disk and infect the adjacent vertebral body (Fig. 4). MRI provides excellent diagnostic specificity for diskitis, osteomyelitis, and epidural abscess (Fig. 5). Computed tomography (CT) can provide a better understanding of the degree of infectious osteodestruction (Fig. 6).

The clinical presentation of cervical vertebral osteomyelitis is nonspecific. Greater than 90% of patients complain of neck pain. Swallowing or respiratory difficulties are reported by Sapico and Montgomerie (41) to occur in approximately 11% of cases with cervical involvement. The frequency of neurologic changes is much higher with cervical vertebral osteomyelitis. Eismont et al. (12) reported paralysis in 82% of their cervical cases, and Stone et al. (48) found that more than one-half of their patients had evidence of neurologic deficits.

Treatment of cervical osteomyelitis is largely surgical due to the risk of catastrophic neurologic deficit that may occur with medical failure. The same principles as outlined for tuberculous infection apply to pyogenic infection. The pathology is usually anterior, and, thus, the surgical approach should be anterior. Following the principles of the Hong Kong tuberculosis experience, surgery should include radi-

cal excision of the involved tissues and immediate reconstruction with autogenous strut graft to restore stability. Anterior cervical plating is contraindicated in the presence of infection due to the adherent nature of bacteria to the foreign body. However, reports have shown some success with plating anteriorly at the time of débridement. Longer follow-up and review are necessary before these techniques can be widely promoted.

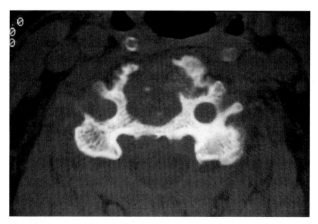

FIGURE 6. Computed tomography axial cut of the same patient shown in Figures 4 and 5 illustrating the degree of bone loss. The patient was treated with anterior decompression and fusion.

CERVICAL SCOLIOSIS

Cervical scoliosis and cervicothoracic scoliosis are rare clinical entities. These deformities can be severely disfiguring and difficult to treat as the deformity progresses. Their presence provokes early recognition and treatment if progression is demonstrated. Cervical spine scoliosis is poorly tolerated by patients due to the inability of the occipital-cervical junction to provide any sort of compensatory curve. These patients will have obvious cosmetic deformity as progression occurs.

All patients with congenital scoliosis should be screened for associated anomalies of the trachea, esophagus, rectum, renal system, and auditory system. MRI of the spine before surgery is recommended to rule out the presence of diastematomyelia or spinal dysraphism. Approximately 50% of patients with congenital scoliosis or cervicothoracic scoliosis have associated Klippel-Feil anomalies of the cervical spine (19,52). When scoliosis is associated with Klippel-Feil abnormalities, a progressive deformity can be severe due to the lack of compensating normal spine above and below the deformity.

Mild asymptomatic curves that progress more than 10 degrees can be treated with simple posterior arthrodesis with or without instrumentation (45). Larger curves may benefit from preoperative skeletal traction for approximately 10 days. Skeletally immature patients with a rigid curve can be treated with facet joint decortication and halo traction for 2 to 3 weeks followed by halo casting for 6 months.

A 30% incidence of laminar aplasia is seen with cervical scoliosis (46). During exposure, extreme caution should be used because the cord and dura are in an unprotected, essentially subcutaneous position. Surgeons must be aware of this possible defect during exposure to prevent dural and cord injury with Cobb elevators or with electrocautery.

METASTATIC TUMOR

Metastatic tumor or primary neoplasias involving the cervical spine commonly produce severe pain (8,17) (Fig. 7). Infiltrating lesions often progress rapidly, producing vertebral body collapse and, potentially, quadriplegia (17,18,26). In the past, surgical treatment of these lesions frequently consisted of laminectomy for decompression, often producing dangerous instability and no improvement in neural function (25,49) (Fig. 8). Severe cervical kyphosis with progressive neurologic involvement may occur when laminectomy is combined with radiation therapy for tumor (36). The

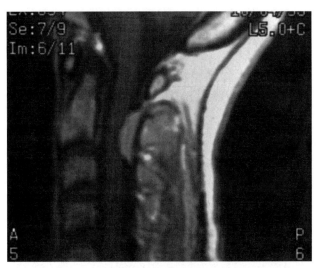

FIGURE 7. Sagittal T1-weighted magnetic resonance image shows a meningioma at the level of C2-3. The patient presented with neck pain and gait disturbance.

necrosis of the vertebral body secondary to radiation therapy, coupled with loss of posterior tethering structures, produces a sharp, angular kyphotic deformity. Once this deformity is recognized, surgical intervention should be expeditious to prevent unrelenting progression. Preoperative cervical traction for reduction should be considered with slow correction. Vertebral body necrosis after radiation therapy may produce

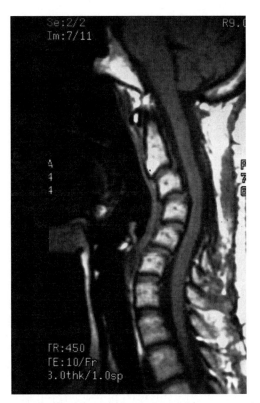

FIGURE 8. Sagittal T1-weighted magnetic resonance image with postlaminectomy kyphosis 6 months after the resection of the tumor seen in Figure 7.

kyphosis without laminectomy. In this setting, with intact posterior elements, the deformity tends to be much more rigid.

Stabilizing operations of the cervical spine can greatly improve the quality of life during the often shortened life expectancy of these patients. The aim of surgery should be to minimize hospitalization time and postoperative bracing needs so that patients can return to as active a life as possible.

POSTLAMINECTOMY KYPHOSIS

The most common cause of kyphosis is iatrogenic, that is, postlaminectomy kyphosis (44). Preventing the development of cervical kyphosis can be accomplished by fusion at the time of laminectomy as well as not using laminectomy in the setting of preoperative cervical kyphosis. In the skeletally immature patient, laminectomy should always be accompanied with posterior arthrodesis. This arthrodesis can be produced by simple ablation of the posterior facets, decortication of the lateral masses, and bone grafting.

In adults, prevention of postlaminectomy kyphosis can be accomplished by close attention to (a) facet integrity and (b) preoperative sagittal contour. Several biomechanical studies have demonstrated the importance of minimizing the extent of facet removal during laminectomy of the cervical spine. Zdeblick et al. (56) found that removal of greater than 50% of the bony facet markedly reduced the stability in flexion and torsion of the cervical spine. Saito et al. (39), using finite element analysis, demonstrated that resection of one or more spinous processes or posterior ligaments resulted in a transfer of tensile stresses to the facets. Failure of the facets to resist this tensile load was primarily responsible for the development of postlaminectomy deformity. Raynor et al. (37) showed that resistance to vertebral body shear load was significantly reduced following bilateral facetectomy of greater than 50%. Raynor additionally demonstrated good exposure of the nerve root from its axilla distally for up to 5 mm by removing 50% of the medial facet joint.

Clinical reports of postlaminectomy kyphosis support the need to minimize facet resection and avoid laminectomy as an isolated procedure in patients with instability or kyphotic sagittal alignment. Herkowitz (20) reported a 25% incidence of kyphosis at an average 2-year follow-up in patients with bilateral facetectomies. Callahan et al. (10) demonstrated in their series of 25 patients with postlaminectomy deformity an association of instability with age younger than 25 years, fracture-dislocation, and laminectomy com-

bined with foraminotomy or extensive facet resection. Epstein (15) additionally supported the concept of maintaining facet integrity by recommending that two-thirds of the facet remain intact during foraminal decompression.

The occurrence of kyphosis is much greater in the skeletally immature patient than in adults (11,28,52). Yasuoka et al. (54) reported postlaminectomy deformity in 46% (12 of 26) of the patients who were younger than 15 years of age at the time of surgery. An isolated laminectomy in an adult patient is usually insufficient to produce instability if the facet resection has been minimized (15). Postoperative kyphosis occurs less frequently after surgery for degenerative conditions than after surgery for a cervical tumor or ossification of the posterior longitudinal ligament (32). A C-2 laminectomy is also highly associated with a postoperative kyphosis, as is removal of the muscular insertions at the C-2 spinous process (25).

ETIOLOGIES OF CLINICAL FAILURE FOR CERVICAL DEFORMITY SURGERY

Clinical failure following cervical deformity surgery may manifest itself in many different ways for patients, including pain, myelopathy, and increasing deformity. Pseudarthrosis is a common mechanism of clinical failure. Certain risk factors for pseudarthrosis may be eliminated or controlled, including cigarette smoking, choice of bone graft material, number of motion segments fused, and restoration of sagittal and coronal balance.

Clinical studies by Brown et al. (7) and An et al. (1) have found smoking to impair the healing of spinal fusions. Nonunion rates increase two- to fourfold in patients who use tobacco products. Every effort should be made to ensure that the patient stops smoking before surgery and eliminates all nicotine products. The choice of bone graft material is preferably autogenous, although obtaining autogenous graft has been associated with complications, including donor site morbidity (i.e., pain, infection, hemorrhage, and nerve damage). Despite donor site morbidity, increased operating room time, and increased blood loss, autologous bone graft remains the gold standard and should be used after thorough decortication.

Another potential source of clinical failure for cervical deformity surgery is the development of degenerative changes or instability above or below the fusion site, or both. This can lead to development of late neurologic symptoms of the juxtafused segments (4,43). Altered biomechanics from the rigid fused segment

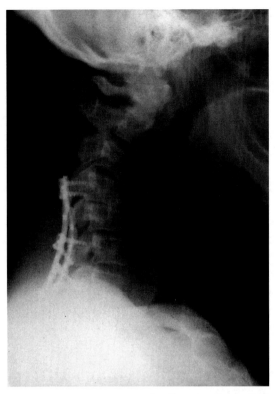

FIGURE 9. One-year postoperative lateral radiograph showing junctional kyphosis above a fusion that does not extend to the superior-most aspect of the laminectomy.

place increased stress on adjacent motion segments. To minimize degenerative changes at adjacent motion segments, the surgeon must avoid ending the fusion at segments with compromised ligamentous attachments to the spinous processes and lamina. Every effort should be made to protect the facet capsule and preserve the facet articular cartilage. The disk itself should not be touched with electrocautery, and the anulus and anterior longitudinal ligament should be preserved. The number of motion segments to be incorporated should include the minimum number necessary to treat the pathology. The fewer motion segments fused, the less stress on adjacent segments and decreased chance for nonunion. Bohlman et al. (4) demonstrated increased nonunion rates as the number of motion segments fused increases.

Avoidance of pseudarthrosis and implant failure additionally relies on maximizing sagittal and coronal correction to minimize spinal instability. The use of preoperative skeletal traction using either a halo device or skull tongs should be considered. Some deformities are rigid and even painful. Any improvement of deformity preoperatively potentially makes the procedure technically easier. Vertebral subluxation and increasing kyphosis are often seen with incomplete correction of kyphotic deformity following an isolated posterior cervical fusion. In this setting of posterior fusion with

inadequate reduction of the kyphotic deformity, the graft is under tension and may be less likely to fuse (9).

Instrumentation failure is usually a result of inability to achieve a solid arthrodesis. All implants eventually fail if fusion is not achieved. Plate and screw fixation of the cervical spine can be used anteriorly and posteriorly for deformity surgery. Such devices help to obtain immediate rigid fixation and promote fusion by minimizing host bone–graft interface motion. Instrumentation should always incorporate all levels that have been potentially destabilized, that is, laminectomy, to prevent a junctional area of instability (Fig. 9). These internal fixation devices may additionally limit the degree of external immobilization that is necessary in the postoperative period. This can greatly improve patient comfort and, ultimately, patient satisfaction.

EVALUATING THE FAILED CERVICAL DEFORMITY PATIENT

The surgeon should begin with a very careful evaluation of the patient's history, including preoperative symptoms, their duration, and their nature. If pain is the presenting problem, the surgeon must determine whether a pain-free interval has ever been present. Careful questioning about preoperative neurologic status, Nurick grade, and whether this has improved or declined since the procedure was performed is essential. Did the patient experience a postoperative complication? Is he or she involved in litigation regarding a preoperative or postoperative claim? These answers can greatly affect patient outcome and reliability.

A thorough physical examination with careful attention to upper motor neuron signs, atrophy, sensory loss, reflexes, weakness, and nonorganic signs is fundamental. Clinical failure may be due to other unrecognized pathologic diseases, such as rheumatoid arthritis with stage IV myelopathy. A careful review of all diagnostic and imaging studies performed before the last surgery is essential to understanding the degree of preoperative deformity and neural element compression.

New imaging studies are essential for the determination of a revision surgery plan. Assessing whether the deformity was ever corrected, or if it has recurred, is fundamental to understanding the etiology of the failure. Plain x-rays as well as flexion and extension views are necessary to determine evidence of nonunion, instability, or junctional problems (Fig. 10). MRI with gadolinium can be helpful in evaluating the new onset

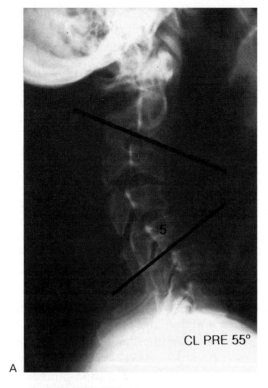

A

CL PRE 55°

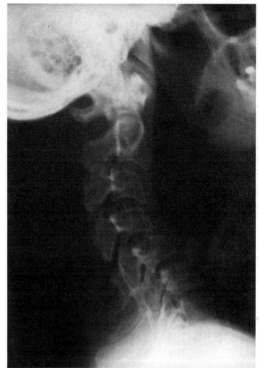

B

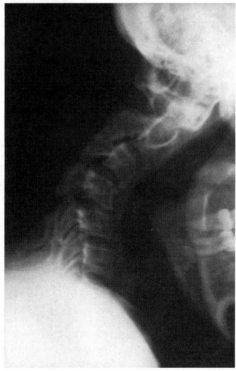

C

FIGURE 10. A: Lateral radiograph in neutral position of patient 1 year following cervical laminectomy from C-2 to C-4. **B:** Lateral radiograph of same patient in extension. Note the lack of correction of the deformity. **C:** Lateral radiograph of the same patient in flexion. Note the degree of widening posteriorly at C3-4.

of neural element compression and junctional disk disease. Myelography with postmyelogram CT scan is an essential study to determine nerve root compression and degree of cord compression in patients with radicular complaints and myelopathy (Fig. 11). All of these studies must be carefully compared with the preoperative studies to determine all possible mechanisms of failure and levels of surgical intervention.

Revision deformity surgery of the cervical spine should not be considered until all conservative options have been exhausted. The surgeon must be able to confidently correlate the patient's symptoms with definable imaging pathology. The high complication rate, risk of serious neurologic injury, and potential for surgical inability to relieve symptoms must be discussed thoroughly with the patient preoperatively.

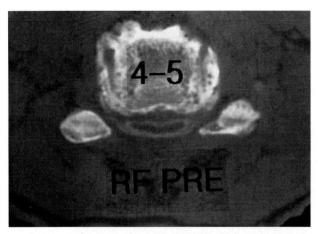

FIGURE 11. Postmyelogram computed tomography axial cut of a patient seen in follow-up with postlaminectomy kyphosis and myelopathy. Note the degree of cord flattening despite the absence of posterior elements.

TREATMENT OF KYPHOTIC DEFORMITY

Kyphotic deformity of the cervical spine can be quite difficult to treat. As discussed previously, the use of preoperative traction can be a very important component of preoperative treatment. Many surgeons believe that the best surgical approach to kyphosis surgery is anterior with multilevel corpectomies or diskectomies and strut grafting (51,56). For one- or two-level corpectomies, an autogenous iliac crest strut graft is used, whereas autogenous fibular strut graft is used for three or more levels. The obvious advantage of anterior strut grafting is the loading of the graft and construct in compression. Posterior scar tissue obscures landmarks, and the potential for dural and spinal cord injury is high. Adequate kyphotic correction may not be obtainable without anterior release. With an isolated posterior approach to kyphotic deformity correction, the bone graft is under tension and may be less likely to fuse (9).

If cervical myelopathy is present in the setting of kyphotic deformity, posterior management alone may not sufficiently decompress the spinal cord. With kyphotic deformity the spinal cord may be draped over the kyphotic segments anteriorly, leading to anterior cord ischemia and tension. Isolated posterior decompression in this setting usually does not correct the sagittal kyphotic deformity enough to relieve the anterior cord compression and may result in progression of kyphosis. Anterior diskectomy in isolation at the kyphotic segments may help restore lordotic sagittal contour but does not always effectively eliminate midline osteophytes of the vertebral bodies. Careful review of preoperative CT

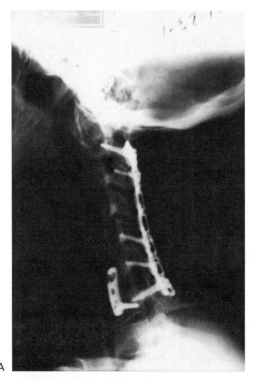
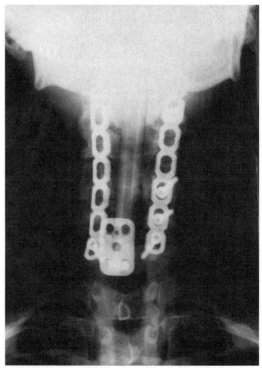

FIGURE 12.   A, B: One-year postoperative anteroposterior and lateral radiographs following correction of postlaminectomy kyphosis with anterior fibular strut graft with buttress plate at the distal end. Posterior fixation is with lateral mass plates with pedicle screws in C-2 and C-7 for maximal fixation.

scans, especially postmyelogram CT scans, can help determine the extent of posterior vertebral body compression versus multiple level osteophytic spurring at the disk level. Multiple level corpectomy is often required to decompress the cord adequately and restore lordosis if the osteophytes extend behind the vertebral bodies centrally. Additionally, care must be taken to preserve the posterior longitudinal ligament, which acts as the center of motion when the correction of the kyphotic deformity is performed. Preserving the posterior longitudinal ligament also prevents sudden lengthening of the neural elements during correction.

After multiple-level corpectomies and anterior strut grafting in the postlaminectomy setting, 360 degrees of instability has been created. In patients who were treated with autogenous fibular strut grafting, we have included a small anterior plate distally to prevent graft kick-out. This plate has two screws in the lowest remaining vertebral body and then extends proximally 3 to 4 cm with no proximal fixation in the graft. It simply acts as a buttress at the inferior graft-body junction site. We additionally add a posterior instrumented fusion in cases that involve three or more corpectomy levels. This additional fixation is thought to decrease graft dislodgment, settling, and nonunion (Fig. 12). Postoperatively, all patients are treated in a halo for 6 to 12 weeks.

Intraoperative monitoring of spinal cord function is essential for kyphosis correction surgery. Baseline levels of cord function before positioning are essential in cases of myelopathy. Continual monitoring throughout the case enables careful attention to neuromonitoring signals during reduction of the kyphotic deformity.

CONCLUSION

Cervical deformity is a complex and difficult problem for spine surgeons to treat effectively and safely. Failed deformity surgery of the cervical spine presents a higher level of difficulty for the spine surgeon. Understanding the etiology of previous surgical failure and new treatment options can be a challenge. The commonest form of cervical deformity requiring revision surgery is postlaminectomy kyphotic instability. Technically, this condition is best treated with anterior correction and arthrodesis. This type of surgery is at high risk for complications due to the degree of instability and revision nature of the procedure. Correct diagnosis and understanding of the etiology of the previous surgical failure depend on careful history taking and physical examination.

Care must be taken to plan the procedure thoughtfully before the operation, with adequate imaging techniques that correlate the symptoms with the diagnosis.

REFERENCES

1. An HS, Lynch K, Toth J. Prospective comparison of autograft vs. allograft for adult posterolateral lumbar spine fusion: differences among freeze dried, frozen, and mixed grafts. *J Spinal Disord* 1995;8:131–135.
2. Bohlman HH. Acute fractures and dislocations of the cervical spine. An analysis of three hundred hospitalized patients and review of the literature. *J Bone Joint Surg Am* 1979;61A:1119–1142.
3. Bohlman HH. Surgical management of cervical spine fractures and dislocations. The American Academy of Orthopedic Surgeons, Instructional Course Lectures. St. Louis: Mosby, 1985;34:163–187.
4. Bohlman HH, Emery SE, Goodfellow DB, et al. Robinson anterior cervical discectomy and arthrodesis for cervical radiculopathy. *J Bone Joint Surg Am* 1993;75:1298–1307.
5. Bridwell KH. Sagittal spinal balance—Symposium No. 1. Presented at the AAOS Section IV Scoliosis Research Society, New Orleans, February 1994.
6. Breig A. *Adverse mechanical tension in the central nervous system*, 2nd ed. New York: John Wiley and Sons, 1978:264.
7. Brown WC, Orme TJ, Richardson HD. The rate of pseudarthrosis (surgical nonunion) in patients who are smokers and patients who are nonsmokers: a comparison study. *Spine* 1986;11:942–943.
8. Bucy PC. The treatment of malignant tumors of the spine: a review. *Neurology* 1963;13:938–944.
9. Butler JC, Whitecloud TS. Postlaminectomy kyphosis: causes and surgical management. *Orthop Clin North Am* 1992;23:505–511.
10. Callahan RA, Johnson RM, Margolis RN, et al. Cervical facet fusion for control of instability after laminectomy. *J Bone Joint Surg Am* 1977;59A:991–1002.
11. Cattell HS, Clark GL Jr. Cervical kyphosis and instability following multiple laminectomies in children. *J Bone Joint Surg Am* 1967;49:713–720.
12. Eismont FJ, Bohlman HH, Soni PL, et al. Pyogenic and fungal vertebral osteomyelitis with paralysis. *J Bone Joint Surg Am* 1983;65A:19–29.
13. Eismont FJ, Montero C. Infections of the spine. In: Davidoff RA, ed. *Handbook of the spinal cord*, vol 5. New York: Marcel Dekker Inc, 1987:411.
14. Endress C, Guyot DR, Fata J, et al. Cervical osteomyelitis due to IV heroin use: radiograph findings in 14 patients. *AJR Am J Roentgenol* 1990;155:333–335.
15. Epstein JA. The surgical management of cervical spinal stenosis, spondylosis and myeloradiculopathy by means of the posterior approach. *Spine* 1988;13:864–869.

16. Fellander M. Paraplegia in spondylitis: results of operative treatment. *Paraplegia* 1975;13:75–88.

17. Harrington KD. Metastatic disease of the spine, current concepts review. *J Bone Joint Surg Am* 1986;68A:1110–1115.

18. Harrington KD. Anterior decompression and stabilization of the spine as a treatment for vertebral collapse and spinal cord compression from metastatic malignancy. *Clin Orthop* 1988;233:177–197.

19. Hensinger RN, Lang JR, MacEwen GD. Klippel-Feil syndrome: a constellation of associated anomalies. *J Bone Joint Surg Am* 1984;66A:403–411.

20. Herkowitz HN. A comparison of anterior cervical fusion, cervical laminectomy, and cervical laminoplasty for the surgical management of multiple level spondylitic radiculopathy. *Spine* 1988;13:774–780.

21. Herkowitz HN, Rothman RH. Subacute instability of the cervical spine. *Spine* 1984;9:348–357.

22. Hodgson AR, Stock FE, Fang HSY, et al. Anterior spinal fusion: the operative approach and pathologic findings in 412 patients with Potts disease of the spine. *Br J Surg* 1960;48:172.

23. Hodgson AR. An approach to the cervical spine (C3 to C7). *Clin Orthop Rel Res* 1965;39:129.

24. Hsu LCS, Leong JCY. Tuberculosis of the lower cervical spine (C2 to C7): report on 40 cases. *J Bone Joint Surg Br* 1984;66:1.

25. Katsumi Y, Honma T, Nakamura T. Analysis of cervical instability resulting from laminectomies for removal of spinal cord tumor. *Spine* 1989;13:1171–1176.

26. Kennady JC, Stern WE. Metastatic neoplasms of the vertebral column producing compression of the spinal cord. *Am J Surg* 1962;104:155–168.

27. Koppel BS, Tuchman AJ, Mangiardi JR, et al. Epidural spinal infection in intravenous drug abusers. *Arch Neurol* 1988;45:1331–1337.

28. Lonstein JE. Post-laminectomy kyphosis. *Clin Orthop* 1977;128:93–100.

29. Malanski SK, Ludanski S. Pyogenic infection of the spine. *Clin Orthop* 1991;272:58–66.

30. McAfee PC, Bohlman HH. One-stage anterior cervical decompression and posterior stabilization with circumferential arthrodesis. A study of twenty-four patients who had a traumatic or a neoplastic lesion. *J Bone Joint Surg Am* 1989;71A:78–88.

31. Medical Research Council Working Party on Tuberculosis of the Spine. A 10 year assessment of controlled trial comparing débridement and anterior spinal fusion in the management of tuberculosis of the spine in patients in standard chemotherapy in Hong Kong. *J Bone Joint Surg Br* 1982;64:393.

32. Mikawa Y, Shikata J, Yamamuro T. Spinal deformity and instability after multilevel cervical laminectomy. *Spine* 1987;12:6–11.

33. Morgan TH, Wharton GW, Austin GN. The results of laminectomy in patients with incomplete spinal cord injuries. *J Bone Joint Surg Am* 1970;52A:822.

34. Pal GP, Sherk HH. The vertical stability of the cervical spine. *Spine* 1988;13:447–449.

35. Parke WN, Rothman RH, Brown MD. The pharyngovertebral veins: an anatomic rationale for Grisel's syndrome. *J Bone Joint Surg Am* 1984;66A:568–574.

36. Perese DM. Treatment of metastatic extradural spinal cord tumors. A series of thirty cases. *Cancer* 1958;11:214–221.

37. Raynor RB, Pugh J, Shapiro I. Cervical facetectomy and its effect on spine strength. *J Neurosurg* 1985;63:278–282.

38. Ross PM, Fleming JL. Vertebral body osteomyelitis: spectrum and natural history: a retrospective analysis of 37 cases. *Clin Orthop* 1976;118:190–198.

39. Saito T, Yammanuro T, Khikata J, et al. Analysis and prevention of spinal column deformity following cervical laminectomy. Pathogenic analysis of post laminectomy deformity. *Spine* 1991;16:494–502.

40. Sapico FL, Montgomerie JZ. Pyogenic vertebral osteomyelitis: a review of nine cases and review of the literature. *Rev Infect Dis* 1979;1:754–776.

41. Sapico FL, Montgomerie JZ. Vertebral osteomyelitis. *Infect Dis Clin North Am* 1990;4:539–550.

42. Scrimgeour EM, Kaven J, Gajdusek DC. Spinal tuberculosis: the commonest cause of non-traumatic paraplegia in Papua New Guinea. *Trop Geogr Med* 1987;39:218–221.

43. Shinomiya K, Okamoto A, Kamikozuru M, et al. An analysis of failures in primary cervical anterior spinal cord decompression and fusion. *J Spinal Disord* 1993;6:277–288.

44. Sim FH, Svien HJ, Bickel WJ, et al. Swan neck deformity following extensive cervical laminectomy. *J Bone Joint Surg Am* 1974;56A:564–580.

45. Smith MD. Congenital scoliosis of the cervical or cervicothoracic spine. *Orthop Clin North Am* 1994;25:301–310.

46. Smith MD, Lonstein JE, Winter RB. Congenital cervicothoracic scoliosis. A long-term follow-up study. *Orthop Trans* 1992;16:165–170.

47. Stauffer ES, Kelly EG. Fracture dislocations of the cervical spine. Instability and recurrent deformity following treatment by interbody fusion. *J Bone Joint Surg Am* 1977;59A:45–48.

48. Stone JL, Cybulski GR, Rodriguez J, et al. Anterior cervical débridement and strut grafting for osteomyelitis of the cervical spine. *J Neurosurg* 1989;70:879–883.

49. Tachdijian MO, Matson DD. Orthopedic aspects of intra-spinal tumors in children. *J Bone Joint Surg Am* 1965;47A:223–248.

50. Waldvogel FA, Medoff G, Swartz MN. Osteomyelitis: a review of clinical features, therapeutic considerations and unusual aspects. *N Engl J Med* 1970;282:198–206.

51. Whitecloud TS, LaRocca H. Fibular strut graft in reconstructive surgery of the cervical spine. *Spine* 1976;1:33–43.

52. Winter RB, Moe JH, Lonstein JE. The incidence of Klippel-Feil syndrome in patients with congenital scoliosis and kyphosis. *Spine* 1984;9:363–366.

53. Reference deleted.

54. Yasuoka S, Peterson HA, MacCarty CS. Incidence of spinal column deformity after multilevel laminectomy in children and adults. *J Neurosurg* 1982;57:441–445.

55. Reference deleted.

56. Zdeblick TA, Warden KE, McCabe R, et al. Cervical stability after foraminotomy. *J Bone Joint Surg Am* 1992;721:22–27.

5

CERVICAL SPINE: TRAUMA

K. DANIEL RIEW, WILLIAM O. SHAFFER, AND ERIC J. GRAHAM

AVOIDING REVISION SURGERY

Fracture Identification

The most important step in avoiding revision surgery following trauma to the cervical spine is to identify all existing injuries correctly. Generally, observations in the operating room reveal more detail than the best preoperative workup; however, proper preoperative planning is necessary to ensure optimal surgical outcome. Discovering a concomitant spinal injury, whether intraoperatively or postoperatively, that was missed in the initial evaluation may result in either a poor outcome or an unnecessary reoperation. A thorough history, physical examination, and radiologic workup are essential for a proper evaluation of the injured patient.

To identify all of the injuries that a patient sustained, one must first obtain a detailed history concerning the mechanism of injury. Following a motor vehicle collision, it is helpful to document the magnitude, speed, and direction of impact and to note the use of any restraining devices such as airbags and seat belts. For example, if a head-on collision has occurred between a subcompact and a large, four-wheel drive vehicle, the individual in the latter vehicle will likely have fewer injuries. Was the patient wearing a seat belt? Was he or she hit from behind or on the side? Did the head hit the windshield? Did the car roll over? Was the vehicle totaled? Did any other associated injuries occur? These are all important elements that help the surgeon piece together the magnitude of the injuries suffered by the patient. The loss of consciousness, degree of head trauma, and severity of concomitant injuries are associated with the degree of trauma to the cervical spine (50).

It is also important to keep in mind that not all fractures are simple traumatic fractures but can be pathologic fractures due to tumor, infection, metabolic, or inflammatory disease. The patient may give a history of nonmechanical neck pain that antedated the traumatic event. Alternatively, the severity of the fracture may not be consistent with the type of trauma that the patient sustained. Finally, the radiologic workup may suggest something other than a common fracture.

After obtaining a detailed history, one must carefully and thoroughly examine the patient. Significant injuries to the spine are manifested by tenderness to palpation of the spinous processes. In the cervical spine, one can palpate the carotid tubercle and other transverse processes located medial to the sternocleidomastoid muscle. Patients with muscular or ligamentous strains often have tenderness to palpation, and the location of maximal tenderness can direct the surgeon to examine the radiographs carefully in that particular region of the spine. Cooperative patients are relatively easy to examine because motor and sensory skills and reflexes can be tested. However, motor strength may be blunted secondary to pain. If a patient is obtunded, one can focus on the bulbocavernosus reflex and Babinski's sign. The absence of a bulbocavernosus reflex suggests that the patient is in spinal shock with or without severe damage to the cauda equina (10). If the patient exhibits hyperreflexia, clonus, a positive Hoffmann's sign, or an extensor Babinski's response, the spinal cord may be compressed or a significant brain injury may have occurred.

A full radiologic workup of the cervical trauma patient complements the history and physical examination. Adequate plain x-rays visualizing the C-7 to T-1 level are mandatory (3,28,60,67,103,121). An open mouth anteroposterior view of the C1-2 area is crucial, as the most commonly missed fractures are those of the atlantoaxial articulation and occipitoatlantal articulation (82,94,111,130) (Fig. 1). In the presence of one spinal fracture, another associated spinal fracture is quite common (36,56,73,92,115). This is especially true for atlantoaxial injuries (82,126). If attention is focused only on the most obvious injury, a more subtle injury may be overlooked (76).

If the patient does not require emergent surgery, a thorough radiologic evaluation of the entire cervical spine should be performed before any operation. Unambiguous preoperative radiographic studies facilitate a successful decompression. Exploratory surgery to identify compression intraoperatively can result in the unnecessary removal of stabilizing structures, further destabilizing the already traumatized cervical

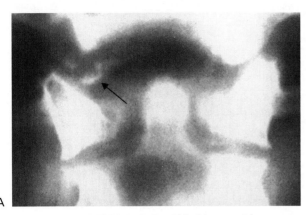
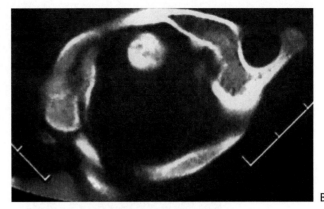

FIGURE 1. A, B: This 32-year-old woman complained of upper cervical pain after a motor vehicle collision. Her plain x-rays were not particularly helpful. She has an occipital condylar fracture (*arrow*) with some displacement of the fragment but relatively smooth occiput to C-1 articulation.

spine (13,12,17,37,95,112). With today's advanced imaging technology, "exploratory" surgery of the cervical spine should rarely, if ever, be performed.

If the patient is unconscious, full thoracic, lumbar, and pelvic x-rays must be obtained. In addition to plain cervical radiographs, it may be necessary to obtain a computed tomogram (CT), magnetic resonance image (MRI), or CT myelogram (CTM). Specific recommendations about which of these tests is necessary or even cost effective vary in the literature.

As long as time permits, we prefer a CT or an MRI, or both, before surgical intervention. These additional studies should not unduly delay an operative procedure that may potentially restore an incomplete neurologic deficit, however. In our trauma centers, if a cervical spine fracture is suspected and plain x-rays are difficult to obtain, a high-speed spiral CT of the C-spine is obtained to identify the extent of the injury. This allows excellent reconstructions in the coronal and sagittal plain.

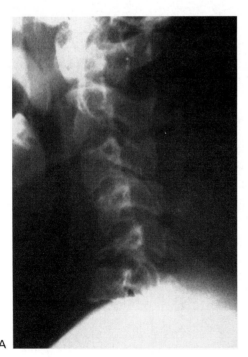
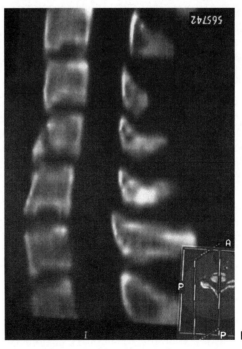

FIGURE 2. An 18-year-old male who jumped into a farm pond headfirst and was stuck in the pond bed submersed below water. He had a teardrop fracture with marked displacement of the C-5 body into the neural canal and destruction of the posterior elements of C5-6. **A:** The patient presented with shoulder shrug only and respiratory depression. **B:** The alignment of the cervical spine after reduction and cervical tong traction. Computed tomography reconstruction shows excellent alignment of the neural canal and decompression of the cord. The patient improved to a C-5 motor level with deltoid, biceps, and respiratory function return. (*continued*)

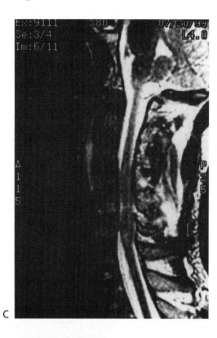

FIGURE 2. (*continued*) **C:** The magnetic resonance image shows the injury to the spinal cord with hematomyelia and swelling of the cord from C3-4 to C5-6.

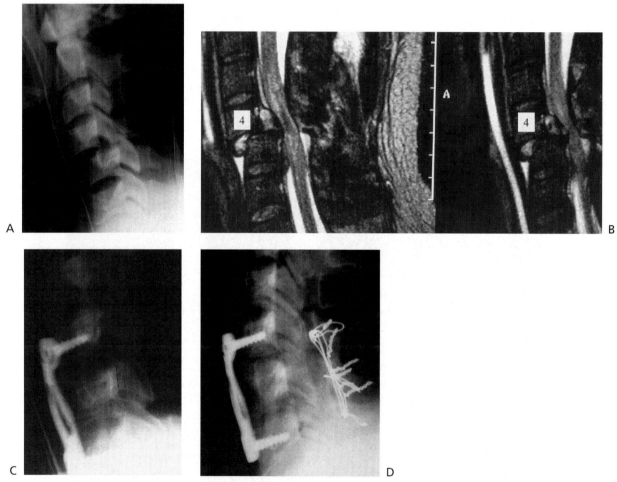

FIGURE 3. A: This patient had a bilateral facet dislocation along with a small facet fracture at C4-5. Closed reduction was unsuccessful. **B:** The magnetic resonance image demonstrates a disk herniation at C4-5 as well as at C5-6. The patient underwent emergent anterior diskectomy and arthrodesis. **C:** Intraoperative radiographs following the anterior procedure demonstrated persistent subluxation at C4-5 that could not be reduced despite multiple attempts. The patient was therefore turned prone and underwent posterior reduction and wiring. **D:** Following completion of the posterior surgery, the small fractured facet fragment was noted to block complete reduction. If a facet fractures and the fragment is not attached to any soft tissues, it is usually impossible to reduce closed or even with an open anterior approach. A posterior procedure alone would not have addressed the herniated disks.

Decompression

Alignment of the cervical spine is paramount, and reduction can be accomplished in the emergency room in most cases. Reduction through cervical traction decompresses the neural elements in many cases (13,38,49,76) (Fig. 2). After reduction, the spine should be further assessed for residual cord or root impingement. At the initial operation, residual neural compression should be corrected (15,20). A revision decompression usually means operating through scar tissue; the preferred approach to avoid a difficult revision procedure is to perform a complete decompression at the time of the index operation.

If the patient has a dislocated facet, a simple fusion without relocation of the facets yields suboptimal results. A persistently dislocated facet may cause or exacerbate radiculopathy, myelopathy, or paralysis (18,14,22,108). Revision is frequently extensive and difficult. The selected approach must allow complete reduction of the dislocation. If delayed until revision surgery, anatomic reduction is difficult or even impossible to obtain (Fig. 3).

In burst fractures, all fragments that cause neural compression must be removed before the column support is reconstructed (65,129,139). If the patient's associated injuries or medical condition preclude a complete decompression, repeat decompression and stabilization should be executed in a timely fashion. Beyond 2 weeks, exuberant scar formation makes the procedure more technically demanding (Fig. 4).

Spinal Alignment

Although there are numerous reports regarding sagittal alignment in the thoracolumbar spine, the impor-

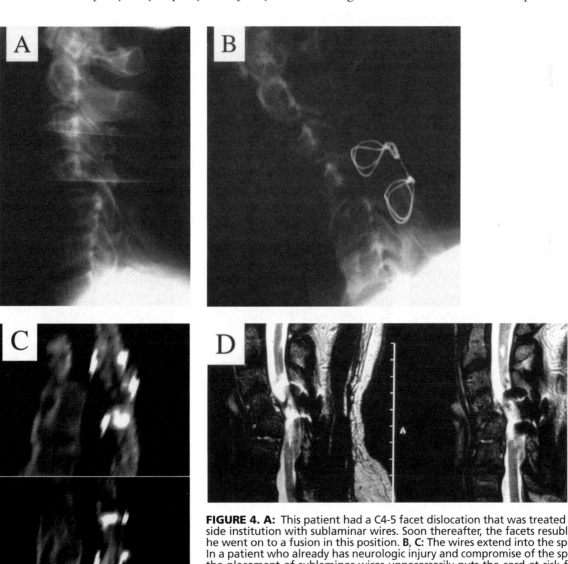

FIGURE 4. A: This patient had a C4-5 facet dislocation that was treated at an outside institution with sublaminar wires. Soon thereafter, the facets resubluxed, and he went on to a fusion in this position. **B, C:** The wires extend into the spinal canal. In a patient who already has neurologic injury and compromise of the spinal canal, the placement of sublaminar wires unnecessarily puts the cord at risk for further injury. **D:** The patient's magnetic resonance image several years after the index procedure shows persistent subluxation and cord compromise. Because of persistent neurologic deficits, he was treated with a three-column osteotomy and corpectomy of C-5 and reduction and realignment of the dislocated C4-5 facet. The malunion was taken down posteriorly, and bone graft was added, followed by placement of a spinous process cable. (*continued*)

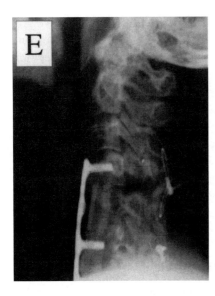
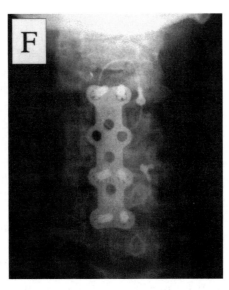

FIGURE 4. (*continued*) E, F: We then performed an anterior corpectomy and osteotomy. Although the patient is now reduced, one can see that he still has a mild kyphosis. This could have been corrected by going back posteriorly and tightening up the spinous process cable. It was believed, however, that the patient had adequate decompression of the cord and that the alignment was acceptable. He improved by one Nurick grade.

tance of sagittal alignment in the cervical spine is debatable (117,132,144). After an extensive laminectomy, residual sagittal plane kyphosis can lead to neurologic deficits. A postoperative spine that is left in poor sagittal alignment may have a greater tendency to develop a transition syndrome at the level adjacent to the fused segment. In the anterior spine, it is important to obtain an anatomic anterior column support to allow as normal an alignment as possible. If the patient has an unstable three-column injury fixed with too large a graft, the entire segment can become overly distracted (33). This may result in greater instability until solid arthrodesis is achieved (Fig. 5). Alternatively, an undersized graft or one that collapses can result in kyphosis at the fractured segment.

Instrumentation

In cases that necessitate anterior decompression, anterior column support with bone grafting and appropriate stabilizing instrumentation is usually required (2,114,119). If posterior decompression is performed, the spine is further destabilized, and bone graft and internal fixation are mandatory to provide adequate stability to the spine until the bone graft is incorporated (5). Adequate instrumentation helps to maintain the reduction after decompression of an unstable fracture or dislocation. Although posterior cervical wiring is an excellent technique to augment an anterior arthrodesis, wiring alone provides adequate stability only in cases of facet dislocations without any concomitant

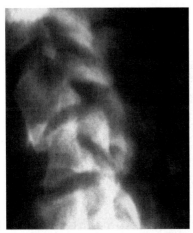
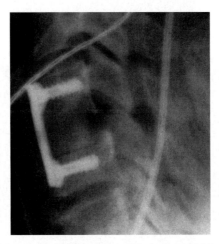
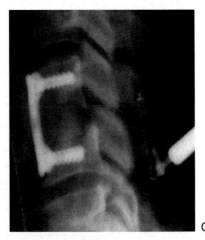

A,B

C

FIGURE 5. A, B, C: This patient had a C4-5 facet dislocation, which was reduced with tong traction at an outside institution. He apparently was then lost to follow-up and presented a few months later with neck pain and radiculopathy. He had bridging bone anteriorly at the dislocated segment **(A)**. An anterior cervical diskectomy and fusion was performed. The intraoperative radiograph demonstrates that he is slightly overdistracted and still not completely reduced. He then underwent posterior spinous process cabling and bone grafting. This case demonstrates the ease with which one can place a graft that is too large in a patient with osteoligamentous injury. In addition, it may be advisable to perform a circumferential fusion in patients who are chronically dislocated, noncompliant, or not likely to fuse due to tobacco abuse or medications.

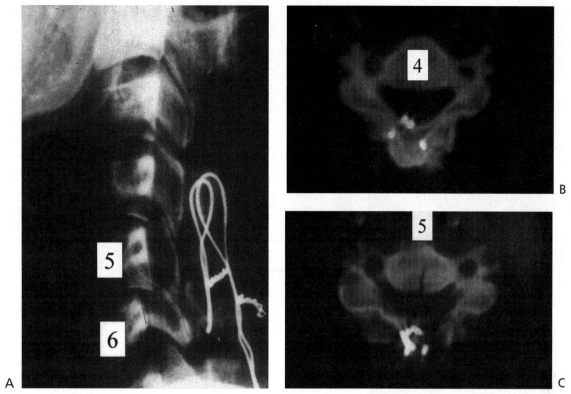

FIGURE 6. A, B, C: This patient had a teardrop fracture of C-5 and retrolisthesis of C-5 on C-6. The outside surgeon used sublaminar wires in this individual, who apparently already had a neurologic deficit. The postoperative CT scans show obvious fractures of the posterior elements, as expected for a retrolisthesed teardrop fracture. In the presence of neurologic deficits and posterior element fractures, sublaminar and spinous process wires are a poor choice of fixation. In addition, the patient was fused from C-4 down to C-7. Ideally, he should have been treated with a corpectomy of C-5 to remove the fracture fragments and circumferential fusion from C-4 to C-6. Rigid fixation is the preferred choice for unstable injuries.

fractures. In the presence of posterior element fractures, the use of wires often necessitates the inclusion of uninvolved segments that could be spared with more rigid instrumentation. Alternatively, patients may need to be immobilized in a halo vest, whereas a collar might suffice with the more rigid instrumentation. Finally, sublaminar wires can place the already traumatized spinal cord at risk and should almost never be used in trauma situations (Fig. 6). The more unstable reductions are prone to displacement even with a halo vest (8,71,107). If a patient is treated with a corpectomy without instrumentation, it is likely to displace despite halo vest immobilization; therefore, instrumentation provides additional support during healing. One example of this is a severe teardrop fracture dislocation, which disrupts all three columns. If a patient is treated with a corpectomy alone, it is likely to displace despite instrumentation or halo vest immobilization (Fig. 7). Severe injuries may require instrumentation circumferentially to prevent postoperative displacement (33,89,93) (Fig. 8).

When instrumenting the cervical spine, one must try to avoid disrupting a normal adjacent level. For anterior instrumentation, the screws should be placed in the midportion of the vertebral body. If a screw is placed within a couple of millimeters of the adjacent disk space, there is a risk of the screws displacing into the adjacent disk space if the graft subsides (19) (Fig. 9). This may necessitate removal of the instrumentation at a later date followed by an extension of the fusion into the next level. Long corpectomies that involve two or more segments or corpectomies in conjunction with posterior instability are at risk for displacement even with anterior instrumentation (32,48,127). Although this situation has only been reported in degenerative conditions, the likelihood of failure is also increased in traumatic conditions in which posterior instability is common. As the graft extrudes, it can further displace the anterior cervical plate. With an extension force, the screws lose bony purchase and the graft extrudes, breaking the anterior lip of the inferior vertebra (Fig. 10). Alternatively, an axial load drives the screws and the graft into the inferior vertebra and adjacent disk space (Fig. 11). In either case, the patient may complain of severe dysphagia or experience respiratory embarrassment. This can occur despite halo vest immobilization, as a halo vest does not prevent axial load to the cervical spine.

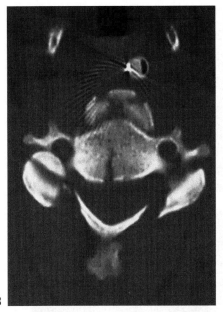
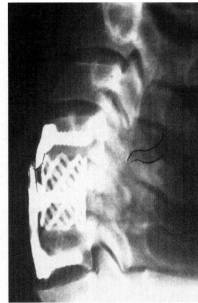
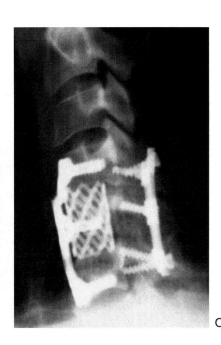

A,B

C

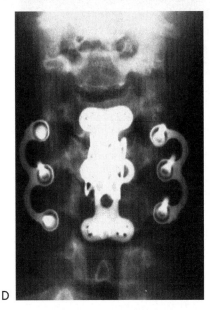

D

FIGURE 7. A 34-year-old was involved in a motor vehicle accident and suffered a teardrop fracture with immediate quadriplegia. **A:** Marked displacement of the C-5 body into the neural canal occurred, with the teardrop fracture sitting well in front of the superior aspect of the body. Marked comminution and multiple posterior and anterior element fractures occurred. The patient was treated with an anterior corpectomy with osteosynthesis, with a titanium metal mesh cage and anterior cervical plate. A planned posterior cervical fusion and wiring could not be accomplished because of the patient's unstable medical condition. He was treated in a halo. **B:** Several months later, he hit his head against a windshield and had neck pain. A lateral x-ray showed a fracture of the anterior cervical plate with impaction of the cage and plate into the inferior body. Because of the fracture of the plate, the revision was approached as a posterior cervical lateral mass plating and fusion. **C, D:** The x-rays show adequate healing of the corpectomy site. The patient's symptoms stabilized.

When using posterior instrumentation, care must be taken to avoid disrupting the interspinous and supraspinous ligaments at the adjacent segments. If lateral mass plates and screws are used, care must be taken to avoid placing the screws into or too near the adjacent facet joints. Following a posterior spinal fusion, increased stress is already placed on the adjacent segments. If these levels are further destabilized by iatrogenic injury of the ligamentous or facet complex, an early adjacent segment disease may result, necessitating an extension of the fusion to incorporate that level (23,136) (Fig. 12). Intraoperative x-rays should be obtained to confirm proper placement of screws. Exposure, decortication, or graft placement at segments outside of the intended levels of fusion should be avoided, as they can lead to partial fusion or graft impingement at that segment (63) (Fig. 13). In the younger patient,

stripping the periosteum off an uninvolved segment likely results in an iatrogenic autofusion.

Immobilization

The type of immobilization that is required following surgery is dependent on numerous factors. First, the quality of the patient's bone must be assessed. The more osteoporotic the bone, the more rigid the immobilization must be until the bone finally heals (39,40,64). Even if a patient with severely osteoporotic bone undergoes an instrumented multilevel corpectomy and halo vest immobilization, there is still the risk of graft subsidence with or without fracture of the inferior vertebra. It may be advisable to perform a circumferential fusion with posterior instrumentation in such patients to prevent this type of complication.

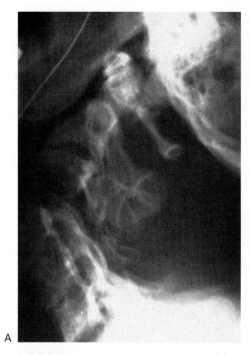

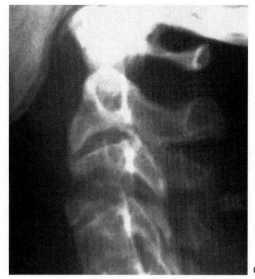

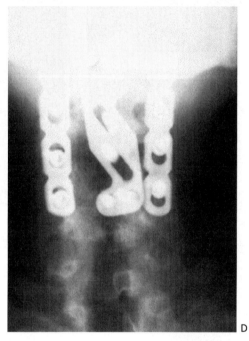

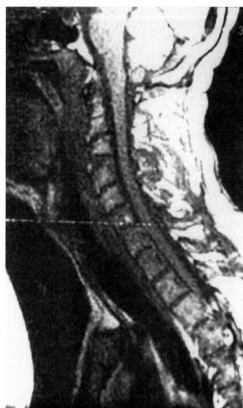

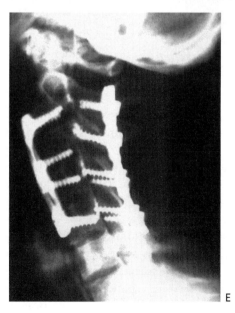

FIGURE 8. A: A 35-year-old man with ankylosing spondylitis was found on the street with flail extremities after being beaten. He was brought to St. Louis University Hospital with a respirator-dependent quadriplegia without even shoulder shrug activity. He had a 60-degree deformity through the C3-4 disk space with marked displacement of the cervical spine. **B:** Immediate halo traction was applied. At this time, the patient regained a flicker of toe motion. **C:** Magnetic resonance image of the injury through the ankylosed disk space with bleeding into the neural canal but minimal spinal cord swelling and injury. **D, E:** The patient underwent emergent posterior stabilization and anterior plate fixation. Two years later, he regained all function, including independent community ambulation and use of motor control of the hands and lower extremities.

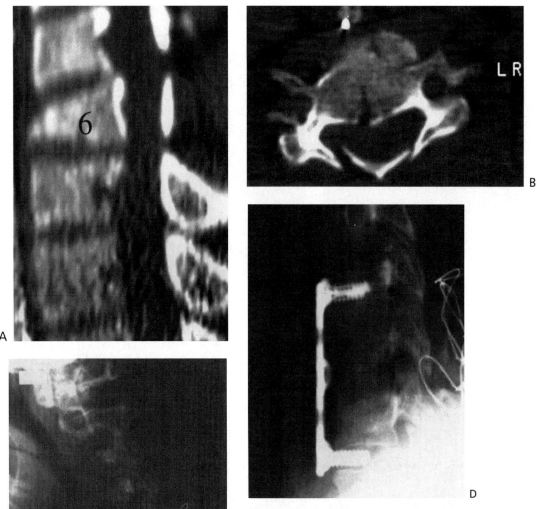

FIGURE 9. A 28-year-old Bosnian refugee who was involved in a motor vehicle accident. This patient experienced a burst fracture of C-6 with an incomplete quadriplegia. **A:** X-ray shows the improved alignment in halo traction. **B:** This figure shows the degree of comminution of the body on computed tomography. The impaction of the posterior lamina into the neural canal further compromised the neural canal in addition to the anterior body. **C:** The patient was treated with an anterior corpectomy, plating, and posterior wiring. **D:** At 6 months postoperatively, the patient's neurologic condition had improved. However, it was noted that there was further collapse of the graft and the lower screws had eroded into the endplate, necessitating early anterior plate removal. A posterior plate with more rigid immobilization might have prevented this complication.

Second, the patient's compliance with the postoperative regimen needs to be assessed. If the patient is prone to substance abuse, it would be prudent to provide maximal internal fixation anteriorly and posteriorly while supplementing this with a halo vest. Third, the reliability of the internal fixation determines the type of external fixation that is required. If a few cycles of flexion, extension, or rotation are likely to displace the graft and the hardware, a two-poster brace or a halo vest should be applied. Even with adequate fixation, comorbidities such as ankylosing spondylitis might require supplementation with a halo.

A halo is recommended if the patient has undergone either an anterior or posterior procedure alone in the presence of a three-column injury (33,71,93). Anterior fixation alone may be adequate for the treatment of a three-column injury (33), assuming that the alignment is anatomic and the patient is adequately immobilized during the healing period. Because a three-column injury is unstable in flexion or hyperextension, immobilization that prevents this motion is essential. The same can be said about these injuries that are treated with posterior instrumentation alone.

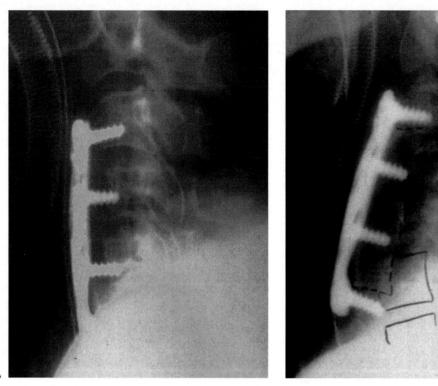

FIGURE 10. A, B: This patient had a long graft placed at an outside institution with a plate. The screws appear to be short. In extension, the plate pulls out of the inferior vertebra. Screws into the graft only serve to weaken it without decreasing the risk of pullout.

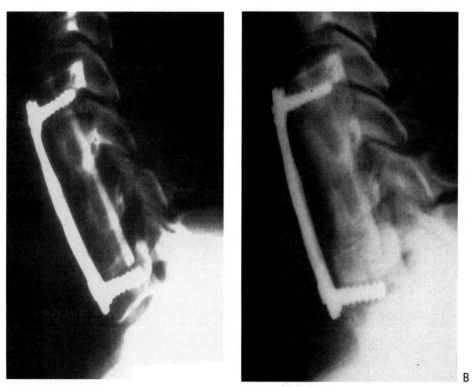

FIGURE 11. A: This patient had a two-level corpectomy and placement of an allograft fibula. **B:** Over the next year, as his graft matured and finally fused, it settled and pushed the plate into the next disk space. This was associated with severe axial neck pain that required a fusion of the next disk space. In flexion, the graft and plate fail by collapsing the inferior vertebra.

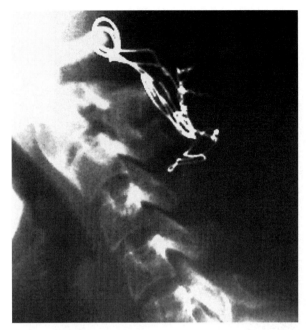

FIGURE 12. Two years after C1-3 fusion, one can see mild junctional kyphosis at C3-4. This is most likely due to partial disruption of the C3-4 ligamentous complex at the index procedure. Care must be taken not to expose or disrupt uninvolved segments.

If these injuries are treated with circumferential fusion and there is rigid fixation into nonosteoporotic bone in an otherwise compliant and reliable patient, a soft collar may be adequate immobilization (72). In a paraplegic or quadriplegic individual, we believe

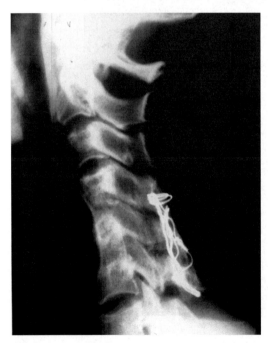

FIGURE 13. This patient had a posterior fusion from C-4 to C-6. One can see that some fusion mass is extended above and below the fused posterior segments. The surgeon must take great care to prevent extension of the fusion into unintended segments.

that every effort should be made to maximize the internal fixation to allow the patient to be immobilized in a soft collar. A patient who is already encumbered by profound neurologic deficits can thereby avoid further limitations on activities of daily living. In addition, maximal fixation and bone grafting decrease the probability of performing multiple operations on an individual who is prone to postoperative depression.

OPERATIVE APPROACH FOR REVISION SURGERY

Anterior Approach

The exposure of the anterior cervical spine can be as easy in revision surgery as it is in the primary procedure if the spine is approached on the contralateral side. Most surgeons have a definite preference for approaching the anterior spine exclusively through either the left or the right side. Those who favor the left side cite the more reliable course of the recurrent laryngeal nerve. Those who prefer the right side believe that it is easier than the left-sided one for right-handed surgeons. Although the danger to the recurrent laryngeal nerve is real with revision surgery, the ease of exposure through the unoperated side supersedes the small risk of inadvertent injury to the nerve.

We recommend against using the contralateral (unoperated) side if there is any question about the integrity of the recurrent laryngeal nerve following the index procedure. If the preoperative evaluation reveals a palsy of the recurrent laryngeal nerve, an exposure on the contralateral side endangers the remaining recurrent laryngeal nerve. Bilateral recurrent laryngeal nerve palsies necessitate a permanent tracheostomy.

During the exposure, scar encases the previous anterior instrumentation, the uncovertebral joints, and other landmarks. The key to establishing the midline is to identify virgin disk spaces at the rostral and caudal ends of the exposure. From this midline, an electrocautery can be used to strip the scar off of the anterior vertebra. As the dissection proceeds laterally, it is possible to identify the uncovertebral joints at the lateral margins of the diskectomy or corpectomy sites. The graft rarely spans the entire width of the decompression. The remaining uncovertebral joints are identified and exposed. Intraoperative anteroposterior and lateral x-rays can provide confirmation of the appropriate surgical levels.

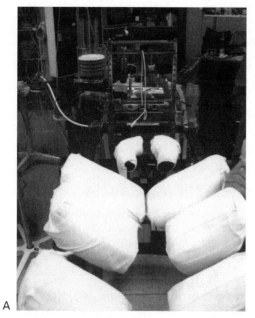

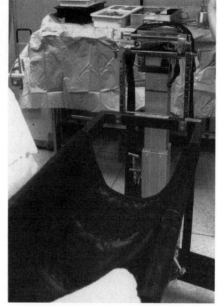

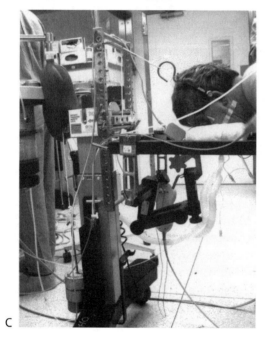

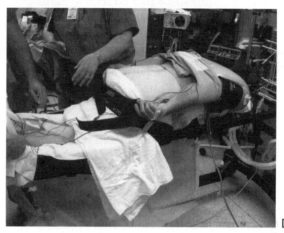

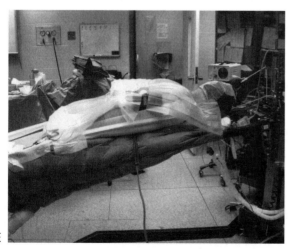

FIGURE 14. At Barnes-Jewish Hospital, an Orthopedic Systems, Inc. (Union City, Calif.) frame is used to place the patient in a reverse Trendelenburg's position for posterior cervical procedures. **A:** Three sets of chest and abdomen resting blocks are used. At the foot end of the table, a sling allows the legs to be placed lower than the body such that the blood can pool in the large capacitance vessels of the legs. In addition, the foot end of the table is placed on the last rung of the connecting bar **(B)**, and the head end is on the highest rung **(C)**. This allows maximal tilting of the table. A second connecting bar is placed above the table to allow for suspension of the Gardner-Wells tongs apparatus. The patient is placed into 15 to 20 lb of skull tong traction. The traction keeps the head in place, and the Mayfield headrest barely touches the face. It is there in case the Gardner-Wells tongs or the weights fail accidentally. Because the patient is going to be tilted in a reverse Trendelenburg's position, he or she needs to be secured with a strap that goes below the buttocks and is secured to the table above the lowest resting blocks that support the anterior iliac crest. **D:** The arms are secured by placing a sheet underneath and around with tapes holding them in place. Finally, the arms are taped down to decrease the posterior neck skin fold, and a warming blanket is taped to the undersurface of the table **(E)**. Because the patient loses the most body heat through the ventral surface and warm air rises, placement of the blanket on the undersurface keeps the patient quite warm. The table is also tilted at approximately 15 to 20 degrees. Care should be taken not to pull on the shoulders excessively, as a brachial plexopathy can occur. Spinal cord monitoring should be used for these procedures to detect early brachial plexus stretch. If the monitoring demonstrates such a finding, the table is leveled out, and the tapes are loosened.

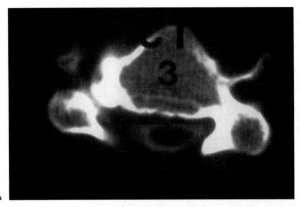
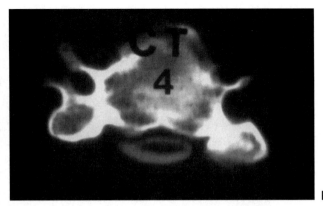

A   B

FIGURE 15. A, B: Postmyelogram computed tomography images of a patient who has had laminectomies. At C-3, all of the neural elements lie ventral to the remaining posterior elements. However, at C-4, the dura is dorsal to the remaining bony elements. At this level, great care must be taken to prevent injury to the exposed dura and cord.

Posterior Spine

Exposure of the posterior spine in a patient without laminectomy is relatively straightforward (Fig. 14). If the surgery is performed acutely, care must be taken not to depress or move the fractured fragments, especially if there is a concomitant laminar fracture or instability of the cervical segment. Electrocautery and sharp scalpel dissection are safer than the use of a periosteal elevator. One needs to adhere to the midline between the paraspinal muscles to minimize bleeding and trauma to the muscles.

The exposure of the previously laminectomized spine is significantly more difficult with increased potential complications. It is critical to examine the preoperative radiographs, especially the postmyelogram CT. This study readily identifies the relationship between the posterior dura and the remaining facets and lateral masses (Fig. 15). The dorsal dura usually lies ventral to the remaining lateral bony elements. If the dura protrudes dorsal to the remaining bony elements, there are fewer landmarks to guide the depth of the dissection. The most rostral and caudal spinous processes and laminae of the fusion mass should be exposed first. The remaining lateral bony elements of the laminectomized segments are subsequently exposed. Once the borders of the previous laminectomy have been thoroughly identified, these bony landmarks guide the depth of the dissection over the laminectomy site.

Radiology

In traumatic situations, the initial procedure is often performed on an emergent basis with limited preoperative studies. The preoperative planning for a revision procedure requires more extensive imaging. Instru-

mentation artifacts, metallic debris artifacts, and scar tissue compromise the preoperative radiologic evaluation in revision spine surgery. To adequately assess the extent of surgery required, a number of radiologic studies are necessary. Despite advances in imaging afforded by the new MRI machines, a cervical myelogram and CT scan can still yield invaluable information that is often missed on MRIs (35). Because most trauma surgery uses instrumentation to stabilize the spine, metallic artifacts can distort MRI images, even when titanium instrumentation is used. This artifact can be difficult to distinguish from residual bony compression (90,127) and can hide residual bony impingement on the soft tissues. In this situation, CTM helps to differentiate metal reaction from residual compression. The CT is arguably the best modality to assess bone stock and to determine the success of fusion with concurrent instrumentation. Although polytomograms are useful for this purpose, their role has declined in favor of the two-dimensionally reconstructed CT image. One-millimeter orthogonal cuts provide high-quality sagittal and coronal reconstruction. The CTM allows for improved visualization of stenosis at the neural foramen. It also is better at showing the differences between disk herniation versus a bony spur (122,142). In addition, the CT best defines the relationship between the dural sac and the bony elements. Two- or three-dimensionally reconstructed CT images provide additional insight during preoperative planning. In some cases, reconstructed CT images can show that a patient's anatomy is not amenable to certain procedures such as a C1-2 transarticular screw (35) (Fig. 16).

On the other hand, the MRI has distinct advantages. It is able to detect and follow posttraumatic soft tissue changes such as a syrinx (75). Also readily identified are cord signal changes and myelomalacia

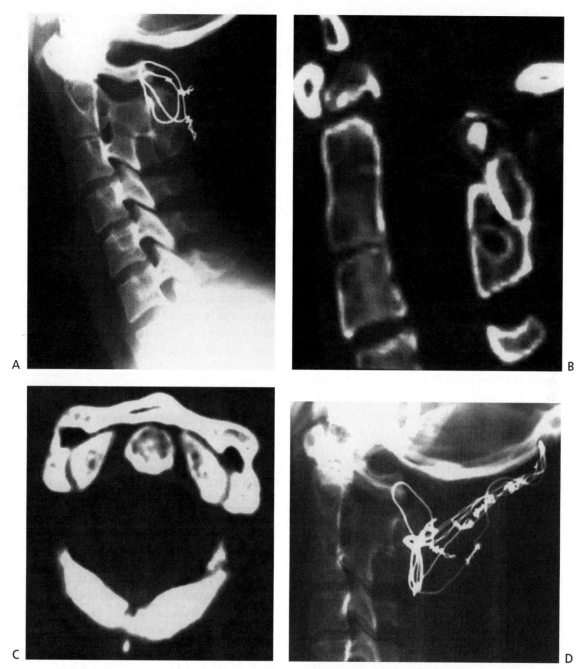

FIGURE 16. This 17-year-old girl had undergone three previous attempts at C1-2 and C2-3 fusion for an os odontoideum versus a nonhealed dens fracture. She presented with a broken wire at C1-2 and reasonable maintenance of alignment of the C1-2 articulation, although the extension view showed that she was quite unstable. The C2-3 was fused from her previous surgical attempts. **A:** Because of ongoing neck pain and instability, we evaluated her for a C1-2 transarticular screw fixation. However, **(B)** and **(C)** show an unusual congenital abnormality with persistent foramen ovalis into the body of C-1, with the vertebral artery literally in the path of C1-2 articulation transarticular screws. **D:** She was treated with an occiput to C2-3 fusion.

that are associated with a poorer prognosis for neurologic recovery (123).

Flexion/extension laterals of the cervical spine are important to obtain before surgery to determine the chance of instability at the injury site or at an adjacent level (39). This obviously is unnecessary and ill advised in cases in which obvious gross instability already exists (7). In such cases, the White stretch test is safer in acute or subacute situations. The surgeon supervises traction applied through Gardner-Wells tongs or a head halter. We prefer either tongs or a halo ring. Starting at 10 lb, one gradually adds weight in 5- to 10-lb increments, up to a maximum of one-third the patient's body weight. After each 10-lb increment the patient is reexamined and radiographs are obtained. Any change in the neurologic examination suggests a positive sign of instability. The surgeon should observe for overdistraction through the injury level, which also indicates instability. Oblique or pillar views help to confirm correct placement of lateral mass screws and to assess the integrity of the facet fusion mass. They are useful in determining if a facet dislocation has been successfully reduced and identify fractures of the pedicles and lateral masses. Finally, they provide an alternative to CT or MRI in assessing the fusion mass following an anterior arthrodesis.

SPECIFIC PROBLEMS

Kyphosis

Postlaminectomy Kyphosis

The principle of spinal trauma surgery is to decompress all neural elements and to stabilize the spine (6,27,96,120). Accordingly, a laminectomy without a spinal fusion is rarely indicated. A patient in whom a postlaminectomy kyphosis develops, with or without subluxation, presents a unique problem to the spine surgeon (69). An anterior decompressive procedure is typically indicated to decompress the spinal cord that is draped over the fixed kyphotic vertebral segments (135,140). After anterior and posterior decompression, the spine becomes highly unstable (34,91,104,134). The laminectomy disrupts the posterior part of the ring, whereas the corpectomy disrupts the anterior part. This results in two disconnected sides that are held together only by soft tissues (Fig. 17). Even with

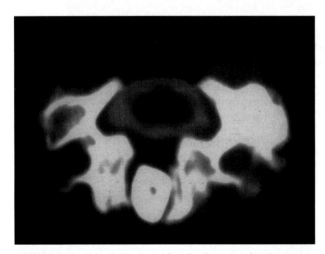

FIGURE 17. This patient, who had a postlaminectomy kyphosis and myelopathy, underwent an anterior cervical corpectomy and arthrodesis. Note that the left and right halves of the spine are only connected by soft tissues. This results in an extremely unstable state with poor rotational stability. These patients should undergo anterior as well as posterior instrumentation.

concurrent bone grafting and anterior cervical plating, the entire construct remains markedly unstable and prone to displacement not only with flexion/extension but also with rotational movements of the neck (99,100). These patients require circumferential spinal fusion with instrumentation. The efficacy of a halo vest is poor in preventing graft-related complications in this situation (71,104).

Kyphosis without Previous Laminectomy

If the kyphosis is due to ligamentous instability alone, a simple procedure consisting of a posterior arthrodesis and lateral mass plates or spinous process wires may suffice (13,23,25,26,30,41,63,98,109,110). More commonly, the kyphosis results in cord compression and necessitates an anterior decompression (Fig. 18). If the kyphosis is secondary to a collapsed anterior cervical graft, an anterior revision procedure is also usually necessary (11). Replacement of a collapsed structural graft restores cervical lordosis. Any remaining anterior compression should be addressed at the same time. If no neural compression is present anteriorly and the kyphosis is minimal, a posterior wiring or plate stabilization provides excellent support (15,63,110).

Adjacent Level Disease

If a transition syndrome develops after a previous arthrodesis, special considerations must be addressed. Arthrodesis of a level that is adjacent to a long fusion segment is at increased risk for pseudarthrosis (19). We recommend the use of instrumentation for such cases. The surgical dissection is usually more extensive for these revisions because instrumentation from the first procedure generally exists. The old instrumentation must be removed, allowing placement of the new cervical plate. If the patient does not have a solid arthrodesis across the old segment, the new plate should encompass the new and pseudarthrosis levels. However, if successful arthrodesis of the index procedure has occurred, a short plate across the newly operated level is enough support.

Infection

Osteomyelitis rarely complicates cervical spinal procedures, as demonstrated by the paucity of reports in the literature. If an infection occurs, removal of the hardware and graft followed by débridement and irrigation is essential before replacement of a fresh graft and instrumentation with fixation into uninvolved segments. If osteo-

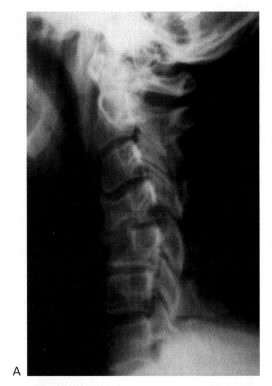

A

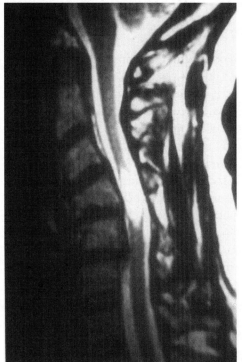

B

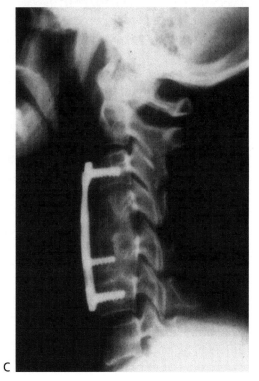

C

FIGURE 18. This patient was involved in a motor vehicle accident several years before her presentation. She was apparently treated with some type of immobilization but without surgical intervention. She presented with a syrinx and cervical kyphosis. She had symptoms and signs of a myeloradiculopathy that were believed to be due to a compressed cord as well as the syrinx. Her degenerated segments were C3-4, C4-5, and C5-6 **(A, B)**. A two-level corpectomy to decompress C-4 and C-5 and realign the kyphosis might have been complicated by graft extrusion or a fracture of the C-6 vertebra. Alternatively, she could have been treated with an anterior as well as a posterior arthrodesis. We elected to treat her with a corpectomy of C-4 and a diskectomy at C5-6 to distribute the load. At final follow-up, she achieved a solid arthrodesis and had significant resolution of her symptoms without having her syrinx drained. Her alignment, although not perfect, was also improved **(C)**. A combination of corpectomy and diskectomy can be used to distribute the load while keeping the number of healing endplates to four.

myelitis occurs anteriorly without abscess formation, graft collapse, or graft extrusion, treatment with antibiotics alone may abate the disease process (29,61). If the graft or hardware threatens extrusion or collapse, the surgeon can supplement fixation with revision surgery anteriorly or posteriorly (70,74). If anterior débridement is necessary, we recommend a revision graft and instrumentation, with the option of posterior fixation, with or without supplemental strut grafting and halo fixation. However, if concern about future collapse exists and anterior débridement is not absolutely indicated, a posterior augmentation procedure is preferable. Leaving surgical wounds open to drain and heal by secondary intention in the setting of spinal infection is rarely indicated (34,51).

Hardware Complications

Anterior Instrumentation

Loose screws dislodged from an anterior cervical plate pose a significant risk for esophageal laceration; therefore, screw removal is usually necessary. A loose screw may be associated with a pseudarthrosis, and addressing the pseudarthrosis at the time of hardware removal and reinstrumentation often becomes necessary. Screw breakage also suggests pseudarthrosis. Although this is rarely seen with modern instrumentation, the patient may require revision surgery (79,128). Plate breakage is also a rare phenomenon. Unlike a dislodged screw, a broken plate may not necessarily pose an overt risk to the patient, as scar tissue envelops the plate within a few weeks after the initial surgery. Flexion/extension views confirm proper hardware placement and ensure that sharp surfaces do not pose a risk to the surrounding soft tissues. If the patient has an asymptomatic pseudarthrosis, revision surgery usually is not warranted. If surgery becomes necessary, posterior wiring can often suffice. If there is obvious instability, the entire plate and graft construct may need to be removed and a circumferential procedure may be necessary (53,104).

Posterior Instrumentation

As in the anterior spine, plate breakage or screw loosening with instrumentation is often a sign of pseudarthrosis. Whereas vital structures are at risk if the hardware fails in the anterior spine, these risks often do not apply to the posterior spine. If the patient is asymptomatic, revision surgery can be avoided. However, if the entire construct is at risk of collapse, early revision surgery is advisable. If possible, an anterior approach is preferred, because one avoids operating through a previously scarred surgical bed. The anterior approach is especially preferred in the patient who was previously treated with a laminectomy, spinal fusion, and lateral mass plates that have subsequently displaced and gone on to pseudarthrosis.

If a lateral mass or pedicle screw causes injury or irritation to the nerve root, it needs to be removed. One should usually avoid using lateral mass screws at the C-7 and T-1 levels because the lateral masses are quite thin in most individuals (138). It is preferable to use pedicle screws after performing a laminotomy to identify the location of the pedicles at C-7 and T-1 (1,4). Placing a flat elevator into the facet joint can help establish the appropriate sagittal angulation for lateral mass screw placement. Intraoperative fluoroscopy can also be used. An alternative to screws at C-7 and T-1 is mini-sublaminar hooks that are especially designed for cervical placement. Additionally, wires are often a safe, effective, and easy option when the spinous processes are intact (25,55,68).

Graft Displacement

Graft Extrusion

Graft extrusion is a reported complication in a small percentage of unplated anterior cervical diskectomy and arthrodesis procedures (44,86,106). If a plate is used following a one- or two-level diskectomy, extrusion is rare or nonexistent. However, a study has demonstrated that long corpectomies instrumented with an anterior cervical plate can still extrude at the inferior margin (19,127). If the extrusion is minimal and the esophagus and trachea are not compromised, it may be possible to treat the patient in a halo vest, assuming that the graft has extruded but not impacted on the inferior vertebra (35,125). In this case, the mechanism of extrusion was an extension moment, which the halo effectively prevents (31,107). If the graft has completely extruded, revision surgery becomes mandatory. A longer bone graft is needed because the inferior vertebra usually becomes impacted (107). If the graft has displaced into the next disk space, a subtotal corpectomy needs to be performed on the fractured vertebra. Occasionally, the graft impacts through the inferior vertebra but appears to be stable. In this situation, revision surgery can be performed from the posterior aspect alone (29). If no anterior neural compression occurs, the surgeon can use lateral mass plates with or without spinous process wires to perform a posterior cervical fusion incorporating the adjacent levels (80).

If the inferior vertebra requires subtotal corpectomy and supplemental grafting, several options exist. Because the construct is usually a three- or four-level corpectomy, an allograft fibula or titanium mesh Harms cage can be used for the anterior portion of the procedure (31,50,66,105). The iliac crest autograft that had been used in the anterior spine can then be used for a posterior augmentation or used to fill a titanium mesh Harms cage with instrumentation. If the original anterior cervical graft had been a fibula, options are more limited. Although it is possible to harvest the contralateral fibula, the associated morbidity to an ambulatory patient may be significant. An alternative option is to use a freeze-dried allograft or a Harms cage filled with autologous bone for the anterior procedure and the fibula autograft for the posterior fusion. The fibula can be split in half and wired to the lateral masses or spinous processes.

Graft Intrusion

Graft intrusion may be associated with neurologic injury. If an intrusion of the graft occurs but the patient sustains no neurologic deficit, the graft should be repositioned to prevent further intrusion (29). If the intrusion is minimal, stable, and asymptomatic, a reasonable alternative is immobilization in a halo vest. Graft intrusion can usually be avoided by leaving an adequate posterior ledge in the caudal and rostral vertebrae to block posterior displacement (14,18).

Methylmethacrylate

Methylmethacrylate has no role in the treatment of acute cervical spine trauma fixation, save for pathologic fractures. Although they did not specifically address the cervical spine, McAfee et al. (87) have shown that methylmethacrylate has a high rate of failure within 1 year of surgery. If the life expectancy is less than a few months, it may be a reasonable option for short segment fixation. Allograft bone is readily available and is more likely to provide a much better construct than is methylmethacrylate. The bone-cement interface loosens with continued neck motion, increasing the instability with time. Despite rigid instrumentation, subsequent motion results in eventual construct failure (42,87). If methylmethacrylate has been used in a previous procedure, it needs to be removed in its entirety during the revision procedure to prepare the remaining bone for grafting.

Pseudarthrosis

As discussed in Anterior Instrumentation, most patients with an asymptomatic pseudarthrosis can be treated conservatively. If the patient is symptomatic or graft extrusion is imminent, a revision becomes necessary. If a pseudarthrosis occurs after a previous anterior procedure, the two revision options are a repeat grafting anteriorly versus augmentation of the fusion posteriorly (81,141). Although repeat anterior grafting can be successful, we prefer the posterior approach. Posterior wiring and supplemental autograft usually result not only in a posterior fusion but also in the eventual incorporation of the anterior pseudarthrotic graft (141). If the patient was treated initially with a laminectomy, lateral mass plating is necessary.

Patients with a pseudarthrosis following a previous posterior procedure can be effectively treated with an anterior arthrodesis (Fig. 19). Provided that the posterior cervical spine was successfully fixed with spinous process wires and autograft, one can usually use allograft in the front. The intact spinous process wires prevent flexion, and anterior bone graft and plating prevent extension. We routinely augment lateral mass plates with spinous process cables, as long as the spinous processes are intact. This "belts and suspenders" approach allows us to use unicortical lateral mass screws. Additionally, if a pseudarthrosis develops, the lateral mass screws are likely to fail before the cables. This allows an anterior-only revision procedure.

Revision Surgery of Upper Cervical Spine Fractures

Fractures of the Odontoid

If an odontoid screw construct develops a pseudarthrosis, we recommend posterior spinal fusion of the C1-2 joint. Ideally, this is performed before the odontoid screw breaks. The C1-2 fixation can be performed using either a Brooks or a Gallie technique, but our preference is to perform a Magerl C1-2 transarticular screw fixation (24,52,62,83,85).

Odontoid fractures can be treated posteriorly in numerous ways. If the C-1 arches are completely intact, C1-2 wiring is a well-accepted technique (57,58). If the C-1 arch is fractured or incompetent, occipital-cervical fusion with halo vest immobilization is one option (43,77,133). Alternatively, C1-2 transarticular screws can be used to augment wiring techniques. Careful evaluation of the C1-2 articulation for congenital anomalies is imperative. In addition, this technique obviates the need for occipital cervical fusion in patients with a concomitant Jefferson's fracture or an incompetent C-1 posterior arch (Fig. 20). Careful preoperative planning and intraoperative fluoroscopy are necessary to prevent injury to the vertebral artery. One alternative may be to place only one screw in the patient's nondominant vertebral artery side and augment it with traditional wiring techniques. Most commonly, the left artery is the dominant one in right-handed people and is often larger on the cervical MRI. If the cervical MRI is equivocal, magnetic resonance angiography or traditional angiography can demonstrate the dominant vertebral artery. A transarticular screw helps to control rotatory motion and stabilizes the spine such that halo vest immobilization is usually not necessary (54,83,131).

If a nonunion has developed after posterior wiring alone, revision surgery can be performed using transarticular screw fixation. With careful dissection, the C1-2 joint can be exposed and decorticated and bone graft can be placed into the joint. New image-guided systems are available that may allow for safer and more

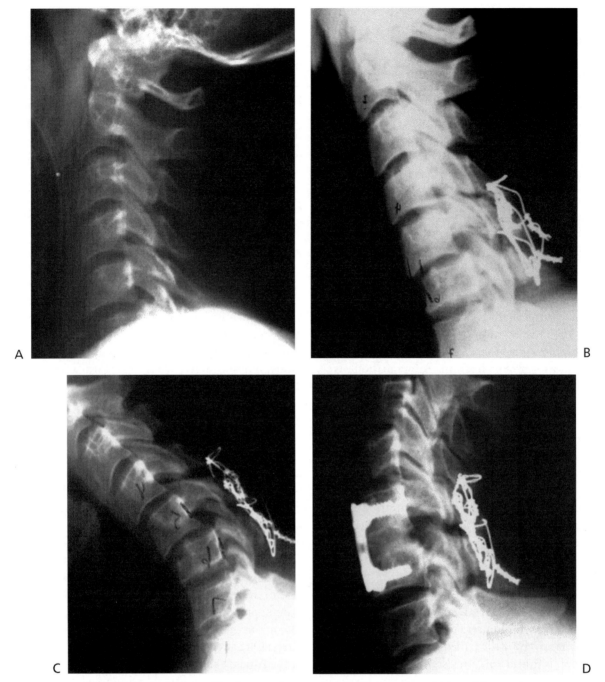

FIGURE 19. A 22-year-old college student was involved in a motor vehicle accident and experienced fractures of the C-5 facet and pedicle, resulting in subluxation of the C4-5 as well as the C5-6 facets. **A:** He was treated in halo traction and had improvement in alignment of unilateral facet subluxation but continued to have significant radicular pain. **B:** He was treated with a C4-6 posterior wiring and fusion, but there was a residual spondylolisthesis at C5-6. A circumferential fusion at C5-6 may have realigned the broken C-5 facet and avoided arthrodesis of the C4-5 level. **C:** One and a half years later, he presented to St. Louis University Hospital and was noted to have continued motion at the C5-6 level with an increase in the spondylolisthesis at C5-6. **D:** He underwent an anterior cervical diskectomy and fusion. Posterior wiring was not revised.

accurate placement of screws. To date, however, our experience with image guidance systems has not convinced us to use the technique on a routine basis.

If the patient presents with a pseudarthrosis of a transarticular screw fixation procedure, the screws may be broken, and the fracture may have completely displaced. If an obvious pseudarthrosis is present but the screws remain intact, a revision surgery is still recommended. CT scan with two- or three-dimensionally reconstructed images can help to determine if a screw with a larger diameter can be passed through the channel of the previous screw. The old screws should be removed and replaced with a larger diameter screw and fresh bone graft (Fig. 21). The bone graft should

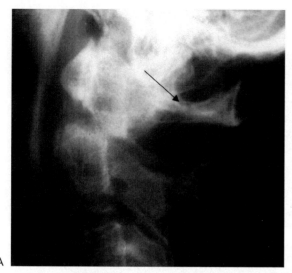
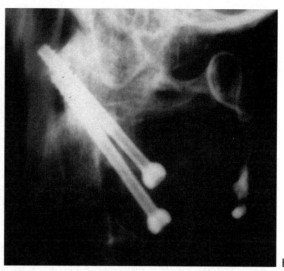

A

B

FIGURE 20. A: This octogenarian had a Jefferson's fracture as well as a displaced type II odontoid fracture. Arrow points to fracture through C1 ring. He was treated at an outside institution with a halo vest for several weeks but did not heal completely. He was then transferred to Barnes-Jewish Hospital where an operative attempt was made to reduce the odontoid fracture. A complete reduction could not be made despite the fact that he still had motion across the fracture site. **B:** He underwent transarticular screw fixation and wiring of bone graft. The fracture site at C-1 was also supplemented with bone graft, as it had not healed. At final follow-up, he achieved a solid arthrodesis of both fragments. Although the initial halo vest treatment is often recommended for this combination of fractures, performing this procedure at the outset can obviate the need for prolonged cervical immobilization.

be wired to C-1 and C-2 using a Magerl, Brooks, or Gallie technique. If a revision of the transarticular screws and C1-2 wires is too risky, or if the patient has failed more than one attempt at a fusion of the C1-2 segment, extending the fusion to the base of the skull should be considered (127). An alternative would be to perform an anterior C1-2 transarticular fusion (24,45,46,52,83,131).

Pseudarthrosis of a previous occipital cervical fusion may pose more of a challenge. If wire fusion was previously used, occipital plate fixation (116) or wiring techniques with rod systems can be used as a salvage procedure. Because a number of bends are needed to accommodate the occipital cervical junction, titanium lateral mass plates are not advisable. The brittle metal usually fatigues after repeated bending moments are applied. Currently, we use a titanium rod/plate system. The plate portion of the instrumentation is fixed to the skull, and the rod is contoured to the upper cervical region. Side attachments to the rod allow fixation of the rod to the upper cervical spine. This obviates the need for complex three-dimensional bends, which are necessary using the straight plate systems. Regardless of the type of plate used, the top of the plate should abut the base of the inion proximally. Below the inion, 8- to 10-mm fully threaded bicortical screws are used, whereas, at the level of the inion, unicortical 12- to 16-mm holes are drilled, measured, and then tapped before placing the screws (110). A total of six to

eight well-placed screws in the skull appear to be adequate. Under fluoroscopic control, 14- to 16-mm screws can be placed into the lateral mass or pedicle of C-2. In addition, wires can be placed into the skull or the spinous process of C-2 to secure the bone graft from the skull to C-2.

A number of studies have attempted to look at the safe placement of screws into the skull (59,143). The midsagittal sinus torcula needs to be avoided. The best screw purchase is below the level of the inion lateral to the midline. This area is devoid of a major sinus. More importantly, the thick cortical bone accepts a large screw with solid purchase.

An alternative technique is to use a rod secured to the skull with wires. The Southwick technique uses a U-shaped rod contoured to the lordotic convolution of the skull and into the cervical spine (47,102,118). One report noted successful treatment of rheumatoid patients with a contoured metal rod without bone grafting (97). Although we believe that all trauma patients should undergo arthrodesis, the loop may be a useful adjunct to stabilize the occipital cervical region.

Nonunion of a Hangman's Fracture

A hangman's fracture that is operatively fixed and subsequently develops a pseudarthrosis may require C1-3 fusion. This can often be achieved with standard wiring techniques (21,84,124,137). If transarticular

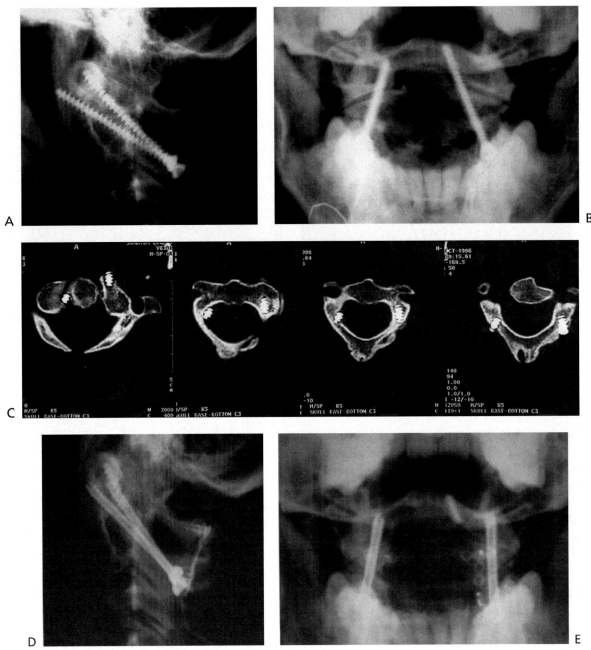

FIGURE 21. This patient underwent C1-2 transarticular screw fixation at an outside institution. **A:** The patient does not have a fusion, and one of the screws is broken. **B:** The open mouth odontoid view demonstrates that the right-sided screw is not across the joint. **C:** The magnetic resonance image demonstrates that the right-sided screw is also in the spinal canal. The patient was treated with removal of the old screws and replacement with larger diameter screws. The central portion of the posterior arch of C-1 was missing, and therefore we could not wire the graft in place. We therefore used small phalangeal plates to secure the lateral aspects of C-1 to C-2 and in addition placed bone graft underneath this plate as well as over the sides. Bone graft was also placed into the C1-2 joint. **D, E:** The patient went on to a solid arthrodesis despite her history of tobacco abuse.

screws are used, careful preoperative imaging and planing are necessary to determine the course of the vertebral artery. The vertebral artery often displaces anteriorly, avoiding the path of the screw. The fracture should be reduced as anatomically as possible. If one of the vertebral arteries already is compromised secondary to the fracture, damage to the opposite vertebral artery will result in a basilar stroke (101).

Revision of Lower Cervical Spine Fractures

Burst Fracture

In patients with burst fractures who are treated operatively, a malunion can develop with kyphosis and angulation with or without a pseudarthrosis. If the patient is asymptomatic, no further surgery may be

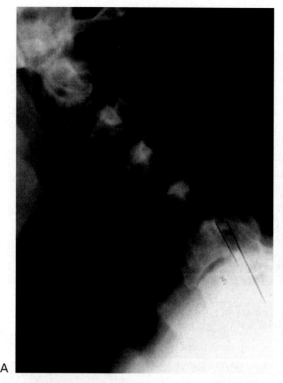

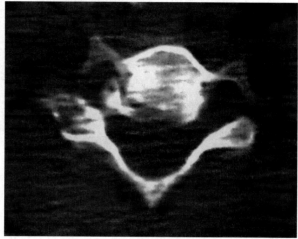

A   B

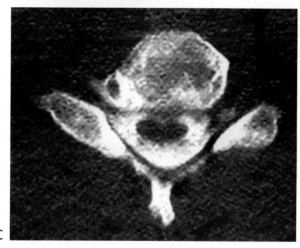

C

FIGURE 22. A 30-year-old woman involved in a motor vehicle accident suffered a unilateral facet fracture of C6-7. This was treated in a halo vest with healing of the facet fracture, and the patient did reasonably well with some mild residual numbness in the thumb and index finger. She presented 30 months later with increasing pain in the involved right arm and increasing numbness and tingling in the right arm. **A:** This x-ray shows the stable nature of her C6-7 articulation and narrowing of the disk space with a mild spondylolisthesis at that level. **B:** The initial trauma computed tomography scan shows the fracture of her facet. **C:** The healed facet at 30 months with marked foraminal stenosis on the involved side. Her revision consisted of a keyhole foraminotomy and decompression of the root with resolution of her radicular pain and, for the most part, resolution of her thumb and index finger numbness.

necessary or advisable. If, however, persistent or progressive neurologic deficits are present, surgery may be beneficial.

These patients can usually undergo a repeat decompression using standard corpectomy techniques. If no facet fusion is present posteriorly, the malalignment can be corrected using a larger graft and plating the entire construct. Posterior stabilization should be strongly considered in more unstable fracture patterns. If a facet fusion is present, a circumferential osteotomy may be necessary to decompress and realign the spine properly.

Facet Dislocations

A malunion of a facet dislocation or an unreduced facet dislocation can sometimes be revised posteri-

orly if only a posterior fusion exists (113,114). However, if ankylosis of the anterior spine is present, an anterior and posterior procedure may be required to realign the spine adequately. Typically, patients who have a solid fusion do not exhibit radiculopathy, but this is not always the case. If the patient is fused in a dislocated position such that the nerve remains kinked, (s)he may have persistent radiculopathy even in the presence of a solid malunion. If the alignment is acceptable and the repair is solid, a simple keyhole foraminotomy may successfully treat the radiculopathy that is related to a displaced but healed unilateral facet fracture (9) (Fig. 22). In a young patient with severe malalignment, however, consideration should be given to performing a realignment procedure. An indication for an anterior-posterior procedure is the

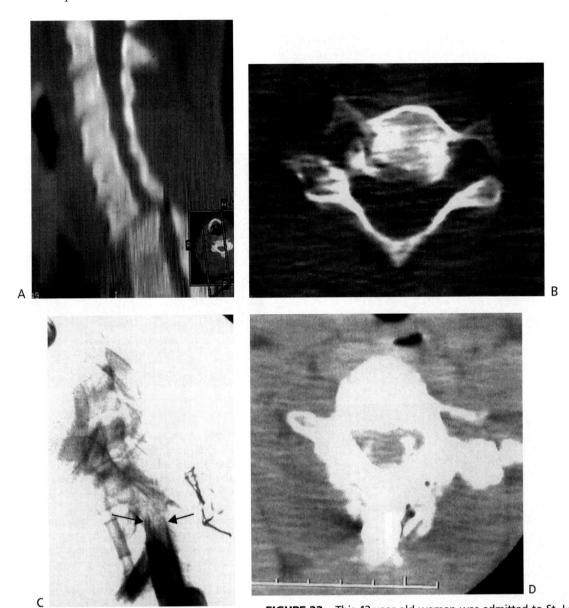

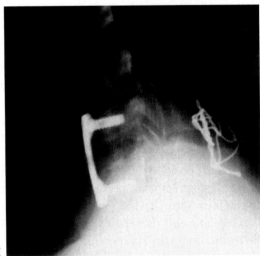

FIGURE 23. This 42-year-old woman was admitted to St. Louis University Hospital with an incomplete anterior cord syndrome. While wrestling with her husband, she was placed in a full-Nelson headlock. They both heard an audible crack from her neck. She had sudden neck pain and electrical sensation throughout her entire body. **A, B:** She was noted to have a bilateral facet dislocation at C6-7. She underwent a posterior wiring and arthrodesis at C6-7. Postoperatively, her neurologic examination was stable, with no numbness and only mild residual weakness in her lower extremities. The second day postoperatively, during mobilization, the patient had sudden recurrence of her quadriplegia. **C:** A myelogram demonstrated a complete block at C6-7. **D:** The post-myelogram computed tomograph showed a central disk herniation with impingement on the spinal cord. She was taken emergently to the operating room and underwent an anterior cervical diskectomy and fusion with an anterior plate. The use of wires posteriorly allows enough "play" such that the anterior diskectomy and arthrodesis can be performed. She fortunately had complete resolution of her quadriplegia. **E:** One-year follow-up results of the fusion after plate osteosynthesis.

presence of a partial neurologic deficit. Loss of neural function below the level of the dislocation must be treated aggressively if neurologic recovery is to be expected. Even late decompressions in these cases have been associated with recovery of root as well as cord function (7,16,78) (Fig. 23).

Anterior-Posterior Revision Surgery

If it has been determined that a combined approach is necessary, the surgeon must decide whether to go anteriorly or posteriorly first (80). A number of advantages are obtained by performing the posterior procedure first. After releasing all of the facet joints that have fused, one can use the triple Bohlman technique of spinous process wiring with iliac crest graft on either side of the spinous processes (13,88). One can then perform an anterior decompression and placement of a strut graft to restore the normal lordotic curve. Lateral mass plates should not be used in this case because their rigidity inhibits the ability to perform the anterior reduction maneuver. After diskectomy and osteophytectomy are performed from the anterior side, the spine is released in all columns. One can then place a structural graft in the anterior column, thereby reducing the kyphotic angulation. At this point an anterior cervical plate can be placed (Fig. 23). Rarely, the posterior column may be too loose after both procedures. This may require a return to the posterior side to tighten up the spinous process wires.

If the anterior decompression is approached first in a patient who is circumferentially fused in kyphosis, the graft is placed into the decompression site while the spine is still in a kyphotic alignment. The subsequent posterior procedure, which restores the lordotic alignment, may result in a poorly fitting anterior graft or possibly even extrusion. In a kyphotic and malunited spine that has ankylosed anteriorly and has been fused posteriorly without reduction, the anterior and the posterior areas need to be released before the kyphosis can be corrected. On the other hand, if only the anterior longitudinal ligament and anterior osteophytes have ankylosed, these can easily be released from a simple anterior approach.

REFERENCES

1. Abumi K, Itoh H, Taneichi H, et al. Transpedicular screw fixation for traumatic lesions of the middle and lower cervical spine: descriptions of the technique and preliminary report. *J Spinal Disord* 1994;7:19.
2. Aebi M, Zuber K, Marchesi D. Treatment of cervical spine injuries with anterior plating. *Spine* 1991;16:538.
3. Allen BL, Ferguson RL, Lehmann TR, et al. A mechanistic classification of closed, indirect fractures and dislocations of the lower cervical spine. *Spine* 1982;7:1.
4. An HS, Gordin R, Renner K. Anatomic considerations for plate-screw fixation of the cervical spine. *Spine* 1991;16:548.
5. An HS. Posterior instrumentation of the cervical spine. In: An HS, Cotler JM, eds. *Spinal instrumentation*. Baltimore: Williams & Wilkins, 1992:33–47.
6. Anderson LD, Stivers BR, Park WI III. Multiple level anterior cervical spine fusion. A report of sixteen cases. *J Trauma* 1974;14:653.
7. Anderson PA, Bohlman HH. Anterior decompression and arthrodesis of the cervical spine: long term motor involvement: II. Improvement in incomplete traumatic quadriplegia. *J Bone Joint Surg Am* 1992;74A:671.
8. Anderson PA, Budorrick TE. Failure of halo vest to prevent in vivo motion in patients with injured cervical spines. *Spine* 1991;16:501.
9. Anderson PA, Henley MB, Grady MS. Post cervical arthrodesis using AO reconstruction plates. *Spine* 1991;16:72.
10. Benson DR, Keenan TL. Evaluation and treatment of trauma to the vertebral column. *Instr Course Lect* 1990; 39:578.
11. Bernard TN, Whitecloud TS. Cervical spondylotic myelopathy and myeloradiculopathy: anterior decompression and stabilization with autogenous fibular strut graft. *Clin Orthop* 1987;221:149.
12. Bohlman HH. Cervical spondylosis with moderate to severe myelopathy: a report of seventeen cases treated by Robinson anterior cervical discectomy and fusion. *Spine* 1977;2:151.
13. Bohlman HH. Acute fractures and dislocations of the cervical spine: an analysis of 300 hospitalized patients and review of the literature. *J Bone Joint Surg Am* 1979; 61A:119.
14. Bohlman HH. Indications for late anterior decompression and fusion for cervical spinal cord injuries. In: Tator CH, ed. *Early management of acute cervical spinal cord injury. Seminars in neurologic surgery.* New York: Raven Press, 1982:315–333.
15. Bohlman HH. Surgical management of cervical spine fractures and dislocations. *Instr Course Lect* 1985;34:163.
16. Bohlman HH, Anderson PA. Anterior decompression and arthrodesis of the cervical spine: long term motor involvement: I. Improvement in incomplete traumatic quadriplegia. *J Bone Joint Surg Am* 1992;74A:659.
17. Bohlman HH, Ducker TB. Spine and spinal cord injuries. In: Rothman RH, Simeone FA, eds. *The spine*, 3rd ed. Philadelphia: WB Saunders, 1992:973.
18. Bohlman HH, Eismont FJ. Surgical techniques of anterior decompression and fusion for spinal cord injuries. *Clin Orthop* 1981;154:57.
19. Bohlman HH, Emery SE, Goodfellow D, et al. Robinson anterior cervical diskectomy and arthrodesis for cervical radiculopathy. *J Bone Joint Surg Am* 1993;75A:1298.
20. Bolesta MJ, Bohlman HH. Late complications of cervical fractures and dislocation and their management. In:

Frymoyer JW, ed. *The adult spine.* New York: Raven Press, 1991:1297–1316.

21. Borne GM, Bedou GL, Pinaudeau M. Treatment of pedicular fractures of the axis. A clinical study and screw fixation techniques. *J Neurosurg* 1984;60:88.

22. Brackman R, Vinten P. Unilateral facet interlocking in the lower cervical spine. *J Bone Joint Surg Br* 1967;49B:249.

23. Bridwell KH. Where to stop the fusion distally in adult scoliosis: L4, L5, or the sacrum? *Instr Course Lect* 1996; 45:101–107.

24. Brooks AL, Jenkins EB. Atlanto-axial arthrodesis by the wedge-compression method. *J Bone Joint Surg Am* 1978; 60A:279.

25. Cahill DW, Bellegarrigue R, Ducker TB. Bilateral facet to spinous process fusion: a new technique for posterior spinal fusion after trauma. *Neurosurgery* 1983;13:1.

26. Callahan RA, Johnson RM, Margolis RN, et al. Cervical facet fusion for control of instability following laminectomy. *J Bone Joint Surg Am* 1977;59A:991.

27. Capen D, Garland DE, Waters RL. Surgical stabilization of the cervical spine. A comparative analysis of anterior and posterior spine fusions. *Clin Orthop* 1985;196:229–237.

28. Clark CR, Ingram CM, El Khoury GY, et al. Radiographic evaluation of the cervical spine injuries. *Spine* 1988;13:742.

29. Cloward RB. Complications of anterior cervical disc operation and their treatment. *Surgery* 1971;69:175.

30. Coe JD, Warden KE, Sutterlin CE, et al. Biomechanical evaluation of cervical spinal stabilization methods in a human cadaveric model. *Spine* 1989;14:1123.

31. Cotler JM, Star AM. Complications of spinal fusion. In: Cotler JM, Cotler HB, eds. *Spinal fusions: science and technique.* New York: Springer-Verlag, 1990:361–387.

32. Curtin SL, Heller JG. Multi-level anterior cervical reconstruction: pseudarthrosis and complication rates. *Orthop Trans* 1996;20:26.

33. Cybulski GR, Douglas RA, Meyer PA, et al. Complication in three-column cervical spine injury requiring anterior-posterior stabilization. *Spine* 1991;16:253.

34. Dernbach PD, Gomez H, Hahn J. Primary closure of infected spinal wounds. *Neurosurgery* 1990;26:707.

35. Devlin VJ, Anderson PA. Revision cervical spine surgery. In: Margulies JY, Aebi M, Farcy JPC, eds. *Revision spine surgery.* St. Louis: Mosby, 1999;52–88.

36. Dickman CA, Hadley MN, Browner C, et al. Neurosurgical management of acute atlas-axis combination fractures. *J Neurosurg* 1989;70:45.

37. Doppman JL, Girton M. Angiographic study of the effect of laminectomy in the presence of acute anterior epidural masses. *J Neurosurg* 1976;45:195.

38. Ducker TB, Russo GL, Bellegarrique R, et al. Complete sensorimotor paralysis after cord injury: mortality, recovery, and therapeutic implications. *J Trauma* 1979; 19:837.

39. Dvorak J, Froehlich D, Penning L, et al. Functional radiographic diagnosis of the cervical spine: flexion/extension. *Spine* 1988;13:748.

40. Dvorak MF, Fischer CG. Revision spine surgery in the presence of osteoporosis. In: Margulies JY, Aebi M, Farcy JPC, eds. *Revision spine surgery.* St. Louis: Mosby, 1999:646–655.

41. Edwards CC, Matz SO, Levine AM. The oblique wiring technique for rotational injuries of the cervical spine. *Orthop Trans* 1986;10:455.

42. Eismont FJ, Bohlman HH. Posterior methylmethacrylate fixation for cervical trauma. *Spine* 1981;6:347.

43. Elia M, Mazzara JT, Fielding JW. Onlay technique for occipitocervical fusion. *Clin Orthop* 1992;280:170.

44. Esperson JO, Buhl M, Eriksen EF. Treatment of cervical disease using Cloward's technique. 1. General results and effects of different operative methods and complication in 1106 patients. *Acta Neurochir (Wien)* 1984;70:97.

45. Esses SI, Bednar DA. Screw fixation of odontoid fractures and nonunions. *Spine* 1991;16:483.

46. Etter C, Coscia M, Jaberg H, et al. Direct anterior fixation of dens fractures with a cannulated screw system. *Spine* 1991;16:25.

47. Fehlings MG, Errico T, Cooper P. Occipitocervical fusion with a 5 millimeter malleable rod and segmental fixation. *Neurosurgery* 1993;32:198.

48. Foley KT, Smith MM, Wiles DA. Anterior cervical plating does not prevent strut graft displacement in multilevel cervical corpectomy. *Orthop Trans* 1998–1999;22:512.

49. Frankel HL, Hancock DO, Hyslop G, et al. The value of postural reduction in the initial management of closed injuries of the spine with paraplegia and tetraplegia. *Paraplegia* 1969;7:179.

50. Freidberg SR, Gumley GJ, Pfeifer BA, et al. Vascularized fibula graft to replace resected cervical vertebral bodies. *J Neurosurg* 1989;71:283.

51. Gaines DL, Moe JH, Bocklage J. Management of wound infections following Harrington instrumentation and spine fusion. *J Bone Joint Surg Am* 1970;52:404.

52. Gallie WE. Skeletal traction in the treatment of fractures and dislocation of the cervical spine. *Am J Surg* 1939;46:495.

53. Garvey TA, Eismont FJ, Roberti LJ. Anterior decompression, structural bone grafting and Caspar plate stabilization for unstable cervical spine fractures and/or dislocation. *Spine* 1992;17:431.

54. Grob D, Jeanneret B, Aebi M, et al. Atlantoaxial fusion with transarticular screw fixation. *J Bone Joint Surg Br* 1991;73B:972.

55. Grob D, Magerl F. Dorsal spondylosis of the cervical spine using a hooked plate. *Orthopaedics* 1987;16:66.

56. Hadley MN, Dickman CA, Browner CM, et al. Acute traumatic atlas fractures: management and long term outcome. *Neurosurgery* 1988;23:31.

57. Hadra BE. The classic wiring of the vertebra as a means of immobilization in fracture and Potts disease. *Clin Orthop* 1975;112:4.

58. Hadra BE. Wiring of the spinous process in injury and Potts disease. *Orthopaedics Assoc* 1981;4:206.

59. Haher TR. Occipital screw pullout strength: a biomechanical investigation of occipital morphology. *J Spinal Cord Med* 1996;19:118.

60. Harris JH. Acute injuries of the spine. *Semin Roentgenol* 1978;13:53.

61. Heller JG. Postoperative infections of the spine. In: Rothman RH, Simeone FA, eds. *The spine*, 3rd ed. Philadelphia: WB Saunders, 1992:1817.

62. Heller JG, Carlson GD, Abitol JJ, et al. Anatomic comparison of the Roy-Camille and Magerl techniques for screw placement in the lower cervical spin. *Spine* 1991; 16:552.

63. Heller JG, Silcox DH III. Post laminectomy instability of the cervical spine. In: Frymoyer JW, Ducker TB, Hadler NM, et al. (eds). *The adult spine: principles and practice*, 2nd ed. Philadelphia: Lippincott–Raven Publishers, 1997:1413.

64. Hu S. Internal fixation in the osteoporotic spine. *Spine* 1997;22(245):43.

65. Hu SS, Capen DA, Rimoldi RL, et al. The effect of surgical decompression on neurologic outcome after lumbar fractures. *Clin Orthop* 1993;288:166.

66. Hughes SS, Pringle T, Phillips FM, et al. Multilevel cervical corpectomy and fibular strut grafting: intermediate clinical and radiographic followup. *Orthop Trans* 1996;20(2):432.

67. Jacobs B. Cervical fracture and dislocation (C3–C7). *Clin Orthop* 1975;109:18.

68. Jeanneret B, Magerl F, Halterward E, et al. Posterior stabilization of the cervical spine with hook plates. *Spine* 1991;16:56.

69. Jodoin A, Gillet P, Dupuis PR, et al. Surgical treatment of posttraumatic kyphosis: a report of sixteen cases. *Can J Surg* 1989;32(1):36.

70. Keller RB, Pappas AM. Infections after spinal fusion using internal fixation instruments. *Orthop Clin North Am* 1972;3:99.

71. Kostuik JP. Indications for the use of the halo immobilization. *Clin Orthop* 1981; Jan–Feb(154):46–50.

72. Law MD, Bernhardt M, White AA. Cervical spondylotic myelopathy: a review of surgical indications and decision making. *Yale J Biol Med* 1993;66:165.

73. Lee C, Rogers LF, Woodring JH. Fractures of the craniovertebral junction associated with other fractures of the spine: overlooked entity? *Appl Nurs Res* 1994;5:775.

74. Leventhal MR. Surgical approaches in the treatment of spinal infections. *Spine: State of the Art Reviews* 1989;3: 419.

75. Levi ADO, Sonntag VKH. Management of posttraumatic syringomyelia using an expansile duraplasty. A case report. *Spine* 1998;23(1):128.

76. Levine AM, Edwards CC. Complications in the treatment of acute spinal injury. *Orthop Clin North Am* 1986;17(1):183.

77. Levine AM, Edwards CC. Fractures of the atlas. *J Bone Joint Surg Am* 1991;73A:680.

78. Ljunggren BM, Al Refai M, Sharma S, et al. Functional recovery after near complete traumatic deficit of the cervical cord lasting more than twenty-four hours. *Br J Neurosurg* 1992;6(4):375.

79. Lowery GL, McDonough RF. The significance of hardware failure in anterior cervical plate fixation: patients with two to seven year follow-up. *Spine* 1998;23:181.

80. Lowery GL, McDonough RF. Revision cervical spine surgery: anterior, posterior or both. In: Margulies JY, Aebi M, Farcy JPC, eds. *Revision spine surgery.* St. Louis: Mosby, 1999:252–270.

81. Lowery GL, Swant ML, McDonough RF. Surgical revision for failed anterior cervical fusions. *Spine* 1995;20: 2436.

82. MacDonald RL, Schwartz ML, Mirich D, et al. Diagnosis of cervical spine injury in motor vehicle crash victims: how many X-rays are enough? *J Trauma* 1990;30:392.

83. Magerl F, Seeman PS. Stable posterior fusion of the atlas and axis by transarticular screw fixation. In: Kehr P, Weidner A, eds. *Cervical spine.* New York: Springer-Verlag, 1987.

84. Marar BC. Fracture of the axis arch. *Clin Orthop* 1975; 106:155.

85. Marcotte P, Dickman CA, Sonntag VK. Posterior atlantoaxial facet screw fixation. *J Neurosurg* 1993;79:234.

86. Mayfield FH. Cervical spondylosis: a comparison of the anterior and posterior approaches. *Clin Neurosurg* 1966;13:181.

87. McAfee P, Bohlman HH, Ducker T. Failure of stabilization of the spine with methylmethacrylate. *J Bone Joint Surg Am* 1986;68A:1145.

88. McAfee PC, Bohlman HH, Wilson WL. The triple wire fixation technique for stabilization of acute cervical fracture-dislocations: a biomechanical analysis. *Trans Orthop* 1985;9:142.

89. McLain RF, Aretakis A, Moseley TA, et al. Subaxial cervical dissociation. *Spine* 1994;19:653.

90. Meeks L, Goodrich A, Toro V. Magnetic resonance imaging artifacts after anterior cervical diskectomy and fusion: a cadaveric study. *Orthop Trans* 1994;8(2):329.

91. Mikawa FH, Shikata J, Yamamuro T. Spinal deformity and instability after multilevel cervical laminectomy. *Spine* 1987;12:6.

92. Mirvis SE, Young JWR, Lim C, et al. Hangman's fracture: radiologic assessment in twenty-seven cases. *Radiology* 1987;163:713.

93. Mirza S, Moquin R, Anderson PA. Stabilizing properties of the halo-vest. *Orthop Trans* 1994;18:697.

94. Mitsui H. A new operation for atlantoaxial arthrodesis. *J Bone Joint Surg Br* 1984;66B:422.

95. Morgan FH, Wharton GW, Austin GH. The results of laminectomy in patients with incomplete spinal cord injuries. *Paraplegia* 1971;9:14.

96. Morgan TH, Wharton G, Austin G. The results of laminectomy in patients with incomplete spinal cord injuries. *J Bone Joint Surg Am* 1976;52A:822.

97. Moskovich R, Crockard A, Shott S, et al. Occipitocervical stabilization for myelopathy in patients with rheumatoid arthritis. Implications of not bone-grafting. *J Bone Joint Surg* 2000;82:349.

98. Oro JJ, Watts C. Sublaminar and epilaminar wire fusion: a new technique for posterior subluxation injuries of the lower cervical spine. *Trans Orthop* 1985;9:1985.

99. Pal GP, Sherk HH. The vertical stability of the cervical spine. *Spine* 1988;12:47.

100. Panjabi MM, White AA, Johnson RM. Cervical spine biomechanics as a function of transection of components. *J Biomech* 1975;8:327.

101. Pelker RR, Dorfman GS. Fracture of the axis associated with vertebral artery injury. A case report. *Spine* 1986; 11:621.

102. Ransford AO, Crockard HA, Pozo JL, et al. Craniocervical instability treated by contoured loop fixation. *J Bone Joint Surg Br* 1986;68B:173.

103. Reid DC, Henderson R, Saboe L, et al. Etiology and clinical course of missed spine fractures. *J Trauma* 1987;27:980.

104. Riew KD, Hilibrand AS, Palumbo MA, et al. Anterior cervical corpectomy in post-laminectomy patients. Short-term complications. *J Bone Joint Surg* 1999;81A(7):950.

105. Riew KD, Hilibrand A, Palumbo M, et al. Diagnosing basilar invagination in the rheumatoid patient. The reliability of radiographic criteria. *J Bone Joint Surg* 2001;83A:194.

106. Riley LH, Robinson RA, Johnson KA, et al. The results of anterior interbody fusion of the cervical spine: review of 93 consecutive cases. *J Neurosurg* 1969;30: 127.

107. Rockswold GL, Bergman TA. Halo immobilization and surgical fusion: relative indications and effectiveness in the treatment of 140 cervical spine injuries. *J Trauma* 1990;30(7):893.

108. Rorabeck C, Rock M, Hawkins R, et al. Unilateral facet dislocation of the cervical spine. *Spine* 1987;12: 23.

109. Roy-Camille R, Mazel CH, Saillant G. Treatment of cervical spine injuries by a posterior osteosynthesis with plates and screws. In: Keher P, Weidner A, eds. *Cervical spine I.* New York: Springer-Verlag, 1987:163.

110. Roy-Camille R, Saillant G, Mazel C. Internal fixation of the unstable cervical spine by a posterior osteosynthesis with plates and screws. In: Bailey RW, Sherk HH, eds. *The cervical spine,* 2nd ed. Philadelphia: JB Lippincott Co, 1989:390–403.

111. Schaffer MA, Doris PE. Limitations of the cross-table lateral view in detecting cervical spine injuries: a retrospective analysis. *Ann Emerg Med* 1987;10:508.

112. Schneider RC. The syndrome of acute anterior spinal cord injury. *J Neurosurg* 1955;12:95.

113. Shapiro SA. Management of unilateral locked facet of the cervical spine. *Neurosurgery* 1993;33(5):832.

114. Shapiro SA, Shaffer WO, et al. The Saint Louis University Blunt Trauma Cervical Spine Protocol. Presented to the Missouri Chapter of the American College of Surgeons, June 1999.

115. Shear P, Hugenholtz H, Richard MT. Noncontiguous fractures of the cervical spine. *Can J Neurol Sci* 1987; 14:212.

116. Smith MD, Anderson P, Grady MS. Occipitocervical arthrodesis using contoured plate fixation. An early report on a versatile fixation technique. *Spine* 1993; 18(14):1984.

117. Soreff J. Assessment of the late results of traumatic compression fractures of the thoracolumbar vertebral bodies. Thesis, Karolinska Hospital, Stockholm, Sweden, 1977.

118. Stambough JL, Balderston RA, Grey S. Techniques for occipitocervical fusion in osteopenic patients. *J Spinal Disord* 1990;3:407.

119. Stauffer ES, Kelly EG. Fracture-dislocation of the cervical spine: instability and recurrent deformity following treatment by anterior interbody fusion. *J Bone Joint Surg Am* 1977;59A:45.

120. Stauffer ES, Shields C. Late instability in cervical spine fractures secondary to cervical laminectomy. *Clin Orthop* 1976;119:144.

121. Streitwieser DR, Knopp R, Wales LR, et al. Accuracy of standard radiographic views in detecting cervical spine fractures. *Ann Emerg Med* 1983;12:538.

122. Suk SI, Lee CK, Kim KT, et al. A comparison of computerized tomography (CT), myelo-enhanced CT (MELT) and magnetic resonance imaging (MRI) in diagnosis of spinal stenosis. *J Korean Orthop Assoc* 1991;26(1):6.

123. Takahashi M, Yamashita Y, Sakamoto Y, et al. Chronic cervical compression: clinical significance of increased signal intensity on MR image. *Radiology* 1989;173:219.

124. Termansen NB. Hangman's fracture. *Acta Orthop Scand* 1974;445:529.

125. Tew JM Jr, Mayfield FH. Surgery of the anterior cervical spine: prevention of complications. In: Dunsker SB, ed. *Seminars in neurological surgery: cervical spondylosis.* New York: Raven Press, 1980.

126. Vaccaro AR, An HS, Lin S, et al. Noncontiguous injuries of the spine. *J Spinal Disord* 1992;5:320.

127. Vaccaro AR, Charlton WPH, Cotler JM. Principles of revision surgery following failed cervical spinal injury. In: Margulies JY, Aebi M, Farcy JPC, eds. *Revision spine surgery.* St. Louis: Mosby, 1999:342–353.

128. Van Peteghem PK, Schweigel JF. The fractured cervical spine rendered unstable by anterior cervical fusion. *J Trauma* 1979;19(2):110.

129. Verbiest H. Anterolateral operations for fractures and dislocation of the middle and lower parts of the cervical spine. *J Bone Joint Surg Am* 1969;51:1489.

130. Wales LR, Knopp RK, Morishima MS. Recommendations for evaluation of the acutely injured cervical spine: a clinical radiologic algorithm. *Am Emerg Med* 1980;9:422.

131. Weidner A. Internal fixation with metal plates and screws. In: Bailey RW, Sherk HH, eds. *The cervical spine,* 2nd ed. Philadelphia: JB Lippincott Co, 1989.

132. Wenger DR, Carollo JJ. The mechanics of thoracolumbar fractures stabilized by segmental fixation. *Clin Orthop* 1984;189:89.

133. Werthen SB, Bohlman HH. Occipitocervical fusion. *J Bone Joint Surg Am* 1987;69A:833.

134. White AA, Panjabi MM, Thomas CL. The clinical biomechanics of kyphotic deformities. *Clin Orthop* 1977;128:8.

135. Whitecloud TS, La Rocca H. Fibular strut graft in reconstructive surgery of the cervical spine. *Spine* 1976;1:33.

136. Whitehill R, Stowers SF. Cervical dislocation adjacent to a fused motion segment. Case report. *Spine* 1987;12 (4):396.

137. Williams TG. Hangman's fracture. *J Bone Joint Surg Br* 1975;57B:82.

138. Xu R, Ebraheim NA, Yeasting R, et al. Anatomy of C7 lateral mass and projection of pedicle axis on its posterior aspect. *J Spinal Disord* 1995;8:116.

139. Young B, Brooks WH, Tibbs PA. Anterior decompression and fusion for thoracolumbar fractures with neurologic deficits. *Acta Neurochir* 1981;57:287.

140. Zdeblick TA, Bohlman HH. Cervical kyphosis and myelopathy: treatment by anterior corpectomy and strut grafting. *J Bone Joint Surg Am* 1989;71A:170.

141. Zdeblick TA, Hughes SS, Riew KD, et al. Failed anterior cervical diskectomy and arthrodesis. *J Bone Joint Surg Am* 1997;79A:523.

142. Zinreich SJ, Long DM, Davis R, et al. Three-dimensional CT imaging in postsurgical "failed back" syndrome. *J Comput Assist Tomogr* 1990;14(4):574.

143. Zipnick RI, Merola AA, Gorup J, et al. The occiput: anatomic considerations for internal fixation. *Spine: State of the Art Reviews* 1996;10(2):269.

144. Zou D, Yoo JU, Edwards WT. Mechanics of anatomic reduction of thoracolumbar burst fractures. *Spine* 1993; 18:195.

6

CERVICAL SPINE: TUMOR

ALEXANDER R. VACCARO AND JONATHAN F. ROSENFELD

Tumors of the spine can be classified as primary or metastatic as well as benign or malignant. Although benign neoplasms are more common in the appendicular skeleton, the spine is more often involved with malignant lesions, with metastases outnumbering primary tumors by at least five to one (31). The axial skeleton is the most common site of metastasis after the lung and the liver (22,28). This has been explained by the rich vascular network within and surrounding the vertebral bodies. The red bone marrow and vertebral venous plexus are well-known pathways for breast and prostate cancer metastasis (22). Primary tumors of spinal metastasis are most often located in the breast, prostate, lung, thyroid, kidney, and hematopoietic system (17).

Whether benign or malignant, tumors of the spine can lead to fracture and instability, which in turn can lead to severe pain, neurologic compromise, and/or paralysis (10,23,29,41). Treatment of tumors of the spine has advanced greatly over the past decades, in most cases obviating the need for surgical treatment. Pain can be relieved acutely in many instances through radiation therapy (25). Many tumors, however, are still best treated by primary surgical removal, as instability is not addressed with radiation therapy or chemotherapy (19,20). Surgery produces immediate results, including removal of compressive tumor disease, an increase in stability following reconstruction, and a definitive tissue diagnosis. Initial surgical intervention for tumorous involvement of the cervical spine is useful in cases of mechanical instability, progressive deformity, or impending deformity with the potential for neurologic embarrassment (6). Additional indications include intractable pain that is unresponsive to nonsurgical measures and a worsening neurologic deficit in the presence of documented neural compression.

GENERAL PRINCIPLES

Revision surgery following a failed decompression or stabilization procedure can be divided into acute or delayed reoperations (34). A reoperation in the perioperative period may be for an early infection, hematoma, cerebrospinal fluid leak, incorrect level, graft extrusion, or early instrumentation failure. A delayed reoperation may be necessary in patients who present with radiographic evidence of impending reconstruction failure, progression of symptoms related to tumor proliferation or recurrence, or loss of stability at the previous surgical site.

The cervical spine is considered unstable following a previous tumor decompression and stabilization when it is unable to prevent physiologic loads from causing injury to the neural elements (41). In the case of a noncompressed spinal cord, the decision to revise prior surgery is more difficult and depends on the nature and degree of pathology and the degree of instability that is present. The operative approach, that is, anterior, posterior, or combined procedure, and the type of decompression and stabilization procedure are based on tumor type, location of destruction, degree of instability, experience of the surgical team, anticipated response to surgery, and the patient's overall medical condition (9,17,20,23,28,33).

In general, the aggressiveness of the disease and the initial surgical treatment present a unique clinical situation that may evolve into a myriad of potential complications. These complications can be divided into five broad categories:

- A tumor may have initially been inadequately resected, and the remaining neoplastic tissue may continue to proliferate, resulting in neurologic compromise and instability.
- Surgery may have completely removed the metastatic foci, but because of its aggressive nature, metastatic recurrence may deposit in noncontiguous spinal areas, causing mechanical and neurologic instability.
- Surgical removal of a tumor without reconstruction may have left the spine unstable because of the degree of bony and soft tissue decompression.
- Surgical reconstruction following decompression may not have been adequate biomechanically, resulting in a progressive deformity.
- Reconstruction may be compromised by the use of grafting substances that have the potential to lose their stability as a result of nonhealing (bone grafting exposed to radiation) or early fatigue failure (acrylic cement used in posterior spinal reconstruction).

The goals of a reoperation following surgery for tumors of the cervical spine are to decompress the neural elements if necessary and stabilize the spinal elements. As before any operation, a detailed history and physical examination provide information on the aggressiveness of the tumor disease in terms of its temporal recurrence and its effect on the overall well-being of the patient—that is, the patient's neurologic, nutritional, and emotional status. A thorough understanding of the histology and grade of the tumor is beneficial, with a general understanding of the overall prognosis, before deciding on the degree and complexity of surgical intervention that are necessary to benefit the patient.

The most useful imaging study before revision tumor surgery of the cervical spine is a magnetic resonance image with gadolinium. This study clearly defines the extent of cord and root compression, bony involvement, and scar tissue differentiation in the absence of ferromagnetic interference. Axial computed tomography (CT) with sagittal and coronal reconstruction provides additional information on the degree of bone involvement and its structural competence through bone mineral evaluation, predicting its response to various grafting and instrumentation procedures. Myelography may also be necessary before CT scanning if significant artifact is noted on magnetic resonance scanning. The choice of grafting material, if any; the use of methylmethacrylate; and the type of instrumentation are predicated on the extent of tumor destruction, the viability of the host, and the experience of the treating surgeons. As with all reoperations, the surgical approach may be complicated with abundant scar tissue deposition, which may obscure important neural and vascular structures, making the surgical exposure difficult.

The patient's life expectancy plays an important role in the decision to proceed with a revision operation (10,28), with more aggressive surgery reserved for patients with greater than 6 months to live. In addition, as with the primary procedure, the location of the tumor within the spine dictates the best surgical approach (6,19). Anterior tumors involving the vertebral body are best approached anteriorly, whereas tumors involving the posterior vertebral canal and bony elements are best approached posteriorly.

SURGICAL APPROACH

If an anterior revision surgical approach is selected, the surgeon should preoperatively evaluate the integrity of the vocal cords to determine the function of the right and the left recurrent laryngeal nerves. If both are functioning, the surgeon may wish to approach the cervical spine from the opposite side of the original surgery to avoid injury to the recurrent laryngeal nerve as a result of scarring. If ipsilateral vocal cord paralysis is found, one may choose to reoperate through the previous approach so as to avoid the potential for complete bilateral vocal cord paralysis, with injury to the contralateral recurrent laryngeal nerve (36).

An anterior surgical approach begins with the patient supine on the operating table with a bolster along the upper thoracic spine so as to present the neck more favorably to the surgeon. The chin may be turned slightly away from the surgical site, but rotation must be kept to a minimum to prevent distortion of surgical anatomy. Lower cervical surgery and radiographic exposure may be facilitated with gentle downward traction placed on the shoulders during the operation through tape application or other methods. When operating near the cervicothoracic junction on the left side, one must be cognizant of the presence of the thoracic duct.

A transverse incision can be used for exposure of a planned corpectomy. If a multiple level corpectomy is intended, a longitudinal incision along the anterior border of the sternocleidomastoid muscle should be made. The subsequent surgical dissection is accomplished through the standard anterolateral approach to the cervical spine. After the required decompression is completed, anterior distraction of the vertebral bodies can be accomplished through traction on previously applied cervical tongs or a halo ring or with a vertebral distraction system such as the Caspar device.

The posterior approach to the cervical spine involves placing the patient prone in a reverse Trendelenburg's position (to reduce blood loss), with the head placed on a padded horseshoe or Mayfield pin headrest. The exposure of the posterior elements is routine, with lateral intraoperative radiography confirming the appropriate cervical levels.

INADEQUATE RESECTION

The initial surgical resection of a cervical spine tumor, especially malignant and metastatic lesions, often leaves behind minute or microscopic tumor remnants after decompression. This tumor presence, depending on the tissue type, size, and response to adjunctive treatment, may continue to proliferate, resulting in potential neurologic compromise as well as late instability. A preoperative magnetic resonance image with gadolinium and CT with or without myelography, if necessary, should allow the surgeon

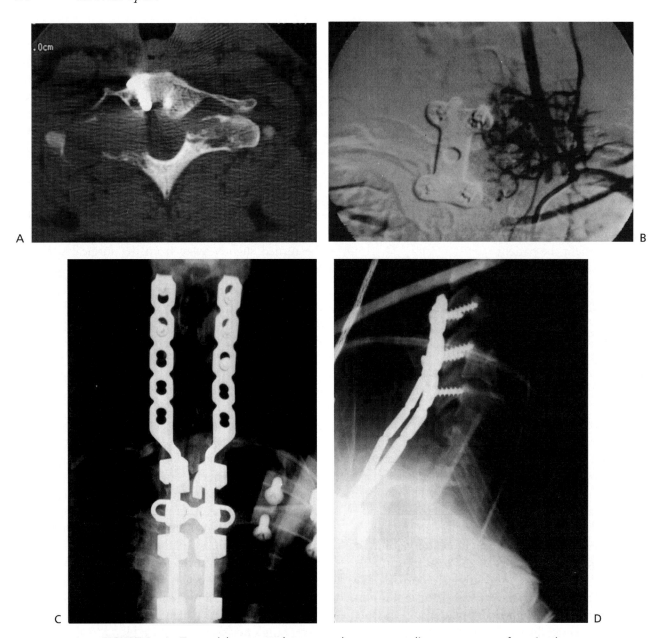

FIGURE 1. **A:** Transaxial computed tomography scan revealing recurrence of an inadequately resected thyroid metastatic lesion of the cervicothoracic junction after a cervical decompression and fusion with instrumentation. **B:** Preoperative vertebral arteriogram revealing the extensive arterial blood supply to the recurrent spinal lesion. Anteroposterior **(C)** and lateral **(D)** radiograph following an extensive anterior decompression with allograft fibula reconstruction followed by posterior segmented plate, screw, and hook reconstruction.

to accurately identify the location and extent of the lesion as well as the optimum operative approach to expose the desired spinal elements (32). Due to the high potential for future imaging needs, titanium implants or other nonferromagnetic devices are desirable for spinal reconstruction to ease visualization of important bony and neurologic structures (1). Such image clarity has been demonstrated in the postoperative period by Hosono et al. (22) with the use of a nonferromagnetic ceramic vertebral body prosthesis implanted in 28 cervical spine tumor patients.

The removal of previously applied instrumentation to gain access to the desired lesion often makes reimplantation at the same spinal elements, especially with screw attachment devices, impossible because of a lack of stability. The surgeon should be aware of this during preoperative planning and determine what vertebral elements can accept a particular spinal device and what material, usually an allograft with or without a metallic adjunctive device, can be used as a spacer if the anterior vertebral elements are removed.

A difficult problem encountered during a revision anterior cervical vertebral decompression is identify-

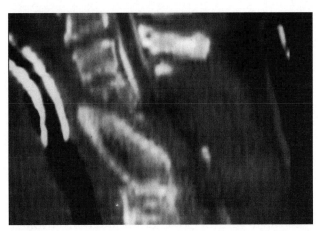

FIGURE 2. Lateral radiograph revealing iliac crest graft extrusion following local recurrence of metastatic prostate cancer.

ing with accuracy the precise location of the vertebral vessels to avoid injury to these structures. This identification is facilitated through the use of a preoperative selective vertebral arteriogram or magnetic resonance angiography.

Due to the morbidity attendant with revision surgery in this class of patients, it is preferable to obtain optimum stabilization of the spinal elements at the time of surgery to avoid the use of cumbersome external immobilization devices such as a halo fixator. This

can be accomplished by performing a circumferential stabilization procedure or using segmental instrumentation posteriorly as well as an internal fixation adjunct to a vertebral body spacer anteriorly (30) (Fig. 1).

RECURRENCE

Tumor recurrence at or immediately adjacent to a site of previous cervical decompression and reconstruction may lead to mechanical instability, pain, and neurologic compromise, as well as loosening and failure of existing internal fixation (2,34,39) (Fig. 2). In a study of vertebral body prosthetic replacements, Hosono et al. (22) noted local tumor recurrence in 24% of their patients, with the largest recurrence rates noted in individuals with thyroid and renal cancer. These findings were thought to be due to the fact that patients with thyroid cancer usually had a prolonged life expectancy and that renal cancer was least responsive to postoperative radiation therapy. In a study by Hammerberg (19) on 56 patients treated for spinal metastases, two required reoperation as a result of same-level recurrence and neurologic complications. Depending on the clinical status of patients and their life expectancy, an aggres-

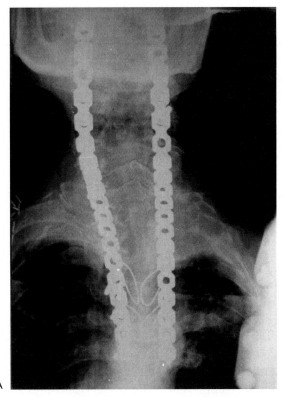

A

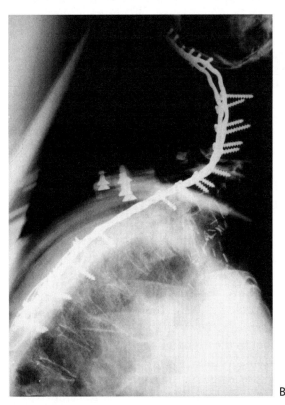

B

FIGURE 3. Anteroposterior **(A)** and lateral **(B)** radiographs following an extensive revision posterior cervical decompression and segmental stabilization for recurrent metastatic breast carcinoma.

sive recurrent lesion may require extensive decompression of the vertebral elements over many segments (Fig. 3). Patients with less than 1 year to live are often not candidates for autogenous bone graft reconstruction in this situation. Instead, synthetic materials, as with a revision decompression for an initial inadequate decompression, can be used to provide immediate support and stability in the postoperative period.

The direct implantation of tumorlytic agents during revision surgery, such as radioactive implants or chemotherapy, is a possible means of suppressing or destroying tumor proliferation while decreasing toxicity on a systemic basis (2). Wang et al. (39) tested a methotrexate-impregnated methylmethacrylate implant in a rabbit model in an effort to decrease the incidence of local recurrence following decompression of spinal metastases. They noted that up to 2 g of methotrexate in 40 g of cement did not alter the biomechanical properties of the cement construct. The continuous release of the drug did not appear to have any systemic toxic effects on the rabbit but did have a significant effect on tumor load. Pulmonary metastases were significantly reduced in proportion to the amount of methotrexate in the acrylic. Extension of this concept to human spinal tumor treatment is theoretically possible and requires further investigation.

In general, patients who present with clinically significant recurrence of tumor should be evaluated as previously described with any proposed revision procedure based on the extent of disease, overall medical condition and life expectancy, and the technical feasibility of the proposed surgical procedure. In general, a rigid spinal construct should be developed with the appropriate fixation devices, usually necessitating a circumferential surgical procedure.

REMOVAL OF TUMOR WITHOUT RECONSTRUCTION

In the majority of surgical tumor procedures that are performed to decompress the cervical neural elements, a stabilization procedure is necessary to prevent instability and early or late deformity with resultant neurologic compromise. Only in rare instances, such as removal of a small intramedullary cervical tumor, is the degree of bony and ligamentous removal minimal without the need for a concomitant stabilization procedure. As long as a thorough understanding of the biomechanics of the cervical spine is appreciated, such a decompression can be performed without an adjunctive fusion procedure. Unfortu-

nately, long-term stability of the cervical spine is not always an important concern at the time of surgical decompression for tumor, with many patients experiencing difficulties with late pain as well as weakness over time because of a loss of stability. One should be cognizant of the fact that if greater than 50% of a facet is removed unilaterally following a cervical laminectomy, a potentially unstable clinical situation exists (9,36). Anytime that an anterior tumorous lesion is removed, a reconstruction and stabilization procedure is warranted (4) (Fig. 4).

Surgical failure rates related to instability are especially high when a posterior laminectomy without fusion is attempted in the decompression of the spinal cord with a tumor located in the anterior vertebral elements (24,25). In fact, the incidence of deformity after laminectomy without reconstruction is highest in the cervical spine (44). The potential for this complication, related to the biomechanics of the cervical spine, is highlighted by a report by Mikawa et al. (27), who found that up to 36% of adults who undergo a decompression for a cervical radiculopathy or myelopathy show postoperative changes in curvature, with a frank spinal deformity developing in 14% of patients. Often, a laminectomy in a patient with a cervical tumor with vertebral body involvement results in a swan neck deformity or localized kyphosis, putting at risk the neurologic integrity of the spinal cord. Herkowitz (21) examined a series of patients who underwent a cervical laminectomy and bilateral partial facetectomy. In this population of patients with cervical degenerative disease, a kyphotic deformity developed in 3 of 12 patients within 2 years of surgery. A reconstruction in this situation usually entails a multilevel cervical corpectomy and grafting procedure followed by a posterior cervical fusion and instrumentation with lateral mass or pedicular fixation (2).

In the setting of a fixed kyphotic deformity, the tented and deformed spinal cord is often dysfunctional as a result of ischemia or myelomalacia. This is important if the surgeon plans to correct the patient's sagittal plane deformity through distraction, which may result in catastrophic loss of neural function. Often, anterior decompression of the tented spinal cord without correction of the sagittal plane deformity followed by a circumferential stabilization procedure is adequate for neurologic recovery (15). If distraction is desired to improve sagittal alignment, a trial of preoperative skeletal traction using a halo ring or cervical tongs should be considered (36). Any correction of the preoperative sagittal alignment in the awake and cooperative

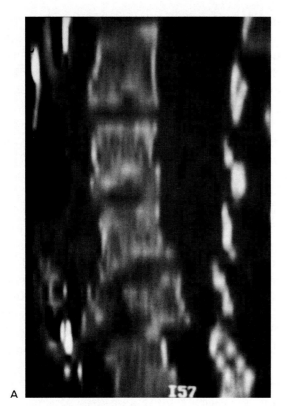
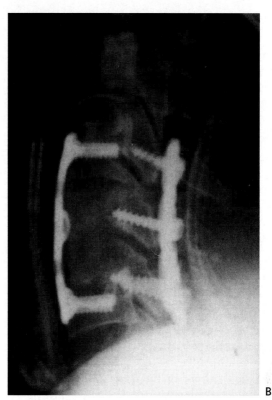

FIGURE 4. A: Computed tomography scan of sagittal reconstruction revealing collapse of the anterior cervical spinal column after previous partial anterior resection without reconstruction of a vertebral metastasis located within the C-5 vertebral body. **B:** Lateral radiograph revealing restoration of normal cervical alignment after an anterior decompression and circumferential reconstruction with instrumentation.

patient greatly facilitates the technical difficulty of the surgical procedure, lessening the risk of neurologic injury.

A combined anterior-posterior cervical decompression and fusion following a failed cervical tumor procedure with deformity provides optimum circumferential stability to allow early rehabilitation without the need for cumbersome external immobilization. In a review of 222 cervical spine fusions for traumatic injury, Capen et al. (7) found no examples of nonunion, loss of reduction, or graft extrusion when a combined or circumferential anterior-posterior fusion was performed. This was in contrast to the occasional reporting of these complications when only a single-stage anterior or posterior procedure was done.

The grafting material used anteriorly in reconstruction procedures after failed surgery is usually a fibular allograft when corpectomies involving three or more levels are performed. Some authors have used a titanium mesh cage filled with allograft or methylmethacrylate for improved early stability (12). An anterior plate may or may not be useful, depending on the length of anterior fusion and the technical difficulty of plate application.

INADEQUATE RECONSTRUCTION WITH PROGRESSIVE DEFORMITY

Previous surgical treatment for a cervical spine tumor may have inadequately reconstructed the spinal column. The immediate consequence is the potential for continued pain as a result of occult instability. As time passes, more significant instability patterns may develop, compromising neurologic function (2,34). Unfortunately, the surgeon is again handicapped by the difficulties of dissecting through scarred tissue planes to expose and remove the previously inserted implants and perform, in some cases, a larger decompression followed by a more extensive reconstruction. If the patient has no objective signs, symptoms, or radiographic evidence of significant spinal cord compromise, a stabilization procedure from the unadulterated side—that is, posteriorly—following an anterior reconstruction may be possible.

GRAFTING MATERIALS

The surgical reconstruction following decompression of cervical spine tumors may be compromised by the use of an improperly selected grafting substance that loosened prematurely or failed to heal and fractured as a result of adjunctive treatment modalities or a prolonged life span. The potential for autogeneic or allogeneic bone graft nonhealing is generally compromised in the immunocompromised patient with malignancy. This is especially true if the grafting procedure is followed by irradiation or chemotherapy (2,5,13,14,17,20). Two common examples of grafting or spacer failures include the use of methylmethacrylate acrylic bone cement in applications that it cannot support or in which it is not properly reinforced and the use of early or large-dose radiation therapy following allograft or autograft reconstruction after decompression. A fatigue fracture within a synthetic grafting composite or nonhealing may lead to significant pain and possible deformity, requiring a subsequent revision procedure (3,16).

Many authors have cited the usefulness of methylmethacrylate in the acute surgical stabilization of the spine following a tumor resection (12,18,20,23,26,30,34,35,38). Biomechanically, when used anteriorly, methylmethacrylate confers immediate and rigid stabilization to the applied spinal segment and maintains this strength for approxi-

mately 16 to 18 weeks *in vivo*, at which time it begins to weaken compared to a healing autogenous bone graft control (38). It is reasonable, therefore, to consider the use of an autogenous graft source in patients with a life expectancy of greater than 5 or 6 months (8,12,18,28,34).

The usefulness of methylmethacrylate is directly related to its application (24,37). Acrylic cement used to supplement a posterior fixation is biomechanically loaded in flexion and tension, stresses in which methylmethacrylate has been shown to be the weakest and most susceptible to fatigue and failure (3,20,40,43). In an *in vivo* canine model (42,43), posterior C4-5 methylmethacrylate and wire constructs lost their mechanical stability within 1 month of application, whereas a comparison bone graft composite was found to be biomechanically equivalent to the control cervical spine at 2 months. Methylmethacrylate is strongest in compression and therefore is most useful in anterior vertebrectomy reconstruction, where it is subject to a compressive load. Metastatic disease most often affects the anterior spinal elements, making such patients with an abbreviated life span and anterior thecal sac compression potential candidates for methylmethacrylate reconstruction.

The strength, ability to withstand bending loads, and longevity of methylmethacrylate fixation are greatly increased when used in conjunction with internal fixation within its substance, such as pins, rods, wires, and screws, and at times alongside bone graft, either autograft or allograft. The viability of the cement construct is also improved substantially when combined with a contiguous stabilizing device (8,11,12,17,19,23). To prevent early failure, it is critical that the internal fixation device be seated in solid, healthy bone, for it is the stability of the metal-bone interface that is predictive of early loosening of methylmethacrylate application (Fig. 5). Although inflammation has not been reported as a complication of acrylic application, the use of cement is not advised, due to its foreign body potential, in contaminated fields such as the transoropharyngeal approach, or in cases of resolved or active infection (10).

In a study of 52 cervical spine fracture-dislocations, Duff et al. (11) concluded that the success of acrylic cement stabilization depended on the stability of the adjunctive internal fixation device used at its junction with the host bone as well as with the bone cement. These authors noted that in applying these principles, only 2 of the 52 patients needed a surgical revision for methylmethacrylate loosening or infection. Dunn (12) reported early failure of anterior cervical methyl-

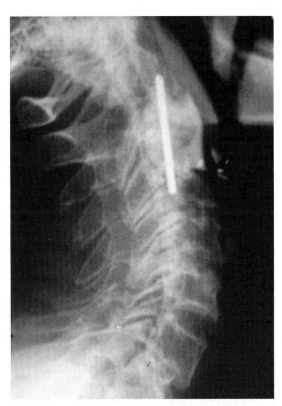

FIGURE 5. Lateral radiograph revealing vertebral body replacement of a breast metastasis lesion with methylmethacrylate cement and Steiman pin fixation with the contiguous vertebral bodies.

methacrylate application for tumor disease in two of ten patients and late failure of posterior application in 2 of 14 patients. One patient from each group required a revision surgical procedure. Halligan and Hubschmann (18) reported on three patients who underwent an anterior cervical corpectomy and stabilization with methylmethacrylate for trauma with late extrusion of their cement graft. Two of the patients experienced erosion of the esophagus with a subsequent infection. McAfee et al. (26) reported on nine cases of methylmethacrylate failure after surgery for metastatic spinal disease. Eight of the nine had radiographic evidence of graft/fixation loosening. All failures occurred at the bone-cement interface, five after an anterior vertebral body replacement and three after posterior stabilization. All failures were the result of biomechanical loosening of the cement construct and were not due to tumor recurrence. The authors noted the need for an extensive surgical exposure as well as the magnitude of the surgical procedure necessary in revising six of the nine patients.

In summary, the need for revision of methylmethacrylate stabilization following decompression for metastatic disease is directly related to the longevity of the patient and the approach used in its application. Many authors find methylmethacrylate useful for anterior stabilization under compression in patients with less than 3 months to live. The use of cement in posterior applications is prone to a high failure rate and should be avoided if possible.

The effects of radiation treatment on the type of grafting procedure, the timing of its application as well as the magnitude of dosage, have been reviewed by several authors. A retrospective analysis was conducted on 25 patients who underwent an anterior vertebrectomy and bone graft fusion for a spinal neoplasm treated with adjunctive radiation therapy (14). Seven patients received preoperative radiation, 13 postoperative radiation, and 5 preoperative as well as postoperative radiation treatment. Twenty-one grafts were autogenous iliac crest, two were autogenous fibula, one an autogenous rib, and one a humeral allograft. At follow-up radiographically, 21 patients had a solid fusion, with four manifesting a pseudoarthrodesis, for a 16% nonunion rate. Two of the four nonunions and 8 of the 21 fusion cases had a posterior surgical stabilization at or before their anterior procedure. The average radiation dose given was found to be significantly higher ($p < .003$) for the nonunion group (4,875 cg vs. 3,518 cg), with all four patients receiving greater than 4,000 cg, one preoperatively and three postoperatively. Only four of the healed fusion cases were irradiated above 4,000 cg. The small sample size prevented statis-

tical analysis of whether graft type or timing of radiotherapy affected solid fusion.

In a rabbit posterior lumbar fusion model with autogenous iliac crest graft performed by Bouchard et al. (5), animals were separated into a control group, a preoperative radiation group, an immediate postoperative radiation group, and a delayed (21-day) postoperative radiation group. Biomechanically, no significant difference was seen between the control and delayed radiation groups. The difference was significant, however, between the control and immediate radiation groups, with the latter being significantly less stiff in extension, flexion, compression, and left lateral bending. The preoperative radiation group was significantly less stiff than the control in extension and compression. Histologically, retarded bone graft healing was most significant in the immediate postoperative radiation group in which only fibrous healing was found, followed by the preoperative radiation group. The authors suggested that at least 3 and preferably 4 to 6 weeks should elapse before the administration of radiation treatment after a posterior fusion procedure.

In a canine autogenous iliac crest model performed by Emery et al. (13), 22 beagles were divided into four subsets, including a control group, a preoperative radiation group, a postoperative day three radiation group, and a delayed (21-day) radiation group. Biomechanically, there was no significant difference between the nonirradiated group, the preoperative radiation group, and the delayed (21-day) postoperative radiation group. A significant decrease in stiffness was found in the postoperative day three irradiation group, and this group also showed the lowest histologic scores for healing, revascularization, and new bone development. Although the delayed (21-day) postoperative radiation group did show slightly decreased histologic scores, it is possible that these would have improved had the dogs been given more than 3 months to heal their grafts.

In summary, the data suggest that a delayed radiation treatment regimen is more advantageous for successful bone graft healing than early postoperative or preoperative treatment. Preoperative radiation treatment, although potentially adversely affecting wound healing, may not significantly prevent bone graft healing to the degree once thought.

CONCLUSION

The initial surgery for cervical spine tumor decompression and reconstruction may eventually fail as a result of the aggressiveness of the disease, poor host tissue viability, or an error in operative decision making. Five common scenarios resulting in the need for subsequent revision cervical surgery have been outlined for the reader. Reoperations are often complicated by the presence of scar tissue, with obscuration of tissue planes making revision surgery technically challenging. The appropriate use of specific imaging modalities allows the surgeon to identify the location and extent of tumor proliferation, scarring, and the location of specific neurovascular elements. The need for revision surgery is predicated on the overall condition and prognosis of the patient, often requiring the use of synthetic materials with adjunctive internal fixation to gain immediate stability without the need for cumbersome external immobilization. When autogeneic or allogeneic bone grafts are used, the harmful effects of perioperative adjunctive radiation or chemotherapy may be realized and if possible temporarily delayed to improve healing success. As with any revision cervical procedure, a circumferential stabilization procedure often results in excellent stability and pain relief, with correction of a preexisting deformity, vitally important in this class of patients.

REFERENCES

1. Alleyne CH, Rodts GE, Haid RW. Corpectomy and stabilization with methylmethacrylate in patients with metastatic disease of the spine: a technical note. *J Spinal Disord* 1995;8(6):439–443.

2. An HS, Balderston RA, Simeone FA. Complications of spinal tumor surgery. In: Balderston RA, An HS, eds. *Complications in spinal surgery.* Philadelphia: WB Saunders, 1991:79–104.

3. Andreshak TG, An HS. Complications of cervical spine surgery. In: An HS, Simpson JM, eds. *Surgery of the cervical spine.* Philadelphia: Williams & Wilkins, 1994:401–426.

4. Atanasiu JP, Badatcheff F, Pidhorz L. Metastatic lesions of the cervical spine: a retrospective analysis of 20 cases. *Spine* 1993;18(10):1279–1284.

5. Bouchard JA, Koka A, Bensusan JS, et al. Effects of irradiation on posterior spinal fusions: a rabbit model. *Spine* 1994;19(16):1836–1841.

6. Cantu RC. Osseous fusion of the cervical, thoracic, and lumbar spine with primary and metastatic spine tumors. In: Sundaresan N, Schmidek HH, Schiller AL, et al., eds. *Tumors of the spine.* Philadelphia: WB Saunders, 1990:446–456.

7. Capen DA, Garland DE, Waters RL. Surgical stabilization of the cervical spine. *Clin Orthop* 1985;196:229–237.

8. Clark CR, Keggi KJ, Panjabi MM. Methylmethacrylate stabilization of the cervical spine. *J Bone Joint Surg* 1984;66-A(1):40–46.

9. Cybulski GR. Methods of surgical stabilization for metastatic disease of the spine. *Neurosurgery* 1989;25(2):240–252.

10. DiLorenzo N, Delfini R, Ciappetta P, et al. Primary tumors of the cervical spine: surgical experience with 38 cases. *Surg Neurol* 1992;38:12–18.

11. Duff TA, Khan A, Corbett JE. Surgical stabilization of cervical spinal fractures using methyl methacrylate. *J Neurosurg* 1992;76:440–443.

12. Dunn EJ. The role of methyl methacrylate in the stabilization and replacement of tumors of the cervical spine: a project of the Cervical Spine Research Society. *Spine* 1977;2(1):15–24.

13. Emery SE, Brazinski MS, Koka A, et al. The biological and biomechanical effects of irradiation on anterior spinal bone grafts in a canine model. *J Bone Joint Surg* 1994;76-A:540–548.

14. Emery SE, Hughes SS, Hungals WA, et al. The fate of anterior vertebral bone grafts in patients irradiated for neoplasm. *Clin Orthop* 1994;300:207–212.

15. Farcey JPC. Revision surgery in late spine instability, including sacral stabilization. In: Holtzman RNN, McCormick PC, Farcy JPC, eds. *Contemporary perspectives in neurosurgery: spinal instability.* Philadelphia: JB Lippincott Co, 1991:489–506.

16. Fielding JW. The status of arthrodesis of the cervical spine: a current concepts review. *J Bone Joint Surg* 1988;70A:1571–1574.

17. Green DA, Garfin SR. Tumors of the cervical spine. In: An HS, Simpson JM, eds. *Surgery of the cervical spine.* Philadelphia: Williams & Wilkins, 1994:307–324.

18. Halligan M, Hubschmann OR. Short-term and long-term failures of anterior polymethylmethacrylate construct with esophageal perforation. *Spine* 1993;18(6):759–761.

19. Hammerberg KW. Surgical treatment of metastatic disease. *Spine* 1992;17(10):1148–1153.

20. Harrington KD. Metastatic disease of the spine. *J Bone Joint Surg* 1986;68A:1110–1115.

21. Herkowitz HN. A comparison of anterior cervical fusion, cervical laminectomy, and cervical laminoplasty for the surgical management of multiple level spondylotic radiculopathy. *Spine* 1988;13:774–780.

22. Hosono N, Yonenobu K, Fuji T, et al. Orthopaedic management of spinal metastases. *Clin Orthop* 1995;312:148–159.

23. Kostuik JP, Errico TJ, Gleason TF, et al. Spinal stabilization of vertebral column tumors. *Spine* 1988;13(3):250–256.

24. Levine AM. Operative techniques for treatment of metastatic disease of the spine. *Semin Spine Surg* 1990;2(3):210–227.

25. Marchesi DG, Boos N, Aebi M. Surgical treatment of tumors of the cervical spine and first two thoracic vertebrae. *J Spinal Disord* 1993;6(6):489–496.

26. McAfee PC, Bohlman HH, Ducker T, et al. Failure of stabilization of the spine with methylmethacrylate: a retrospective analysis of twenty-four cases. *J Bone Joint Surg* 1986;68-A(8):1145–1157.

27. Mikawa Y, Shikata J, Yamamuro T. Spinal deformity and instability after multi-level cervical laminectomy. *Spine* 1987;12(1):6–11.

28. O'Connor MI, Currier BL. Metastatic bone disease: metastatic disease of the spine. *Orthopaedics* 1992;15(5):611–620.

29. Pettine KA, Klassen RA. Osteoid-osteoma and osteoblastoma of the spine. *J Bone Joint Surg* 1986;68A(3):354–361.

30. Rompe JD, Eysel P, Hopf C, et al. Metastatic spinal cord compression—options for surgical treatment. *Acta Neurochir* 1993;123:135–140.

31. Rosenberg A, Schiller AL. Tumorous lesions of the spine: an overview. In: Sundaresan N, Schmidek HH, Schiller AL, eds. *Tumors of the spine.* Philadelphia: WB Saunders, 1990:82–85.

32. Simeone FA. Intraspinal neoplasms. In: Horwitz NH, Rizzoli HV, eds. *Postoperative complications of extracranial neurological surgery.* Baltimore: Williams & Wilkins, 1987:120–137.

33. Smith MD, Phillips WA, Hensinger RN. Complications of fusion to the upper cervical spine. *Spine* 1991;16(7):702–705.

34. Sonntag VKH, Herman JM. Reoperation of the cervical spine for degenerative disease and tumor. *Clin Neurosurg* 1992;39:244–269.

35. Timlin M, Thalgott J, Ameriks J, et al. Management of metastatic tumors to the spine using simple plate fixation. *Am Surg* 1995;61:704–708.

36. Vaccaro AR, Mirkovic S, Bauer RD, et al. Revision lumbar and cervical degenerative spine surgery: indications and techniques. In: Bridwell KH, DeWald RL, eds. *The textbook of spinal surgery,* 2nd ed. Philadelphia: Lippincott–Raven Publishers, 1997:1457–1493.

37. Van den Bent MJ, Oosting J, Wouda EJ, et al. Anterior cervical discectomy with or without fusion with acrylate. *Spine* 1996;21(7):834–840.

38. Wang GJ, Reger SI, Shao ZH, et al. Comparative strength of anterior spinal fixation with bone graft or polymethylmethacrylate. *Clin Orthop* 1984;188:303–308.

39. Wang HM, Galasko CSB, Crank S, et al. Methotrexate loaded acrylic cement in the management of skeletal metastases: biomechanical, biological, and systemic effect. *Clin Orthop* 1995;312:173–186.

40. Weinstein JN, McLain RF. Tumors of the spine. In: Rothman RH, Simeone FA, eds. *The spine,* 3rd ed. Philadelphia: WB Saunders, 1992:1279–1318.

41. White AA III, Panjabi MM. Problems of clinical instability in the human spine. In: White AA III, Panjabi MM, eds. *Clinical biomechanics of the spine.* Philadelphia: JB Lippincott Co, 1978:278–378.

43. Whitehill R, Reger S, Weatherup N, et al. A biomechanical analysis of posterior cervical fusions using polymethylmethacrylate as an instantaneous fusion mass. *Spine* 1983;8(4):368–372.

42. Whitehill R, Barry JC. The evolution of stability in cervical spinal constructs using either autogenous bone graft or methylmethacrylate cement. *Spine* 1985;10(1):32–41.

44. Yasuoka S, Peterson HA, MacCarty CS. Incidence of spinal column deformity after multilevel laminectomy in children and adults. *J Neurosurg* 1982;57:441–445.

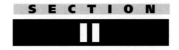

SECTION II

THORACIC SPINE

THORACIC SPINE: EVALUATION

NEILL M. WRIGHT, FARID F. SHAFAIE, AND CARL LAURYSSEN

Evaluation of the patient in whom previous thoracic spine surgery has failed requires an even more thorough history, physical examination, and review of radiologic studies than that of the patient on initial presentation. The spine surgeon needs to ascertain not only if further interventions are warranted but also the initial indications for surgery, the type of surgery performed, the temporal course of the patient's symptoms, and physical and neurologic signs since initial presentation. An approach specific to the evaluation of the patient with a failed thoracic spine is described, with special attention given to findings on history and physical examination, imaging techniques, and a directed differential diagnosis of immediate, early, and late failures.

CLINICAL EVALUATION

History

As the patient with a failed spine by definition has a complicated medical history, the current complaints and physical examination findings must not be viewed in isolation. The medical history obtained from the patient should begin with the initial complaint and symptoms, and, wherever possible, the initial surgeon's notes should be reviewed to confirm physical examination findings. Disorders of bone homeostasis, such as osteopenia and osteoporosis, and medications that affect bone homeostasis, such as diphosphonates, glucocorticoids, and mithramycin (6), should be identified. The patient's response to nonsurgical treatment, including therapy and pharmaceuticals, should be noted. Preoperative radiographs should be obtained and reviewed to appreciate the patient's preoperative spine and to better assess the effects of subsequent surgical intervention.

The patient's previous spinal surgery should also be thoroughly investigated. Not only should the indications for the initial surgery be confirmed, but also whether the patient had the appropriate surgical technique performed. Detailed operative notes should be reviewed to document which surgical approach was used, how much decompression was needed, which vertebral levels were stabilized, and which instrumentation system was implanted. The surgeon should take note of any intraoperative difficulties. Knowledge of intraoperative events not only aids in the diagnosis of the failed spine but can also help warn of potential hazards during revision surgery.

The temporal course of the patient's symptoms since the initial surgery, as well as the current complaints, aids greatly in the diagnosis. The patient who had no immediate benefit from surgery is markedly different from the one who had several months of improvement followed by a steady decline in function. The surgeon should ascertain which symptoms improved or worsened, even transiently, as well as changes in analgesic use and level of activity. The location, character, radiation, intensity, and duration of the patient's pain should also be identified.

Specific history questions with respect to the thoracic spine patient include those relating to motor and sensory functions of the lower extremities, bowel and bladder control, sexual function, gait, stance, and posture. Respiratory control should be carefully assessed, as the thoracic kyphosis, intercostal musculature, and abdominal muscles innervated by the lower thoracic nerve roots all contribute to respiratory capacity. The patient should be questioned about chest, abdominal, and back sensation, although because of overlapping dermatomes, even complete sectioning of a single thoracic nerve root often leaves no sensory deficit. Patients with thoracic nerve root lesions may complain of severe burning dysthesias radiating around the chest wall either unilaterally or bilaterally. These pains are exacerbated by any activity that increases intraspinal pressure, such as coughing, Valsalva maneuvers, and neck flexion (11). The patient should also be questioned about changes in posture and stance, as worsening kyphosis can dramatically interfere with daily activities.

Psychosocial factors should not be overlooked. Several clinical series (44,53) have underscored the prevalence of serious concomitant psychological factors in the failed spine patient population. These factors range from addiction-prone behavior to personality disorders

[*Diagnostic and Statistical Manual*, Fourth Edition (*DSM-IV*) axis II] to frank psychiatric illness (*DSM-IV* axis I). In addition, other series (8) have shown patients on worker's compensation to have a disproportionate rate of failed spine surgery. Although this is not meant to suggest that all patients have formal psychiatric evaluation, the surgeon should consider psychosocial factors, such as coping skills, educational and vocational history, marital history, and general daily pattern of living, to identify patients in whom further psychological examination is indicated.

Physical Examination

On general examination, the spine surgeon should note the overall health of the patient, including nutritional status. The postoperative spine patient is often clinically malnourished (16), with the malnourished state increasing the risk of infection, delayed wound healing, and surgical failure (35). All previous incisions should be carefully examined for signs of infection, dehiscence, or breakdown. The back should be inspected for signs of muscle spasm or local tenderness. Recumbent as well as standing blood pressure measurements should be obtained, as thoracic cord lesions above T-5 may cause impairment of vasomotor control (7). Throughout the examination, the surgeon should observe the patient during various maneuvers, looking for exaggerating behaviors, nonanatomic sensory complaints, or inconsistent performance that suggests the presence of psychosocial factors (43,73).

The stance and posture of the patient should be examined, paying special attention to the amount of thoracic kyphosis and sagittal balance. The current kyphotic curve should be compared to preoperative and prior postoperative visits to assess any significant progression. The surgeon should also look for any thoracic scoliosis. *Adult scoliosis* is defined as a spinal deformity of Cobb angle in the coronal plane of more than 10 degrees (3). The presence of scoliosis, or of progressive kyphosis, raises the suspicion of possible instrumentation or fusion failure or progressive degenerative disease. The patient's spine should also be assessed for range of motion, with pain on motion implying instability.

A detailed neurologic examination is performed. Although the thoracic spinal nerves are more difficult to assess than the cervical or lumbar region, much information can be obtained. On motor examination, the first thoracic nerve can be assessed by testing the functions of the median and ulnar nerves. The patient with an injured first thoracic nerve may have a claw hand deformity from median and ulnar nerve dysfunction. The degree of chest wall excursion on deep breathing helps evaluate intercostal muscle function and the corresponding upper thoracic nerve roots. Intercostal muscle paralysis results in retraction of the costal interspace during inspiration and bulging during coughing or Valsalva maneuvers (11). The strength of the anterior abdominal muscles, including the internal and external obliques, and the transverse and rectus abdomini, can help assess the lower thoracic nerve root function, although all but the rectus abdominis also receive innervation from the first lumbar nerve root via the iliohypogastric and ilioinguinal nerves. The patient may have difficulty arising from the recumbent position if these abdominal muscles are affected. Beevor's sign may be elicited with cord lesions at the T-10 level, with the umbilicus being pulled upward during head flexion against resistance as the intact upper abdominal muscles are unopposed by the weakened lower abdominal muscles (7). A thorough lower extremity motor examination should be performed to assess the thoracic cord as well.

Although the sensory functions of the thoracic nerve roots are more difficult to assess, a careful examination can still provide clues to the nature of the failed spine. The first thoracic sensory dermatome can be assessed from sensation of the medial arm. Unfortunately, sensory disturbances of isolated thoracic nerve roots are often predominantly or completely subjective, with few, if any, physical findings.

An examination of reflexes and gait can also help determine the presence of myelopathy. The injured first thoracic nerve may result in an impaired finger flexor reflex, although this may be preserved with an intact C-8 nerve root. Injury to the first thoracic nerve root often also involves sympathetic nerve fibers coursing upward to join the superior cervical ganglion, with subsequent development of an ipsilateral Horner's syndrome. As the lower six thoracic nerves innervate the anterior abdominal muscles, abdominal reflexes should be assessed. Lesions above T-6 cause a loss of all abdominal reflexes, whereas lesions below T-12 have complete preservation. Lesions at the T-10 level have preservation only of the upper and middle abdominal reflexes (7).

RADIOGRAPHIC IMAGING

Radiographic imaging is an essential adjunct to the evaluation of the patient who has undergone thoracic spine surgery. Many imaging modalities are available for evaluation of the thoracic spine, including conventional radiographs, conventional tomography, myelography, computed tomography (CT), magnetic resonance imaging (MRI), nuclear medicine techniques, thermography, and electrodiagnostic studies.

In recent years, CT and MRI have provided significant advances in the understanding of spinal disorders and have essentially eliminated exploratory spinal surgery. Appropriately ordered diagnostic imaging plays an important role in the correct diagnosis of patients with thoracic spine pathology, as well as subsequent preoperative planning and postoperative evaluation.

Imaging Approach

The spine surgeon and the neuroradiologist should collaborate to determine the optimal imaging modality for each individual case. Comparison with previous spinal radiographic examinations is essential to determine any progression or resolution of the initial pathology. In addition, knowledge of the patient's history, clinical signs and symptoms, and prior surgical procedures is important in evaluating imaging studies. It is useful for radiologists to be familiar with the surgical fixation devices used at their institution and to understand their intended function to properly evaluate the postoperative spine and diagnose any potential complications.

Conventional Plain Film Radiographs

Postoperative imaging with plain film radiography is obtained as a routine follow-up in most patients following spinal surgery. However, a more complete neuroradiology workup is obtained for patients with possible complications or failures of instrumentation. Conventional plain radiographs in the early postoperative period are an inexpensive modality to accurately check for spinal stability, hardware position, restoration of the normal spinal curvature, and reconstruction of the vertebral column. Complex radiographs in the late postoperative period, approximately 9 months to 1 year, provide further data regarding stabilization and bony fusion.

Multiple views of the spine are vital because findings may only be visible in one projection. These findings often provide the initial clue regarding signs of infection, recurrent pathology, or graft failure. In cases of spinal fusion, the lateral and anterior-posterior radiographs are usually sufficient (26). Although pseud-

arthrosis remains difficult to detect accurately and consistently with radiographic imaging, it may be evidenced on plain radiographs by graft displacement, bone resorption, a sclerotic line at the interface between graft and native bone, or a visible halo around implanted instrumentation. Dynamic radiograph films with flexion and extension views are helpful in establishing relative motion in patients who have undergone fusion. Pseudarthrosis should be suspected when flexion/extension views reveal abnormal motion at the level of fusion.

Conventional and Computed Tomography

In some institutions, conventional x-ray polytomography is used to determine the extent of bony fusion. The advantage of conventional tomography is that it can be performed even in the presence of metallic implants. Conventional tomography, with flexion/extension, midline, narrow views, is helpful in confirming the diagnosis of pseudarthrosis. Tomography has better resolution than plain film radiographs in detecting such signs of pseudarthrosis as fracture in the fusion mass, graft displacement or disintegration, or lucency between the graft and native bone.

High-resolution, thin-collimation CT with multiplanar reconstruction further increases the sensitivity of bony spinal fusion detection (25). In addition, spiral examination reconstructions can be performed quickly.

CT remains the imaging modality of choice for visualization of the bony matrix. CT allows for the optimal detection of the amount of bone resected for decompression; the position of implants, including hardware and graft material, postoperatively; implant failure, including migration, breakage, and pullout; the degree of bony fusion; pseudarthrosis; new pathology of the vertebral column; and spinal canal dimensions, especially when facet arthropathy is suspected to contribute to spinal canal stenosis.

The drawbacks of CT remain its inefficiency for scanning large areas of the thoracic spine and the significant image artifact generated by metallic implants. Bone window settings minimize the metallic artifacts from implanted hardware, especially from titanium-based hardware; however, the images can still be less than ideal. Overall, adequate information is usually obtained by CT (26), especially if image reformation is available (63).

Finally, CT can be incorporated into frameless navigational systems that aid in spinal localization during surgery. These systems are particularly useful for evaluating anatomy, assessing the extent of resection, and planning ideal instrumentation placement, preoperatively and intraoperatively (70). These protocols typically use CT to scan the spine in 1-mm, continuous, nonoverlapping slices with a small field of view to produce a high-quality data set, which can then be transferred to the workstation.

Myelography

Myelography is an operator-dependent and invasive study. It uses intrathecal contrast to examine the spinal cord and its nerve root branches with superb spatial and contrast resolution. The spinal cord dimension can be evaluated with respect to the spinal canal and its components, such as the ligaments and facets. Myelography is primarily indicated in a patient who cannot undergo MRI examination, where ferromagnetic appliances interfere with MRI, or in cases in which bone details are important.

Arachnoiditis, pseudomeningocele, and cerebrospinal fluid (CSF) fistulae are some of the postoperative complications that can be visualized with either conventional myelography or CT myelography studies. Conventional myelography with dynamic flexion/extension views provides an accurate assessment in patients with ferromagnetic implants in whom CT and MRI are marred by implant artifact. The cord and proximal nerve roots are profiled by intrathecal contrast, and any compression of these structures can be easily demonstrated.

Drawbacks of myelography remain its invasive nature and its minor potential for causing postmyelographic CSF leaks. Also, although myelogram contrast agents have improved in recent years, certain agents such as iophendylate (Pantopaque) have been implicated in inducing arachnoiditis (12).

Bone Scintigraphy

Bone scintigraphy is an examination of the skeletal system using a bone-seeking radioactively labeled phosphate or phosphonate compound, typically technetium 99m–labeled methylene diphosphonate. Although the exact mechanism of uptake of bone-seeking radiopharmaceuticals remains unclear, the activity of these agents is affected by the vascularity and osteoblastic activity of bone, and they are most actively taken up at sites of active bone formation (24). Some of the indications for this study are detection, staging, and follow-up of metastatic disease; evaluation of osteomyelitis; determination of bone viability or infarction; and detection of pseud-

arthrosis. Although bone scans are extremely sensitive, they are not very specific, and other radiographic modalities and clinical correlation are often required for accurate diagnosis.

Metastatic disease is typically revealed as multiple areas of increased uptake on bone scintigraphy, although some lytic lesions may not be visualized. Osteomyelitis generally results in increased local uptake on bone scans, but a three-phase study with dynamic perfusion, blood pool, and delayed phases is typically required to make an accurate diagnosis. Osteomyelitis cases characteristically demonstrate greater bone isotope activity in delayed images than in earlier phases, in contrast to cases of surrounding cellulitis in which progressive focal bony uptake is not seen. Diagnosis of bone infarction with scintigraphy is highly dependent on the age of the infarct. In newly infarcted bone, areas of reduced uptake are revealed. However, as the bone heals, this is replaced by increased uptake activity at the margins of the infarcted area.

In cases of nonunion or pseudarthrosis, bone scans typically demonstrate increased uptake of technetium and have focal areas of increased activity. One drawback is that these areas of abnormal uptake may be inseparable from bony remodeling or injunction of bony fusion elements. The utility of bone scan in assessing fusion is further limited due to metallic instrumentation attenuating the photons and causing uptake defects, as well as the nonspecificity of the increased uptake. Bone scans become very sensitive if single-photon emission computed tomography is used.

Magnetic Resonance

MRI has emerged as the modality of choice because of its decreased dependence on operator skill, noninvasive nature, superb image quality, excellent soft tissue contrast, lack of ionizing radiation, and direct multiplanar capability. Surface coils allow a reduced field of view with an increased signal-to-noise ratio and decreased imaging time.

Even though MRI provides a poor definition of bony structures, it remains sensitive for detecting fractures, infections, and pseudarthrosis, as well as spine morphology. Pseudarthrosis may be revealed by abnormal intensity of the endplates as manifested by a low signal intensity on T1-weighted images and a high signal intensity on T2-weighted images.

The primary drawback of MR images in evaluating the spine is that ferromagnetic metallic implants can cause significant susceptibility artifacts. The magnetic susceptibility distortion can be severe enough to yield images unreadable. Advances in metallurgy have allowed the use of titanium-based spinal implants that produce relatively less image artifact than stainless steel implants on CT and MRI. However, a substantial MRI artifact remains, even with titanium-based spinal instrumentation (51). The amount of MRI distortion is related to the bulk of the metallic implant, as well as its chemical composition, orientation, and position (51). Motion artifact from cardiac, respiratory, or vascular sources or from CSF pulsations may also degrade the MRI. The use of cardiac gating and presaturation zones may be helpful in these situations.

The standard imaging technique used at our institution requires the placement of surface coils for full coverage of the adult thoracic spine. This protocol includes a T1-weighted sagittal body scout with a vitamin E–impregnated marker placed in the midthoracic region, sagittal and axial T2-weighted turbo spin echo sequences, and sagittal and axial turbo T1-weighted images before and after contrast administration. T1-weighted pulse sequences are useful in detecting lesions of the vertebral body marrow. Gadolinium is helpful in the diagnosis of neoplasm, postoperative fibrosis (61), and intramedullary lesions. Imaging time is approximately 45 minutes, but this varies depending on the number of images acquired. The optimum choice of acquisitions, and other imaging parameters such as slice thickness, depends on the field strength of the magnet, the specific pathologic condition being studied, and specific requirements for imaging quality. Claustrophobic patients can be sedated before the examination.

Thermography

Thermography, or computerized infrared telethermographic imaging, is the technique of composing a thermal map by measuring the infrared radiation emitted from the body surface at room temperature. The primary utility of thermography in clinical disorders is in objectively and quantitatively evaluating the degree of asymmetry in skin temperatures (72), especially between adjacent dermatomes.

Although medical thermography dates back to 1957, when R.N. Lawson described its use in the diagnosis of breast cancer (46), its use in spinal disorders remains controversial. Although more than 1,700 articles on thermography appear in the Cumulative Medical Index, fewer than 30 concerning spinal disorders are from peer-reviewed journals (2). Further, in a survey of the American Academy of Orthopaedic Sur-

geons, fewer than 5% believed thermography to be a valid test for neck and back pain (2). Others believe thermography to be a useful adjuvant test in the diagnosis of nerve root compression syndromes. In one series of more than 100 patients with cervical or lumbosacral disease, thermography was more accurate than conventional myelography in detecting root compression (55) by detecting abnormal heat patterns in the corresponding limb. In thoracic lesions, with their significantly smaller dermatomal representations, the utility of thermography in detecting root compression remains unproven.

In the evaluation of the failed back, thermography may be most useful in the detection of sympathetically maintained pain. Most syndromes of sympathetically maintained pain, such as reflex sympathetic dystrophy or causalgia, involve not only persistent pain but also varying degrees of vasomotor instability with concomitant dermatomal temperature variations. Detection by thermography of a reduction in skin temperature of 1 degree centigrade or more in the region of pain identifies those patients in whom further testing, including sympathetic blockade, should be considered (77). One series of 224 patients with persistent pain that was unconfirmed by physical examination or radiologic study found 19% to have abnormal thermographs; 74% of these patients had sympathetically maintained pain subsequently confirmed by sympathetic blockade (30). Although thermography in the diagnosis of spinal disorders remains controversial, it may be of use in the diagnosis of sympathetic nerve injuries in the postoperative spine patient with otherwise unexplained pain.

Electrodiagnostic Studies

Electromyography and nerve conduction testing have both proved useful in the differentiation of nerve root syndromes from peripheral neuropathies in the postoperative cervical and lumbosacral spine (41,76). However, little evidence exists to support a role for electrodiagnostic testing in the evaluation of disorders of the postoperative thoracic spine, with the exception of lesions of the first thoracic nerve root.

The first thoracic nerve joins into the lower trunk of the brachial plexus, contributing to the median and ulnar nerves (10). An isolated injury to the first thoracic nerve root causes varying weakness in all muscles innervated by the median nerve except the pronator teres and flexor carpi radialis and all muscles innervated by the ulnar nerve except the flexor digitorum profundus III and IV (74). As with evaluations of the cervical spine, careful electromyographic testing of these muscles and examination of the median and ulnar nerves may help differentiate between a peripheral lesion and injury to the first thoracic nerve root.

Although of limited utility, electromyography may help differentiate between peripheral lesions of the intercostal nerves and the upper six thoracic nerve roots by examining the thoracic paraspinal musculature. Denervation potentials recorded from the thoracic paraspinal musculature suggest root injury as the paraspinal muscles are innervated by dorsal rami, whereas the intercostal nerves arise primarily from anterior rami (65). Several clinical reports have demonstrated the ability of thoracic electrodiagnostic studies to diagnose peripheral or mixed neuropathies by exploiting this difference between the intercostal and paraspinal musculature (29,60). The ability of electrodiagnostic methods to assess injury to the upper six thoracic nerve roots postoperatively remains unstudied.

The lower six thoracic nerves pose a significant challenge to electrodiagnostic methods because of anatomic considerations (65). The lower intercostal nerves pass deep to the progressively shorter costal cartilages to enter into the anterior abdominal wall and are not practically accessible for nerve conduction studies. The external and internal oblique, and the transverse abdominis, muscles are diffusely innervated by all six lower thoracic intercostal nerves as well as by the first lumbar nerve root via the iliohypogastric and ilioinguinal nerves, making specific electrodiagnostic testing of individual thoracic nerves difficult. The rectus abdominis is innervated only by the lower six thoracic intercostal nerves. Although electromyography of the rectus abdominis can be used to assess the lower thoracic nerves as a whole, no conclusions can be reached about individual thoracic roots.

ILLUSTRATIVE CASES

Case 1 (Degenerative)

A 70-year-old woman initially presented with a 6-week history of severe pain in the middle back, trouble with balance, and difficulty walking. She also complained of a heavy feeling in both lower extremities. Imaging revealed a herniated thoracic disk at T10-11 with cord effacement. She underwent a decompressive laminectomy at T10-11 at an outside institution without improvement in her symptoms. Six weeks postoperatively, her incision dehisced, requiring a second operation and a course of intravenous antibiotics.

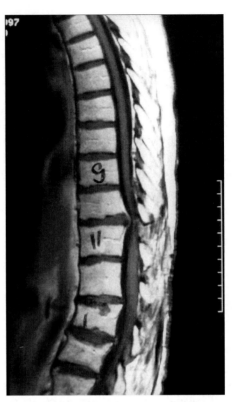

FIGURE 1. (Case 1) Preoperative T-1 sagittal magnetic resonance image showing a large herniated disk at T10-11 as well as the incidental finding of a Schmorl's node in the superior aspect of the L-1 vertebral body. A smaller herniated disk at T9-10 is only evident on more lateral images (not seen here).

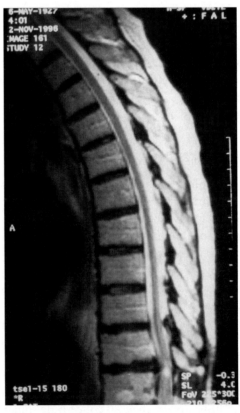

FIGURE 2. (Case 1) Preoperative T-2 sagittal magnetic resonance image showing a herniated disk at T10-11 with signal changes within the cord immediately posterior to the disk.

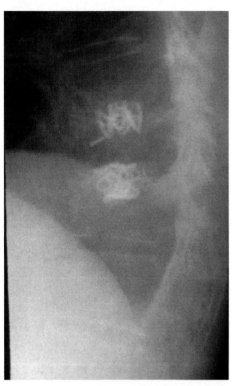

FIGURE 3. (Case 1) Postoperative lateral radiograph showing placement of titanium interbody cages at T10-11 and T9-10.

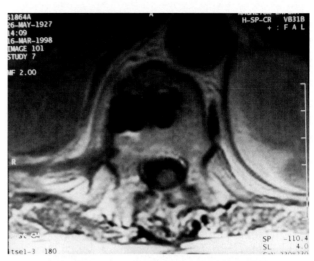

FIGURE 5. (Case 1) Postoperative T-1 (with gadolinium) axial magnetic resonance image showing only trace enhancement around the periphery of the implants.

At the time of presentation to our institution, her walking had deteriorated further, and she now required the assistance of a cane. She also complained of increasing urinary frequency and progressive worsening of her back pain. Physical examination revealed 4+ strength

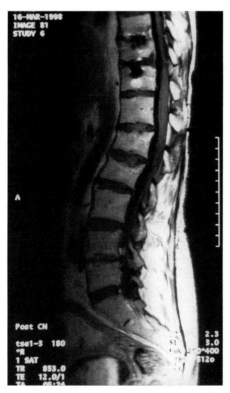

FIGURE 4. (Case 1) Postoperative T-1 (with gadolinium) sagittal magnetic resonance image showing only trace enhancement around the periphery of the implants. Note the minimal interference from the titanium implants. The spinal cord has been completely decompressed.

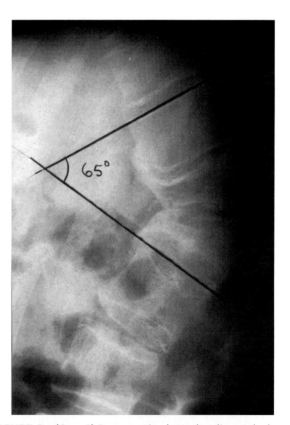

FIGURE 6. (Case 2) Preoperative lateral radiograph showing a significant kyphotic deformity with a Cobb angle of 65 degrees as well as marked deformities of the T-12 and L-1 vertebral bodies.

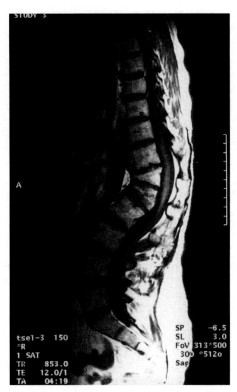

FIGURE 7. (Case 2) Preoperative T-1 sagittal magnetic resonance image.

throughout her lower extremities, with a T-11 sensory level. Her lower extremities were hyperreflexic with positive Babinski's reflexes bilaterally. Her gait was severely spastic, and she was unable to tandem walk.

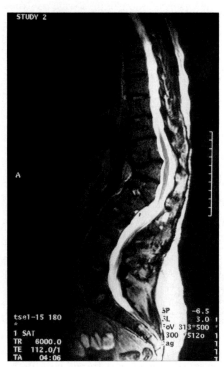

FIGURE 8. (Case 2) Preoperative T-2 sagittal magnetic resonance image.

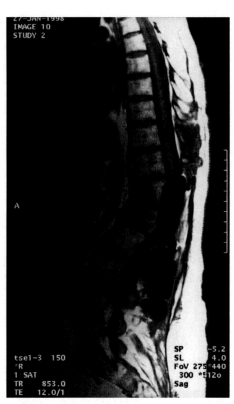

FIGURE 9. (Case 2) Postoperative T-1 sagittal magnetic resonance image showing placement of an anterior strut graft. Note the mild distortion from the posterior titanium instrumentation (sublaminar hooks and rods). However, the cord and disk spaces are still well visualized.

Radiologic evaluation with plain films and MRI revealed a continued significant herniated disk at T10-11 with cord compression, as well as a subtotal posterior decompressive laminectomy at T10-11 (Figs. 1 and 2). A smaller herniated disk at T9-10 was also evident on more lateral images (not shown).

The patient underwent a thoracotomy for anterior T10-11 and T9-10 diskectomies. Two interbody cages were filled with morselized rib and placed at each level (Fig. 3). Postoperative imaging with MRI revealed good decompression of the spinal cord and restoration of the intervertebral disk heights (Figs. 4 and 5). Postoperatively, she has done well, with steady improvement in her myelopathy and significant improvement in her back pain.

Case 2 (Deformity)

This 40-year-old woman initially was involved in a motor vehicle accident 20 years ago and underwent a posterior fusion of T-12 to L-2 at that time. A second motor vehicle accident 1 year ago caused a return of her back pain, which was treated conservatively with analgesics and bracing. Over the past 6 months, however, she has had a marked increase in

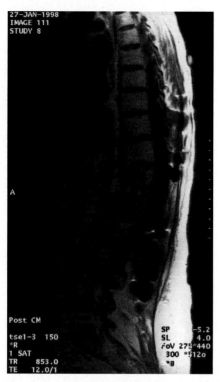

FIGURE 10. (Case 2) Postoperative T-1 (with gadolinium) sagittal magnetic resonance image showing only trace enhancement around the anterior strut graft.

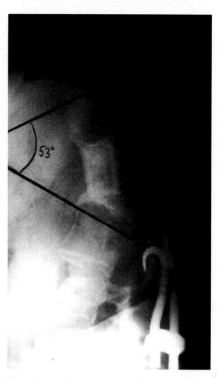

FIGURE 12. (Case 2) Postoperative lateral radiograph showing placement of an anterior strut graft and posterior instrumentation, with a Cobb angle of 53 degrees.

midback pain, as well as sensations of numbness and tingling in the lower extremities.

Her physical examination was essentially unremarkable, with normal motor and sensory function.

Her reflexes and gait were normal with the exception of being unable to tandem walk. Radiologic evaluation with plain films and MRI revealed a significant kyphotic deformity at T-12 to L-1, with a Cobb

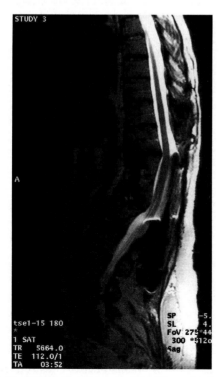

FIGURE 11. (Case 2) Postoperative T-2 sagittal magnetic resonance image.

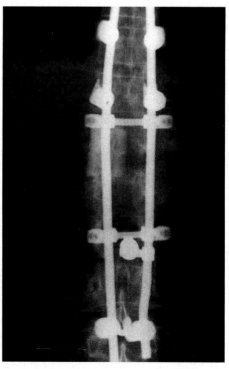

FIGURE 13. (Case 2) Postoperative anteroposterior radiograph.

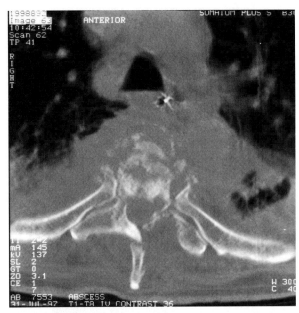

FIGURE 14. (Case 3) Preoperative axial computed tomography scan showing the degree of destruction of the T-5 vertebral body.

angle of 65 degrees (Figs. 6–8). Comparison to prior imaging confirmed a progressive kyphotic deformity of 15 degrees.

The patient underwent a three-stage surgical procedure. Initially, she had a posterior decompressive laminectomy of T-12 and L-1. In addition, osteotomies were made through her previous fusion mass to allow correction of her kyphotic deformity. A thoracotomy was then made, allowing an anterior T-12 to L-1 diskectomy, partial corpectomies of T-

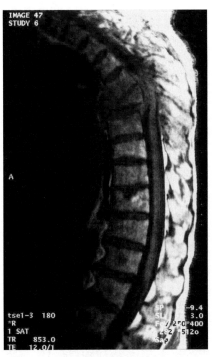

FIGURE 16. (Case 3) Preoperative T-1 sagittal magnetic resonance image showing destruction of the fifth and sixth vertebral bodies, with an associated soft tissue mass anterior and posterior to the vertebral column. The posterior aspect of the soft tissue mass displaces the spinal cord posteriorly.

12 and L-1, correction of her kyphotic deformity, and placement of a tibial strut allograft. Finally, a posterior arthrodesis from T-10 to L-3 was performed using a long construct hook and rod system.

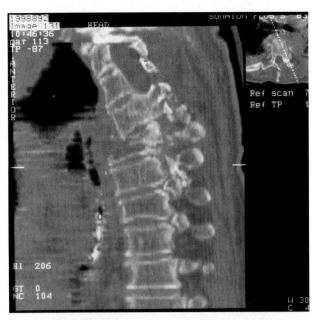

FIGURE 15. (Case 3) Preoperative computed tomography scan with sagittal reconstruction demonstrating almost complete destruction of T-5 and T-6.

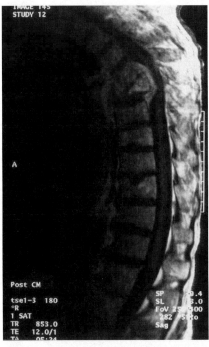

FIGURE 17. (Case 3) Preoperative T-1 (with gadolinium) sagittal magnetic resonance image showing enhancement of the soft tissue mass.

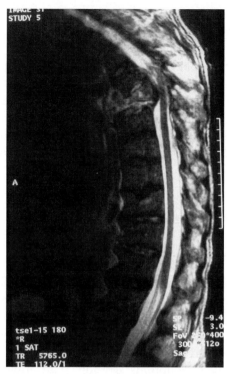

FIGURE 18. (Case 3) Preoperative T-2 sagittal magnetic resonance image. Note the narrowing of the spinal canal immediately posterior to the T5-6 vertebral bodies.

The arthrodesis was supplemented with autologous iliac crest bone.

Postoperative x-rays reveal reasonable long-term correction of her kyphotic deformity, with a Cobb

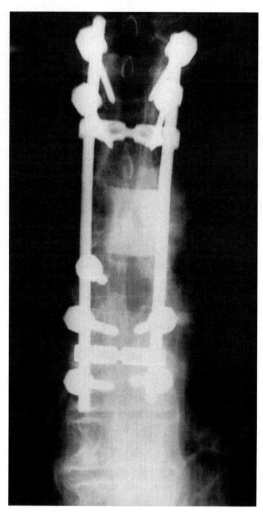

FIGURE 20. (Case 3) Postoperative anteroposterior radiograph.

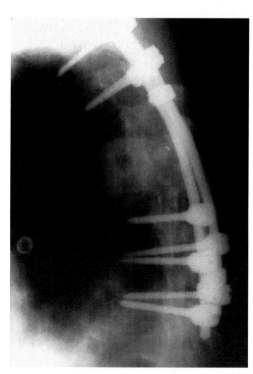

FIGURE 19. (Case 3) Postoperative lateral radiograph showing the anterior strut graft and the posterior pedicle screws and rods.

angle of 53 degrees (Figs. 9–13). She has done well, with significant improvement in her pain.

Case 3 (Infectious)

This 55-year-old man with severe coronary artery disease and chronic obstructive pulmonary disease initially presented with a 6-week history of severe midback pain followed by an acute onset of paraplegia, urinary retention, and a T-5 sensory level. He underwent an emergent posterior decompression of a T5-6 epidural abscess at an outside institution via T4-7 laminectomies and partial vertebrectomies of T-5 and T-6. Bacterial cultures were positive for *Bacteroides fragilis* and *Staphylococcus aureus*. His postoperative course was complicated by sepsis and significant respiratory distress.

On transfer to our institution, his examination was complicated by a septicemic metabolic encephalopathy. His upper extremity strength was 4+/5; his lower extremity strength ranged from 1 to 3/5. He

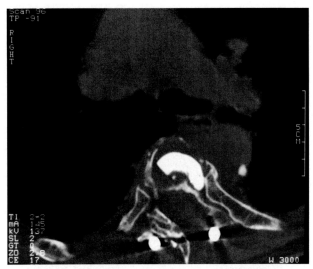

FIGURE 21. (Case 3) Postoperative axial computed tomography scan showing placement of an anterior strut graft and posterior rod instrumentation. Note the scatter effect from the posterior titanium rods.

had a T5-6 sensory level, and his lower extremities were diffusely hyperreflexic, with positive Babinski's reflexes bilaterally. Imaging with plain films, CT (Figs. 14 and 15), and MRI (Figs. 16–18) revealed continued compression and bony destruction.

Due to continued spinal cord compression, he was returned to the operating room, where he underwent proximal extension of his previous decompressive laminectomies to T-3, as well as débridement of the epidural abscess. Corpectomies of T-5 and T-6 were accomplished through a posterolateral approach, and diskectomies of T4-5, T5-6, and T6-7 were performed. He then underwent posterior stabilization

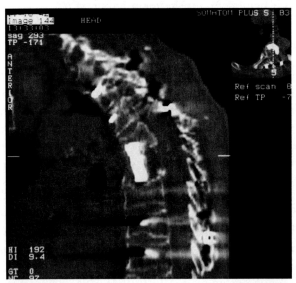

FIGURE 22. (Case 3) Postoperative computed tomography scan with sagittal reconstruction showing correction of the kyphotic deformity. Note again the scatter effect of the posterior instrumentation.

with pedicle screws at T2-3 bilaterally, T-7 on the right, and T8-9 bilaterally. Autologous iliac crest bone supplemented the arthrodesis.

He has done well postoperatively in thoracolumbosacral orthosis bracing. His myelopathy is slowly improving, and he is able to ambulate with the aid of a walker. Postoperative imaging at 1 year with plain films (Figs. 19 and 20) and CT (Figs. 21 and 22) showed correction of his kyphotic deformity and progression of his fusion.

DIFFERENTIAL DIAGNOSIS

Overview

The differential diagnosis of the failed thoracic spine is varied but can be approximately divided into immediate, early, and late failures (Table 1). Patients who fall into the first category have no improvement of their symptoms after surgery, even transiently, or, worse, new symptoms develop. The etiologies of immediate failure include surgical errors or incorrect diagnosis, nonindicated surgery, surgery at the wrong level, inadequate decompression of neural structures, inadequate correction of deformity, iatrogenic instability, psychosocial factors, or foreign body.

Early failures are characterized by initial improvement following surgery, but with deterioration or development of new symptoms starting days to months afterward. The etiology of early failure includes infection, arachnoiditis, epidural fibrosis, recurrent pathology, nerve root injury, or graft migration.

Patients with late failure enjoy improvement in their symptoms after surgery but deteriorate months

TABLE 1. DIFFERENTIAL DIAGNOSIS

Immediate failure
Surgical error
Incorrect diagnosis
Nonindicated surgery
Wrong level
Inadequate decompression
Inadequate correction of deformity
Psychosocial factors
Foreign body
Early failure (days to months)
Infection
Arachnoiditis
Epidural fibrosis
Recurrent pathology
Nerve/root injury
Graft migration
Late failure (months to years)
Instrumentation failure
Instability
Pseudarthrosis

to years later. The etiology of late failure includes instrumentation failure, instability, or pseudarthrosis.

The relative risk of each of the above etiologies of failed thoracic spine cannot be estimated, as few large series of thoracic spine surgery results have been published. Each etiology is instead illustrated by case reports and small reported series of thoracic spine surgeries.

Immediate Failure

Surgical Error

Incorrect diagnosis is a rare but recognized cause of the failed spine surgery syndrome (49). Although the incidence in thoracic surgery is unknown, incorrect diagnoses account for 0.3% of patients with continued pain after lumbar diskectomy (50,58). The differential of entities mimicking root compression or spinal stenosis includes epidural abscesses, osteomyelitis, tumors, arthritic conditions, and peripheral neuropathies (23). Even with the correct diagnosis, an inappropriate surgical procedure can lead to failure. The surgeon must decide whether surgery is indicated, as well as choose the correct surgical approach, degree of decompression, and amount of stabilization that are appropriate for each individual patient.

Surgery at the wrong level or side is fortunately a rare occurrence but is fraught with medicolegal implications. The surgeon must ascertain that the radiographs are labeled correctly preoperatively and that the vertebral level of the lesion is identified accurately. As the thoracic spine is more difficult to visualize accurately with portable radiographs or fluoroscopy than the cervical or lumbar spine, identifying the correct level intraoperatively can be troublesome (57). Preoperative marking with indelible ink injected onto the spinous process of the involved vertebrae can help intraoperative localization, especially in the midthoracic spine.

This localization in the thoracic spine is crucial. Every patient should have a complete anteroposterior and lateral thoracic and lumbar series, as well as an anteroposterior and lateral chest radiograph. These need to be correlated with the patient's MRI or CT, or both, to ensure correct numbering of the lumbar vertebrae.

Inadequate decompression of neural structures and inadequate correction of deformity can also result in immediate failure after thoracic spine surgery. In one series of 225 patients diagnosed with lumbar disk herniation, more than 50% were found to have significant lateral spinal stenosis that required decompression at the time of surgery (13).

Removal of the herniated disk material alone without bony decompression leads to a high rate of failure in these cases.

Inadequate correction of deformity can also result in failed surgery. Even with appropriate correction of thoracic scoliosis, only 75% of patients will have a significant relief of pain (3).

Psychosocial Factors

Several series have identified psychosocial factors as an important predictive factor for failed spine surgery syndrome (8,15,20,44,66). One series of 78 patients (44) with failed backs found more than 12% to have a frank psychiatric illness (*DSM-IV* axis I) and more than 43% to have personality disorders (*DSM-IV* axis II). In addition, nearly 75% misused narcotics. Patients on worker's compensation have also been proven to have a disproportionately high rate of failed spine surgery (8,15,17).

Foreign Body

Foreign bodies left in the surgical site can cause nerve root or cord compression. The surgeon should be judicious with the amount of hemostatic material left in the surgical field. In addition, the placement of free fat grafts or Gelfoam over the decompressed nerve root to stave off the development of epidural scarring can have a deleterious effect by reconstituting the compression (34). Gelfoam also enhances the formation of scar, and its use should be limited.

Early Failure (Days to Months)

Infection

The incidence of postoperative infections in surgery of the thoracic spine, including wound infection, diskitis, osteomyelitis, and frank abscess, has not been well studied, although known risk factors include the use of spinal instrumentation and the posterior approach (40), patient age and nutritional status, and diabetes, cancer, or immunosuppression. Postoperative infection of the surgical site may manifest itself with systemic signs of fever and localized pain, erythema, swelling, rubor, and wound drainage. Laboratory investigation may reveal a normal or increased peripheral white count, and sedimentation rates can be elevated to more than 100 mm per hour (78). However, the sedimentation rate can remain elevated to more than 10 mm per hour, even 6 weeks postoperatively, in up to 38% of spinal surgery patients (64), making the diagnosis of diskitis or osteomyelitis difficult. Although the pain is usually confined to the surrounding tissues with local spasm and tenderness, radicular pain may arise from nerve root compression or irritation. Blood and wound cultures should be obtained before initiation of antibiotic therapy. Needle aspiration should be performed for suspected cases of diskitis or osteomyelitis, although the rate of positive cultures is less than 50% (54). Operative débridement should be considered for patients with persistent signs of infection despite antibiotic treatment and for patients with pustular drainage.

Arachnoiditis

Arachnoiditis is an inflammatory response of the arachnoid membrane with fibroblast proliferation and collagen deposition, resulting in varying degrees of blockage of spinal fluid flow through the subarachnoid space, nerve root clumping, obliteration of nerve root sheaths, and nerve root atrophy (12,78). Although initially recognized as a pathologic reaction of the arachnoid membrane to infection, blood, and injected contrast material, arachnoiditis has increasingly been suspected in cases of failed spine surgery. The incidence of arachnoiditis in the postoperative thoracic spine has not been well studied. Clinically, the progressive encapsulation of the nerve roots by this inflammatory tissue can reproduce the patient's initial radicular pain. Motor deficits are rare, although no consensus exists regarding the clinical syndrome. Typically, the patient's symptoms are worsened by maneuvers that stretch the nerve roots, such as straight-leg raise, sitting, thoracolumbar flexion, and neck flexion.

Diagnosis is based on clinical suspicion and myelographic findings of marked irregularity of contrast filling the thecal sac. Treatment is controversial and is usually reserved for patients with progressive deficits. Shunting of the resulting arachnoid cyst into the pleural or peritoneal cavities has had better clinical outcomes than cyst fenestration alone in the case of progressive neurologic deficit.

Epidural Fibrosis

Recurrent radicular pain caused by fibrosis of the dura mater constitutes one of the leading causes of failed spine surgery syndrome (21), especially in patients with multiple surgeries (22). The thick scarring of the dura mater results in an adherent space-occupying lesion compressing and tethering the underlying nerve root. The temporal relation of developing symptomatic epidural fibrosis to the ini-

tial surgery is variable, occurring from a few months postoperatively to years later.

The primary differential of epidural fibrosis is recurrent disk herniation, as they have similar clinical presentations. Although myelography and CT both help to differentiate epidural scar from recurrent disk fragments, the imaging modality of choice is MRI with and without intravenous gadolinium–diethylenetriamine pentaacetic acid (Gd-DTPA) contrast. More than 6 weeks postoperatively, the accuracy of MRI with and without intravenous Gd-DPTA administration has been shown to be as high as 96% (59) and 100% (32).

The main treatment for epidural fibrosis appears to be prevention, as surgical series of lumbar epidural fibrosis are disappointing. Only 36% of 2,000 patients had a good recovery in one series (71). Although a patient may enjoy a brief improvement, the removal of epidural scar usually stimulates its recurrence. As epidural fibrosis is also caused by chronic irritation due to minor instability, some surgeons recommend a spinal fusion procedure at the time of revision to reduce the rate of scar reformation (22), although this remains extremely controversial.

Recurrent Pathology

The most common cause of the initial recurrence of symptoms in lumbar diskectomy is recurrent herniation (22). In one series of 31 herniated thoracic disks, one patient required reoperation for recurrent herniation 8 months postoperatively (57). Recurrent disk herniation can present with radicular symptoms on either side, or with myelopathy, and may not mimic the initial presentation. MRI is the most sensitive imaging modality to evaluate recurrent disk herniation.

Nerve/Root Injury

Nerve or nerve root injury can produce pain through either neuralgia or through denervation. Partial injury to a nerve root can result in a painful neuralgia along the corresponding dermatome. This pain is often characterized as burning or gnawing in character, present at rest but exacerbated with activity. Diagnostic imaging is unrevealing, except for the presence of varying degrees of arachnoiditis. Spinal nerve blocks can screen for patients in whom a microsurgical dorsal root rhizotomy may be beneficial. One small series of failed lumbar spine patients showed good early results (31).

Injury to the dorsal rami of spinal nerve roots during surgical exposure and retraction can cause denervation atrophy of the paraspinal muscles, with a corresponding decrease in back extensor muscle strength. In one small series of failed back patients, more than 85% of individuals with normal postoperative CT scans were found to have local paraspinal muscle atrophy and dorsal rami lesions on muscle biopsy (62). The consequence of injury to several segmental dorsal rami and subsequent muscle denervation atrophy may be functional instability and chronic pain. Treatment consists only of bracing and physical therapy.

Graft Migration

Bone graft material, whether autograft or allograft, requires several months for fusion and eventual replacement by new bone through a process of creeping substitution. Before incorporation, graft material can be dislodged if it is not secured properly into the fusion site. Significant nerve or cord compression can occur, often requiring emergent reoperation. Grafts in the setting of osteopenia (36) or tumor are especially at risk. In one series of 25 patients undergoing thoracolumbar vertebrectomy and posterior instrumentation for malignant metastatic disease, 16% had graft migration that required reoperation (1). Bone mineral density can be assessed preoperatively with ultrasound and bone densitometry. A lower bone density has been associated with a higher fracture risk (33,48) as well as a higher rate of instrumentation failure (42), with the relative risk ranging from 1.4 to 1.6 per standard deviation decrease in bone mass (47). As osteopenic patients have a low skeletal calcium pool and inadequate dietary calcium, graft incorporation is subject to delay due to competition with the rest of the body for calcium (39). The risk of graft subsidence is also related to the degree of kyphotic correction and the number of segments spanned. Treatment involves repositioning or replacing the graft.

Late Failure (Months to Years)

Instrumentation Failure

Although instrumentation failure rates are minimized by placing supplementary bone graft material at the time of surgery (19) and adequate postoperative immobilization, the incidence is still significant. Instrumentation failure commonly occurs in the setting of pseudarthrosis (38), as the continued stress on the fixation system in the unfused spine eventually results in metal fatigue and failure. Not all

instrumentation failures require reoperation, but all do necessitate careful examination. Patients may present with pain from subsequent instability, symptoms of nerve root or spinal cord compression, or cosmetic deformity, or they may be asymptomatic. Physical examination can reveal local muscle spasm, pain on palpation over the instrumentation site, or visible deformity. Diagnostic imaging with plain radiographs usually reveals the failed instrumentation. Indications for reoperation include instability, compression of neural structures, pain, and cosmesis.

Although the incidence of instrumentation failure in the thoracic spine is not well studied, several case reports describe Harrington rod breakout (37,75), pedicle screw breakage or bending (69), and sublaminar wire breakage (5) in the thoracic spine, most requiring reoperation. A lower bone mineral density has been associated with a higher rate of instrumentation failure from hardware pullout or loosening (39,42). In thoracic scoliosis corrective surgery, large series have reported incidences of rod breakage of 2% (3) to 11% (28), although few patients required reoperation.

Instability

Segmental instability following spinal surgery can result from injury to ligamentous, muscular, or bony structures and has been reported to be the third most common cause of failed lumbar disk surgery, accounting for 18% of failures (23). In the thoracic spine, most reports of postoperative instability occurred after posterior decompressive procedures (52,56), although one case report describes symptomatic spondylolisthesis 3 months after posterolateral thoracic diskectomy (14). However, instability can occur after nearly all spinal surgical procedures. Risk factors for development of postoperative instability include younger age, female sex, preoperative disk space widening, degenerative pathology, magnitude of surgery (23,78), and insufficient paraspinal muscle extensor tone and strength due to neurologic injury or myelopathy. During the initial surgery, care should be taken to prevent extensive removal of or damage to articular facets to minimize the risk of subsequent instability.

Instability typically presents as back pain without a significant radicular component, unless the degree of instability is such that the spinal cord or nerve roots are being compressed. The patient's pain is often aching in nature, aggravated by movement, and is accompanied by physical findings of local muscle spasm, tenderness to palpation, and either restricted or hyperdynamic range of motion. Tension signs are usually absent. Although gross instability with spondylolisthesis or movement on dynamic imaging is readily apparent with plain radiographs, most instability is difficult to confirm with diagnostic imaging. Often the segmental instability does not result in enough translation to be appreciated, even on dynamic imaging. However, radiographic findings suggestive of segmental instability include disk space narrowing and traction spurs.

If instability is suspected, a trial of external bracing may help confirm the diagnosis. Although a 2-week trial of bracing has been proven effective in the diagnosis of lumbar instability (45), its role in thoracic instability remains unproven. However, if the patient has significant improvement in pain with bracing, revision fusion surgery should be considered.

Pseudarthrosis

Failure of implanted graft material to fuse with the vertebral column is the primary cause of pseudarthrosis, defined as the documented failure of solid fusion 1 year after operation (68). Pseudarthrosis may result from physiologic deficiencies of the patient, such as disorders of calcium homeostasis, metabolic disorders of bone formation, or malnutrition (35). Animal studies have shown concurrent or recent radiation to the surgical site to increase the risk of nonunion (9,18). Tobacco use has also been shown to be a major contributing factor to the development of pseudarthrosis (27). Various medications, specifically those that affect bone homeostasis, can lead to pseudarthrosis due to failure of graft integration (67). Surgical errors may encourage pseudarthrosis, including inadequate decortication; inadequate graft size, shape, or material; inadequate internal fixation; or postoperative immobilization.

The incidence of pseudarthrosis in thoracic scoliosis corrective surgery ranges from 0% to 19% (68). Pseudarthrosis developed in nearly 6% of 54 children treated with anterior and posterior fusion of the thoracolumbar junction for spinal deformity in myelomeningocele (4). The clinical presentation of thoracic pseudarthrosis is variable: back pain, midline tenderness, limitation of motion, muscle spasm. Instrumentation failure may also develop in patients with pseudarthrosis. Plain anteroposterior spine radiographs, along with lateral flexion/extension views, can confirm the diagnosis in most cases. A successful fusion shows a continuous trabecular pattern traversing the grafted segment (68). Fine-cut axial CT and three-dimensional CT reconstructions of the fusion site are useful when plain radiographs are ambiguous.

The need for surgical revision for thoracic pseudarthrosis is controversial. The primary indications are instability or intractable pain.

CONCLUSION

Consideration of the patient's clinical symptoms and signs, along with correlation with radiologic studies, is vital for optimal evaluation of each process of infection, neoplasm, or other postoperative complications. In patients in whom recurrent or new symptoms develop after surgery, a more demanding radiographic workup is required than that of normal postoperative imaging. MRI remains the preferred imaging modality for patients with compatible implants.

REFERENCES

1. Akeyson E, McCutcheon I. Single-stage posterior vertebrectomy and replacement combined with posterior instrumentation for spinal metastases. *J Neurosurg* 1996;85:211–220.
2. Ash C, Foster M. Neuromuscular thermography in orthopaedic surgery: a usage poll. *Orthop Rev* 1988;17(6):589–592.
3. Balderston R. Adult scoliosis: the thoracic spine. In: Bridwell K, DeWald R, eds. *Textbook of spinal surgery*, 2nd ed. Philadelphia: Lippincott–Raven Publishers, 1997:715–731.
4. Banta J. Combined anterior and posterior fusion for spinal deformity in myelomeningocele. *Spine* 1990;15(9):946–952.
5. Bernard T, Johnston C, Roberts J, et al. Late complications due to wire breakage in segmental spinal instrumentation. *J Bone Joint Surg Am* 1983;65A(9):1339–1345.
6. Bikle D. Agents that affect bone mineral homeostasis. In: Katzung B, ed. *Basic and clinical pharmacology*, 4th ed. Norwalk: Appleton & Lange, 1989:531–544.
7. Biller J, Brazis P. The localization of lesions affecting the spinal cord. In: Brazis P, Masdeu J, Biller J, eds. *Localization in clinical neurology*, 2nd ed. Boston: Little, Brown and Company, 1990:59–68.
8. Biondi J, Greenberg B. Redecompression and fusion in failed back syndrome patients. *J Spinal Disord* 1990;3(4):362–369.
9. Bonarigo B, Rubin P. Nonunion of pathologic fracture after radiation therapy. *Radiology* 1967;88:889–898.
10. Brazis P. The localization of lesions affecting the cervical, brachial, and lumbosacral plexuses. In: Brazis P, Masdeu J, Biller J, eds. *Localization in clinical neurology*, 2nd ed. Boston: Little, Brown and Company, 1990:43–58.

11. Brazis P. The localization of spinal nerve and root lesions. In: Brazis P, Masdeu J, Biller J, eds. *Localization in clinical neurology*, 2nd ed. Boston: Little, Brown and Company, 1990:59–68.

12. Burton C. Lumbosacral arachnoiditis. *Spine* 1978;3(1): 24–30.

13. Burton C, Kirkaldy-Willis W, Yong-Hing K, et al. Causes of failure of surgery on the lumbar spine. *Clin Orthop* 1981;157:191–199.

14. Curcin A, Lucas P. Spondylolisthesis after posterolateral thoracic discectomy: case report and literature review. *Spine* 1992;17(10):1254–1256.

15. Davis R. A long-term outcome analysis of 984 surgically treated herniated lumbar discs. *J Neurosurg* 1994; 80:415–421.

16. Dick J, Boachie-Adjei O, Wilson M. One stage vs. two stage anterior and posterior spinal reconstruction in adults: comparison of outcomes including nutritional status, complication rates, hospital costs and other factors. *Spine* 1992;18:S310–316.

17. Dvorak J, Vahlensieck M, Fuhrimann P, et al. The outcome of surgery for lumbar disc herniation II: a 4–17 years' follow-up with emphasis on psychosocial aspects. *Spine* 1988;13:1423–1427.

18. Emery S, Brazinski M, Koka A, et al. The biological and biomechanical effects of irradiation on anterior spinal bone grafts in a canine model. *J Bone Joint Surg Am* 1994;76A(4):540–548.

19. Erwin W, Dickson J, Harrington P. Clinical review of patients with broken Harrington rods. *J Bone Joint Surg Am* 1980;62A:1302–1307.

20. Finnegan W, Fenlin J, Marvel J, et al. Results of surgical intervention in the symptomatic multi-operated back patient: analysis of 67 cases followed for three to seven years. *J Bone Joint Surg Am* 1979;61A:1077–1082.

21. Fiume D, Sherkat S, Callovini G, et al. Treatment of the failed back surgery syndrome due to lumbo-sacral epidural fibrosis. *Acta Neurochir* 1995;64S:116–118.

22. Fritsch E, Heisel J, Rupp S. The failed back surgery syndrome: reasons, intraoperative findings, and long-term results: a report of 182 operative treatments. *Spine* 1996;21(5):626–633.

23. Gill K, Frymoyer J. Management of treatment failures after decompressive surgery: surgical alternatives and results. In: Frymoyer J, ed. *The adult spine: principles and practice*, 2nd ed. Philadelphia: Lippincott–Raven Publishers, 1997:2111–2133.

24. Grubb R. Nuclear medicine and positron emission tomography. In: Tindall G, Cooper P, Barrow D, eds. *The practice of neurosurgery*. Baltimore: Williams & Wilkins, 1996:137–157.

25. Reference deleted.

26. Guven O, Yalcin S, Karahan M, et al. Postoperative evaluation of transpedicular screws with computed tomography. *Orthop Rev* 1994;23(6):511–516.

27. Hadley M, Reddy S. Smoking and the human vertebral column: a review of the impact of cigarette use on vertebral bone metabolism and spinal fusion. *Neurosurgery* 1997;41(1):116–124.

28. Harms J, Jeszenszky D, Beele B. Ventral correction of thoracic scoliosis. In: Bridwell K, DeWald R, eds. *The textbook of spinal surgery*, 2nd ed. Philadelphia: Lippincott–Raven Publishers, 1997:611–626.

29. Hayes F, Redmond J, McKenna M. Thoracic polyradiculopathy—abdominal wall swelling and sensory symptoms in diabetes mellitus. *Ir Med J* 1994;87(5):150–151.

30. Hendler N, Uematsu S, Long D. Thermographic validation of physical complaints in "psychogenic pain" patients. *Psychosomatics* 1982;23:283–287.

31. Hoppenstein R. A new approach to the failed, failed back syndrome. *Spine* 1980;5(4):371–379.

32. Hueftle M, Modic M, Ross J. Lumbar spine: postoperative MR imaging with Gd-DTPA. *Radiology* 1988;167: 817–824.

33. Hui S, Slemenda C, Johnston CJ. Age and bone mass as predictors of fracture in a prospective study. *J Clin Invest* 1988;81:1804–1809.

34. Israel Z, Constantini S. Compressive epidural autologous free fat graft in a patient with failed back syndrome: case report. *J Spinal Disord* 1995;8(3):240–242.

35. Jensen J, Jensen T, Smith T, et al. Nutrition in orthopaedic surgery. *J Bone Joint Surg Am* 1982;64:1263–1272.

36. Keppler L, Steffee A, Biscup R. Posterior lumbar interbody fusion with variable screw placement and Isola instrumentation. In: Bridwell K, DeWald R, eds. *The textbook of spinal surgery*, 2nd ed. Philadelphia: Lippincott–Raven Publishers, 1997:1601–1621.

37. Krodel A, Rehmet J, Hamburger C. Spinal cord compression caused by the rod of a Harrington instrumentation device: a late complication in scoliosis surgery. *Eur Spine J* 1997;6(3):208–210.

38. LaGrone M, King H. Idiopathic adolescent scoliosis: indications and expectations. In: Bridwell K, DeWald R, eds. *The textbook of spinal surgery*, 2nd ed. Philadelphia: Lippincott–Raven Publishers, 1997:425–450.

39. Lane J, Cornell C, Barth R, et al. Pathological fractures: Pt II. In: Browner B, Jupiter J, Levine A, et al., eds. *Skeletal trauma: fractures, dislocations, ligamentous injury*. Philadelphia: WB Saunders, 1992:432–441.

40. Levi A, Dickman C, Sonntag V. Management of postoperative infections after spinal instrumentation. *J Neurosurg* 1997;86:975–980.

41. Leyshon A, Kirwan E, Parry CB. Electrical studies in the diagnosis of compression of the lumbar root. *J Bone Joint Surg Br* 1980;63B:71–75.

42. Lim TH, An HS, Hasegawa T, et al. Prediction of fatigue screw loosening in anterior spinal fixation using dual energy x-ray absorptiometry. *Spine* 1995;20(23):2565–2568; discussion 9.

43. Long D. Failed back surgery syndrome. *Neurosurg Clin North Am* 1991;2(4):899–919.

44. Long D, Filtzer D, BenDebba M, et al. Clinical features of the failed-back syndrome. *J Neurosurg* 1988;69:61–71.

45. Markwalder T, Reulen H. Diagnostic approach in instability and irritative state of a "lumbar motion segment" following disc surgery—failed back surgery syndrome. *Acta Neurochir* 1989;99:51–57.

46. Maxwell-Cade C. Principles and practice of clinical thermography. *Radiography* 1968;34(398):23–34.

47. Melton LI, Atkinson E, O'Fallon W, et al. Long-term fracture prediction by bone mineral assessed at different skeletal sites. *J Bone Miner Res* 1993;8:1227–1233.

48. Melton LI, Kan S, Frye M, et al. Epidemiology of vertebral fractures in women. *Am J Epidemiol* 1989;129(5):1000–1011.

49. Mooney V. The failed back—an orthopaedic view. *Int Disabil Studies* 1988;10(1):32–36.

50. North R, Zeidman S. Failed back surgery syndrome. *Cont Neurosurg* 1993;15(4)1–8.

51. Ortiz O, Pait TG, McAllister P, et al. Postoperative magnetic resonance imaging with titanium implants of the thoracic and lumbar spine. *Neurosurgery* 1996;38(4):741–745.

52. Papagelopoulos P, Peterson H, Ebersold M, et al. Spinal column deformity and instability after lumbar or thoracolumbar laminectomy for intraspinal tumors in children and adults. *Spine* 1997;22(4):442–451.

53. Pheasant H, Dyck P. Failed lumbar disc surgery: cause, assessment, treatment. *Clin Orthop* 1982;164:93–109.

54. Pilgaard S. Diskitis following removal of lumbar intervertebral disc. *J Bone Joint Surg Am* 1969;51: 713–716.

55. Pochaczevsky R, Wexler C, Meyers P, et al. Liquid crystal thermography of the spine and extremities. *J Neurosurg* 1982;56:386–395.

56. Rath S, Neff U, Schneider O, et al. Neurosurgical management of thoracic and lumbar vertebral osteomyelitis and discitis in adults: a review of 43 consecutive surgically treated patients. *Neurosurgery* 1996;38(5):926–933.

57. Ridenour T, Haddad S, Hitchon P, et al. Herniated thoracic disks: treatment and outcome. *J Spinal Disord* 1993;6(3):218–224.

58. Reference deleted.

59. Ross J, Masaryk T, Schrader M. MR imaging of the postoperative lumbar spine: assessment with gadopentetate dimeglumine. *AJR Am J Roentgenol* 1990;155:867–872.

60. Schmalstieg E, Peters B, Schochet S, et al. Neuropathy presenting as prolonged dyspnea: case report and review of the literature. *Arch Neurol* 1977;34(8):473–476.

61. Shafaie F, Bundschuh C, Jinkins J. *Postoperative lumbosacral spine.* Philadelphia: WB Saunders, 1996.

62. Sihvonen T, Herno A, Paljarvi L, et al. Local denervation atrophy of paraspinal muscles in postoperative failed back syndrome. *Spine* 1993;18(5):575–581.

63. Slone RM, McEnery KW, Bridwell KH, et al. Fixation techniques and instrumentation used in the thoracic, lumbar, and lumbosacral spine. *Radiol Clin North Am* 1995;33(2):233–265.

64. Slucky A, Eismont F. Spinal infections. In: Bridwell K, DeWald R, eds. *The textbook of spinal surgery,* 2nd ed. Philadelphia: Lippincott–Raven Publishers, 1997;2141–2183.

65. Snell R. *Clinical anatomy for medical students.* Boston: Little, Brown and Company, 1986.

66. Spengler D, Freeman C, Westbrook R, et al. Low-back pain following multiple lumbar spine procedures: failure of initial selection. *Spine* 1989;5:356–360.

67. Starck WJ, Epker BN. Failure of osseointegrated dental implants after diphosphonate therapy for osteoporosis: a case report. *Int J Oral Maxillofac Implants* 1995;10(1):74–78.

68. Steinmann J, Herkowitz H. Pseudarthrosis of the spine. *Clin Orthop* 1992;284:80–90.

69. Stovall DJ, Goodrich A, McDonald A, et al. Pedicle screw instrumentation for unstable thoracolumbar fractures. *J South Orthop Assoc* 1996;5(3):165–173.

70. Reference deleted.

71. Thomalske G, Galow W, Ploke G. Critical comments on a comparison of two series (1000 patients each) of lumbar disc surgery. *Adv Neurosurg* 1977;4:22–27.

72. Uematsu S. Thermography. In: Youmans J, ed. *Neurological surgery,* 3rd ed. Philadelphia: WB Saunders, 1990:500–508.

73. Waddell G, Main C, Morris E. Chronic low-back pain, psychological distress, and illness behavior. *Spine* 1984; 9:209–213.

74. Walton JC. *Aids to the examination of the peripheral nervous system.* London: Bailliere Tindall, 1990.

75. Yosipovitch Z, Robin G, Makin M. Open reduction of unstable thoracolumbar spinal injuries and fixation with Harrington rods. *J Bone Joint Surg Am* 1977;59A(8):1003–1015.

76. Young A, Wynn Parry C. The assessment and management of the failed back, Pt I. *Int Disabil Studies* 1988;10(1):21–24.

77. Young R. Sympathetic nervous system and pain. In: Tindall G, Cooper P, Barrow D, eds. *The practice of neurosurgery.* Baltimore: Williams & Wilkins, 1996;3009–3019.

78. Zeidman S, Long D. Failed back surgery syndrome. In: Menezes A, Sonntag V, eds. *Principles of spinal surgery.* New York: McGraw-Hill, 1996;657–679.

THORACIC SPINE: NONOPERATIVE TREATMENT

LAWRENCE G. LENKE

Surgery for pathology of the thoracic spine differs from that of the lumbar spine in several important ways. Overall, the regional thoracic spine is a more stable entity than the lumbar spine because of the adjoining ribcage and sternum and less motion in the disks throughout. Thus, the incidence of surgery for degenerative disease of the thoracic spine is much less than for the lumbar spine (3,8). The common diagnoses leading to surgical intervention in the thoracic spine include thoracic herniated disks with radiculopathy or myelopathy, fractures or tumors of the thoracic spine imparting spinal instability with or without pain and neurologic impairment, and spinal deformity such as thoracic scoliosis or hyperkyphosis deformities (2,12,15). In addition, the thoracic spine may secondarily require surgery for primary conditions of the cervical spine above or lumbar spine below.

As in any other part of the spine, it is important to perform appropriate surgery on the appropriate patient to produce an optimal result with the first procedure. This chapter investigates various nonoperative treatment regimens of the postoperative thoracic spine.

GENERAL PRINCIPLES

As in any postoperative patient, an initial assessment must include a detailed record of the prior diagnosis, surgical treatment rendered, and pre- and postoperative symptomatology. The clinical and radiographic evaluations of the postoperative thoracic spine are detailed in Chapter 7. This information is essential to plan an appropriate nonoperative management course for these patients. The key elements of the clinical and radiographic assessment include the following: How far postoperative is the patient from the surgery? Are the patient's symptoms improving, static, or intensifying over time? Are obvious structural or neurologic problems present that need to be addressed? To what type of postoperative regimen has the patient been adhering?

This chapter delineates specific nonoperative treatment regimens, such as medications, spinal orthoses, injections, physical therapy, and multidisciplinary pain clinics. Other chapters deal with operative management of the postoperative failed thoracic spine patient.

MEDICATIONS

A variety of medications can be used for the postoperative thoracic spine patient. These include a variety of narcotics, antiinflammatory medications, muscle relaxants, antispasmodics, and tricyclic antidepressant medications. They can be used alone or in combination depending on the symptomatology and any contraindications from principal side effects or adverse drug interactions. It is often important to enlist the help of an internist or a pain management specialist if medications are to be used on a chronic basis (14).

On an acute and limited basis, narcotic medications can be used to control a patient's severe pain syndrome. However, the use of narcotic medications on a chronic basis for nonoperative treatment of any type of spine condition should be avoided. If the postoperative patient is deemed nonoperative and adequate pain control is difficult, referral to a multidisciplinary pain clinic is advised. A more reasonable alternative is the use of one of the myriad nonsteroidal antiinflammatory drugs. A variety of prescription and nonprescription antiinflammatories are available, all with slightly different dosing regimens, efficacies, and side effects. The author tends to recommend that patients choose their own over-the-counter antiinflammatory medications. Discussion regarding the commonest side effect of the gastrointestinal intolerance and irritation must be considered. These medications must be accompanied by some type of oral food intake. Long-term use mandates evaluation of the hepatic and renal systems for rare adverse side effects. The advantage of these medications is that tolerance does not occur and that they can be discontinued without any adverse consequences.

Various muscle relaxants can be used to improve posterior spinal extensor or trapezial myofascial syndromes that can occur after a posterior exposure of

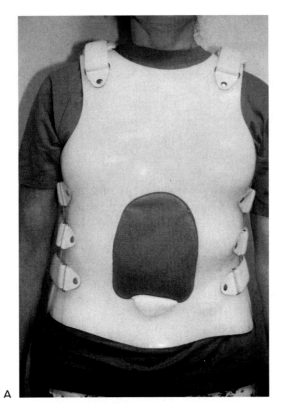
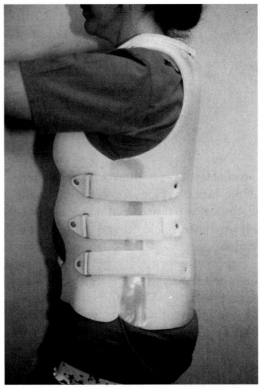

FIGURE 1. **A:** Frontal view of a postoperative thoracic spinal deformity patient wearing an above-the-shoulder thoracolumbosacral orthosis two-piece brace with an anterior abdominal hole present. **B:** Lateral view of the same patient showing the custom-molded fitting of the two-piece brace.

the thoracic spine (5). Similarly, postthoracotomy syndromes may involve scarring or irritation of the latissimus dorsi or serratus anterior musculature after an anterior exposure of the thoracic spine. Intermittent use of various muscle relaxants can help control myofascial syndromes and muscular spasms that can occur in the postoperative patient. Patients must be warned that these medications usually produce drowsiness to varying degrees that may not be well tolerated by patients. They are generally not used on a chronic basis, for if myofascial syndromes or postthoracotomy syndromes are problematic, other techniques (e.g., muscle tissue injections) can be used with a higher degree of short- and long-term success.

Occasionally, the use of antispasmodics is indicated in postoperative thoracic spine patients, especially those with permanent spinal cord injuries that resulted in increased spasticity and lower extremity tone. A neurologist may be quite helpful in deciding on and implementing therapies to overcome this difficult side effect of spinal cord injury. The patient must be counseled that often a decrease in muscle strength may accompany the decrease in spasticity that occurs after the use of antispasmodics. Often the patient and the neurologist or rehabilitation specialist must decide on a tradeoff and balance con-

cerning the amount of medication used on a long-term basis. In a similar vein, tricyclic antidepressants can also be used in these and other patients with severe physical and psychological handicaps following surgical treatment of the thoracic spine secondary to neurocompressive pathology.

SPINAL ORTHOSES

The use of spinal orthoses in the postoperative thoracic spine patient can be quite helpful in the early postoperative period. Spinal orthoses allow for increased trunk and chest stability while muscles and tissues involved in the posterior or anterior surgical approaches, or both, heal. We find early postoperative bracing very useful in patients who have had surgery for increased thoracic kyphosis because of the biomechanical forces acting to dislodge posterior instrumentation, which acts more as a tension band for thoracic hyperkyphosis pathologies. Normally, postoperative bracing for 4 to 7 months is adequate to allow a spinal fusion to mature and to enable the more superficial tissues to heal (Fig. 1).

On a chronic basis, the use of spinal orthoses is of more limited value. They certainly can provide

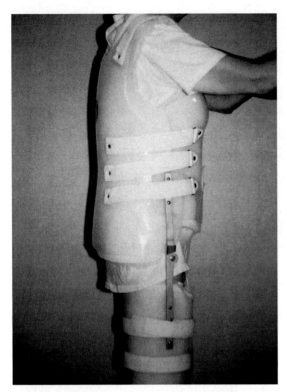

FIGURE 2. Postoperative patient who had a T-2 to the pelvis instrumentation and fusion as well as an osteotomy procedure for marked sagittal imbalance with mild hip flexion contractures. Her postoperative regimen included a thoracolumbosacral orthosis brace with a hinged side cuff that was locked in extension when standing but allowed her to sit with her hip in a 90-degree flexed position.

improved truncal support and stability, but at the cost of muscle and tissue wasting from less intrinsic support being required of the patient. For patients with moderate degrees of spinal instability and medical contraindications to more aggressive surgical stabilization, a spinal orthosis may be an interim measure to improve patient function and lessen pain. If this is the plan, a custom-molded brace that conforms to the body habitus of the patient is the best alternative. Patients with a thinner body habitus are more amenable to receive orthotic support than those with a very large body habitus, in whom control of the thoracic ribcage and, thus, thoracic spine is much more difficult. In an elderly patient with a frail body habitus, the use of a soft shell orthosis may provide adequate support without irritating the often sensitive skin of these older patients. On a short-term basis, an off-the-shelf Jewett-type hyperextension orthosis may be beneficial to provide some cost savings versus custom-molded orthoses. However, we found much better patient compliance and improved support with the use of a custom-molded orthosis for our patients.

In rare circumstances, the use of skeletal traction may be indicated in a patient with a failed thoracic

hyperkyphosis deformity. Normally, this is performed as a preliminary to a redo fusion procedure. In addition, once the spine has reached a more acceptable position, a halo vest–type apparatus can be applied so that posterior surgery can be performed with the patient maintained in the halo vest position by removing the posterior shell of the brace. After surgery, the posterior shell can be reapplied.

Also, in rare circumstances, a spinal orthosis can be attached via one- or two-leg extensions to improve stability of the lumbosacral region. This can be created as a single hip spica vest that is locked or that has a hinge on it that can be locked at either 0 degrees or 90 degrees to allow the patient to stand and sit accordingly. Once again, these are usually reserved for early postoperative patients who require additional support after long spinal fusion procedures of the spine to the pelvis (Fig. 2). However, they can be adjuncts to postoperative management in patients with pain or sagittal alignment problems, or both, that may require additional surgical intervention.

INJECTIONS

Various injection techniques may be helpful in providing pain relief for the postoperative thoracic spine patient (11). Probably the two commonest indications for injection therapy are postoperative myofascial syndromes following posterior approaches to the thoracic spine and postthoracotomy syndromes following an anterior transthoracic or thoracoabdominal approach. We usually have our multidisciplinary pain clinic direct and execute the injections because they have extensive experience in providing injection therapy, and often multiple injections over time are needed to complete a management protocol for these difficult problems.

Trigger point injections are commonly used to treat postoperative myofascial pain syndromes of the posterior spinal extensor musculature. These injections are a combination of a short-acting local anesthetic and a longer-acting steroid mixture that is placed directly into the region of tender muscle trigger points. Patients usually receive an initial favorable response from the short-acting local anesthetic, with a potential long-lasting benefit resulting from the steroid medication. Often other modalities such as medications and physical therapy are required to optimize and continue with the improvements obtained (Fig. 3).

Another difficult postoperative problem that is often aided by injection therapy is postthoracot-

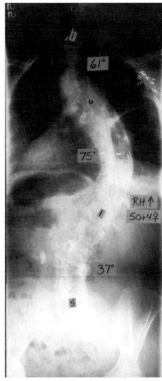

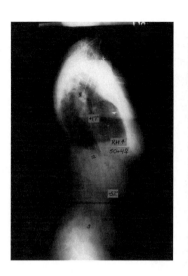

A,B

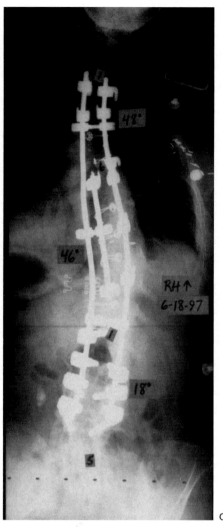

C

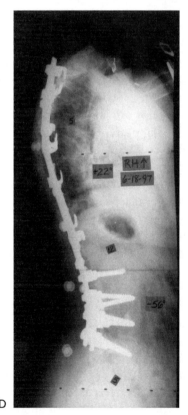

D

FIGURE 3. This 50-year-old woman had progressive double thoracic adult idiopathic scoliosis and significant thoracic axial pain. **A:** Upright coronal x-ray showing a 61-degree upper thoracic and 75-degree main thoracic scoliosis. **B:** Lateral x-ray showing a fairly unremarkable regional and global alignment. She underwent posterior instrumentation and fusion from T-2 to L-4 with segmental spinal instrumentation. **C:** Upright coronal x-ray showing instrumented correction and overall coronal balance. **D:** Postoperative lateral x-ray showing maintenance of her regional and global alignments. Postoperatively, her main complaint was cervical thoracic muscular pain that persisted even up to 1 year after surgery. She underwent a series of cervical thoracic trigger point injections by the pain management service, with successful resolution of her cervical thoracic muscle syndrome.

omy syndrome. This syndrome can occur after either an anterior transthoracic or thoracoscopic approach to the spine is used in surgery. The etiology may be irritation of the intercostal nerves; disruption of the ligaments that attach the rib to the transverse process and vertebral body, which are stretched during a transthoracic exposure of the spine via a rib spreader; or healing with subsequent scar formation in the muscle tissue of the serratus anterior or latissimus dorsi muscles that have been transected to gain open access to the thoracic cavity. Postthoracotomy syndromes appear to occur more often in older patients, who have stiffer chest cavities that tolerate less chest spreading than younger, more flexible chest cavities. Diagnostic and therapeutic injection therapy can be aimed at blocking the intercostal nerves or providing trigger point injections into the musculature involved.

This can be quite a debilitating problem for these patients, who can be cured of their spine pathology but still suffer from this approach-related complication (Fig. 4).

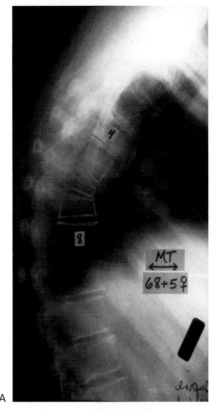

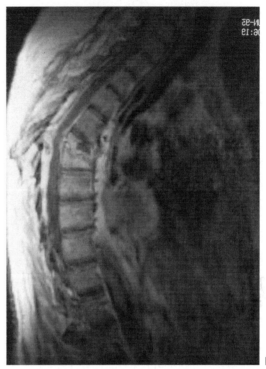

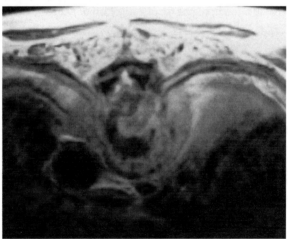

FIGURE 4. This 68-year-old woman presented to our emergency room with the acute onset of paraplegia after a 3-month prodrome of midthoracic back pain. **A:** Supine lateral thoracic radiograph showing a kyphotic deformity centered between T-6 and T-7 with collapse of the T-6 vertebral body noted. **B:** Emergent thoracic magnetic resonance imaging showing destruction of the T6-7 disk, the body of T-6, and the upper endplate of T-7. **C:** The corresponding axial slice at the T6-7 level showing marked narrowing of the spinal canal with a soft tissue mass extending from the boundaries of the vertebral body. Her sedimentation rate at presentation was 98, and her peripheral lymphocyte count was 14,000. Her clinical and radiographic presentation was consistent with spinal osteomyelitis with acute paraplegia. She underwent emergent anterior thoracic débridement and spinal cord decompression followed by an anterior spinal reconstruction with a titanium cage packed with autogenous rib graft. She then was placed prone and underwent an instrumented posterior thoracic fusion for stability after her extensive anterior débridement. (*continued*)

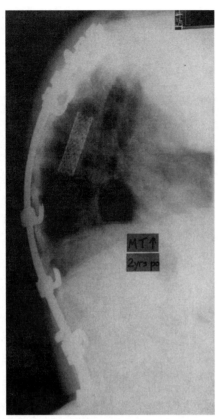
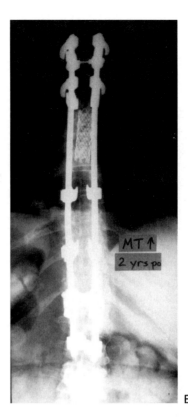

D

E

FIGURE 4. (*continued*) Her 2-year postoperative (**D**) sagittal and (**E**) coronal x-rays show maintenance of appropriate alignment. She regained nearly full neurologic function and was able to walk within 1 week after her surgery. However, for the first 1½ years after surgery, she had a postthoracotomy syndrome that necessitated several hospitalizations and treatment on a continuing basis by the pain management service, with multiple modalities required, including pain medications, physical therapy, and injection therapy. At 2 years after surgery, her symptoms had subsided enough to not require any further pain management services.

PHYSICAL THERAPY

Physical therapy can play an important role for post-operative thoracic spine patients, including those who require revision surgery and some of those who do not (1,4,6,7,10). Physical therapy modalities can be divided into two distinct entities: passive and active. *Passive modalities* are defined as those in which the therapist provides education (13) and direct treatment to the patient, such as massage therapy, electrical stimulation, biotherapy, diathermy, and so forth. These are modalities in which the patient is passive, but they provide direct relief to irritated tissues and joints. In contrast, *active physical therapy protocols* emphasize exercises that stabilize the tissues while promoting flexibility and strength of the muscles. Often a combination of passive and active modalities is required to optimize a patient's condition following spinal surgery.

From a short-term perspective, passive modalities can provide instant relief and satisfaction to the patient with pain. The only drawback is that long-lasting benefits usually do not occur, and thus passive therapy must

continue indefinitely, similar to chiropractic care (1,7). Active physical therapy that emphasizes strengthening and flexibility of the spinal musculature often takes a bit longer to realize true benefits but can be of longer-lasting and permanent value to the patient and relieve his or her discomfort (9). A dedicated and knowledgeable therapist is required to design an individualized treatment program for postoperative patients, who often present quite a challenge to the therapist. The goal of active therapeutic programs is to allow individuals to perform specific exercises at home on an individual basis and to allow them to integrate these exercises into a daily routine of aerobic fitness and a healthier lifestyle. In this respect, these modalities can make a true long-lasting change in the person, not only regarding the spine but also his or her overall health.

MULTIDISCIPLINARY PAIN CLINIC

A multidisciplinary pain clinic can be invaluable in the assessment and treatment of difficult postoperative cases, including those with failed thoracic spine surgery. Multidisciplinary clinics vary from hospital to hospital and institution to institution, but a full-service pain clinic should involve individuals from the following disciplines: anesthesia; physical therapy; occupational therapy; behavioral medicine; psychology or psychiatry, or both; nutritional services; physical medicine and rehabilitation; and neurology. In a multidisciplinary center, they can provide a critical assessment as to the overall emotional and psychological stability of the patients and their chance for either operative or nonoperative cure of their failed thoracic spinal problem. It is imperative that spinal specialists become familiar with the type of pain center that is available for referral and discuss and help direct treatment options for these patients based on assessment of the patient from the spinal surgeon's perspective. In this respect, the pain management team can provide services ranging from trigger point or epidural steroid injections to detoxification from a chronic narcotic abuse problem to coordination of a multidisciplinary evaluation and treatment course for a failed postoperative thoracic spine patient who has been judged to require no further surgery because of a small chance of any success.

CONCLUSION

The failed postoperative thoracic spine patient poses a diagnostic and treatment dilemma to the spinal surgeon. Initially, various operative measures should be discussed and performed if indicated. If prolonged conservative care is needed, that is often best done under the auspices of a multidisciplinary pain clinic. A multidisciplinary team evaluation may also help determine whether further surgery may be of benefit to a specific patient. The following chapters discuss specific surgical interventions that may be indicated for various pathologies involving the postoperative thoracic spine patient.

REFERENCES

1. Anderson R, Meeker WC, Wirick BE, et al. A meta-analysis of clinical trials of spinal manipulation. *J Manipulative Physiol Ther* 1992;15:181–194.

2. Fowles JV, Drummond DS, L'Ecuyer S, et al. Untreated scoliosis in the adult. *Clin Orthop* 1978;134:212–217.

3. Gundewall B, Liljeqvist M, Hansson T. Primary prevention of back symptoms and absence from work. A prospective randomized study among hospital employees. *Spine* 1993;18:587–594.

4. Hadler NM, Curtis P, Gillings DB, et al. A benefit of spinal manipulation as adjunctive therapy for acute low-back pain: a stratified controlled trial. *Spine* 1987;12:702–706.

5. Jackson RP, Simmons EH, Stripinis D. Coronal and sagittal plane spinal deformities correlating with back pain and pulmonary function in adult idiopathic scoliosis. *Spine* 1989;14:1391–1397.

6. Koes BW, Bouter LM, van Mameren H, et al. A blinded randomized clinical trial of manual therapy and physiotherapy for chronic back and neck complaints: physical outcome measures. *J Manipulative Physiol Ther* 1992;15:16–23.

7. Koes BW, Bouter LM, van Mameren H, et al. The effectiveness of manual therapy, physiotherapy, and treatment by the general practitioner for nonspecific back and neck complaints. *Spine* 1992;17:28–35.

8. Lindstrom L, Ohlund C, Eek C, et al. The effect of graded activity on patients with subacute low back pain: a randomized prospective clinical study with an operant conditioning behavioral approach. *Phys Ther* 1992;72:279–293.

9. Lowery WD Jr, Horn TJ, Boden SD, et al. Impairment evaluation based on spinal range of motion in normal subjects. *J Spinal Disord* 1992;5:398–402.

10. Malmivaara A, Hakkinen U, Aro T, et al. The treatment of acute low back pain—bed rest, exercises, or ordinary activity? *N Engl J Med* 1995;332:351–355.

11. Marks RC, Houston T, Thulbourne T. Facet joint injection and facet nerve block: a randomized comparison in 86 patients with chronic low back pain. *Pain* 1992;49:325–328.

12. Ogilvie JW. Adult scoliosis: evaluation and nonsurgical treatment. *Instr Course Lect* 1992;41:251–255.

13. Roland M, Dixon M. Randomized controlled trial of an educational booklet for patients presenting with back pain in general practice. *J R Coll Gen Pract* 1989;39:244–246.

14. Waddell G. Biopsychosocial analysis of low back pain. *Baillieres Clin Rheumatol* 1992;6:523–557.

15. Winter RB, Lonstein JE, Denis F. Pain patterns in adult scoliosis. *Orthop Clin North Am* 1988;19:339–345.

THORACIC SPINE: DEGENERATIVE DISEASE

CHRISTOPHER J. DEWALD

Failed spinal surgery for degenerative disorders of the thoracic spine is dependent on the unique anatomy of the thoracic spine. The thoracic spine is normally kyphotic and functions with a supportive/protective role versus a mobility role. The thoracic disks are narrower than disks in the lumbar spine (53). Rib articulations at each motion segment add to the overall stability and relative stiffness. When degeneration occurs in the thoracic spine, disk height is decreased, but typically this does not lead to segmental instability or sagittal imbalance, because the normal kyphotic sagittal contour is not significantly altered, as it is in the degenerative lumbosacral spine. Due to the preservation of sagittal alignment and the relative lack of motion of the thoracic spine, the severity of degeneration is usually less than the more mobile and lordotic cervical or lumbar spine (2,18,30,47,53). Thus, not unexpectedly, conditions of disk degeneration in the thoracic spine lead much less commonly to symptomatic herniated disks than in the cervical or lumbar spine. In the lumbosacral spine, the stresses associated with the weight-bearing status may change significantly, as seen in lumbar degenerative scoliosis, in which loss of lumbar lordosis and even frank lumbar kyphosis occurs as disk degeneration progresses. In the thoracic spine, loss of disk height produces an increase in the normal kyphotic sagittal alignment and, thus, does not lead to the sagittal balance problems seen in the lumbar spine. Across the thoracolumbar junction, the lower thoracic spine (T11-12) behaves more like the lumbar spine, as these disks are larger and the sagittal alignment is neutral, providing the transition zone from lordosis to kyphosis. Often, the thoracolumbar junction needs to be treated as part of the lumbar spine (29,39,47,59).

As degenerative conditions in the thoracic spine are limited in frequency of occurrences, the incidence of "failed" spine cases for degenerative spinal disorders is limited, especially compared to the lumbosacral spine or cervical spine (24,36,57,65). Conditions that require surgery of the degenerative thoracic spine include decompression of myelopathic or radicular symptoms—that is, thoracic disk herniation (TDH) (1,3,4,8,16,20,23,37,41,43,46,51–53); degenerative

spinal stenosis (2,18,29,30,36,42,47,53,56,63); and stenosis associated with an ossified posterior longitudinal ligament and ossified ligamentum flavum (15,19,34,35,40,54,55,64).

Failed spinal surgeries of the degenerative thoracic spine can be differentiated into four groups: (a) wrong level, (b) wrong patient, (c) inadequate decompression, and (d) segmental instability, unrecognized or postoperative. In addition, postoperative infection/diskitis would also be a cause of a failed surgery involving the thoracic spine, but that is not the subject of this chapter.

WORKUP/ALGORITHM

When an individual presents for examination with continued pain symptoms after undergoing a previous spinal surgery (failed spine), it is important to evaluate the patient logically starting with the initial *preoperative* x-rays, computed tomography myelography (CTM), and/or magnetic resonance imaging (MRI) and to determine what the original pathology was. A careful review of the preoperative examination and operative report is essential. Are the current symptoms the same or different? Is this a continuation of the initial problem or a new problem? Did the patient's condition improve after the initial surgery? For how long or at all? Does the physical examination reveal correlating signs with the initial preoperative radiographic and imaging studies? Were any nonorganic signs present before the initial surgery? Do the imaging studies and x-rays corroborate with the current signs and symptoms? As in all spinal surgeries, but especially the thoracic spine, was the procedure performed on the proper level? Once this initial determination is done, a workup can begin. The workup can be organized according to the algorithm in Figure 1 to determine the most likely cause of the patient's symptoms.

Workup should include a careful history and physical examination, standing and supine radiographs, CTM, and MRI. The postoperative MRI requires

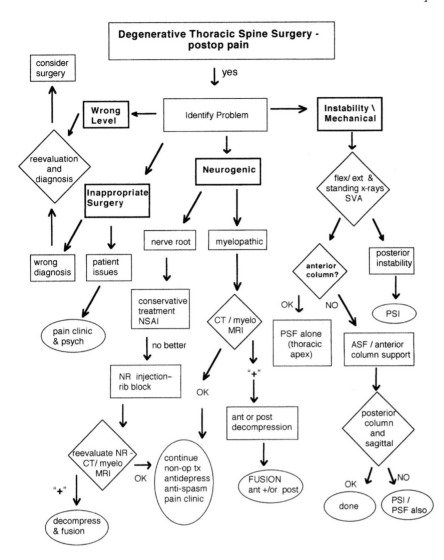

FIGURE 1. Algorithm for the approach and treatment of failed spinal surgery of the degenerative thoracic spine. ASF, anterior spinal fusion; CT, computed tomography; MRI, magnetic resonance imaging; NR, nerve root; NSAI, nonsteroidal antiinflammatory; PSF, posterior spinal fusion; PSI, posterior spinal instrumentation; SVA, sagittal vertical axis.

gadolinium enhancement to help delineate scar from extradural compression (17,42,44,45,58). Dynamic x-rays (flexion/extension) are not as helpful in the thoracic spine as in the lumbar or cervical spine; however, weight-bearing standing x-rays can be quite helpful in evaluating the patient's weight-bearing line or sagittal alignment (or sagittal vertical axis) (57). Myelopathic patients who have undergone decompression may still exhibit signs of myelopathy despite evidence of adequate decompression (53). However, evidence of increasing balance difficulty or uncoordination may require careful reexamination of the spinal cord at the previously operated site as well as the remaining spinal cord.

It is well known that many pseudarthroses of spinal fusions, with or without instrumentation, can be asymptomatic (7,14). This can be particularly understood in the thoracic spine given its relative stiffness and its rib articulations. If a painful pseudarthrosis is apparent, it is likely that an unrecognized segmental instability of the spine is present either anteriorly or posteriorly and must be addressed appropriately from anteriorly, posteriorly, or both (9,57).

WRONG LEVEL

One of the more common errors in spinal surgery is an operative procedure performed at the wrong level (31). The thoracic spine, in particular, is at risk for such a complication, as it is often difficult to determine the level of pathology when either C-2 or the sacrum is not in view on the preoperative imaging studies to count down or up to be certain at which level the pathology exists. One should never assume that the neuroradiologist has numbered levels correctly. One should look for other bony details to help identify the proper level— that is, calcified disks, the twelfth rib, rib abnormalities, and so forth. This is particularly important in the operating room, as the surgeon is frequently limited by the length of spine visualized and the poor quality of the portable operating room radiographs. Postoperative MRI scans of the lumbosacral spine have been found to be accurate at distinguishing recurrent disk from scar tissue (17,44,45,49,58). Although this has been demonstrated with high specificity, we find postoperative MRI scans to be of limited value, especially in the early postoperative period. Currently, we use MRIs as a preliminary noninvasive diagnostic examination (8,39,42). MRI scans remain the study of choice regarding sagittal anatomy and neural anatomy of the spine but due to respiratory motion do not provide superior axial cuts. CTMs are run from either the cistern or up from the lumbar spine and, therefore, can be dilute, making the myelogram more difficult to visualize than the more familiar lumbar spinal myelograms (53). However, the postmyelographic axial CT cuts show superior anatomy of the thoracic dura and bony facets (23,42). It is thus the examination of choice for complex spinal cord compressions and especially in ossified posterior longitudinal ligament conditions (54,63,64). The importance of knowing the anatomy in either the initial or revision situation cannot be overstated. It is easy to find yourself at the wrong level, as intraoperative radiographs make correlation with preoperative MRI or CT difficult.

WRONG PATIENT

Inappropriate Surgery

One of the major causes of "failed back syndrome" is that inappropriate spinal surgeries are being performed initially, a finding that is seen too often. The most common causes include a wrong diagnosis or an inappropriate patient selection (9,50,65). In a review of initial preoperative histories, physical findings, and myelograms in 105 lumbar spinal surgery failures, Fager and Freidberg (9) found that in most of the patients a preoperative pathologic diagnosis of disk rupture or nerve root compression was not substantiated. It is known that abnormalities can be found on CT scans, myelograms, and MRI scans in asymptomatic patients (12,13,62). In the thoracic spine, MRI abnormalities have been reported to be as high as 73% in asymptomatic patients, including TDHs and deformations of the spinal cord (62). Careful evaluation of the original preoperative studies, history, and physical examination are extremely important for all revision cases. Occasionally, spine patients cannot be helped by additional surgery—a lesson hard taught to many young spinal surgeons. In the absence of definable pathology originally or currently, it is the surgeon's role to prevent further

unwarranted surgical procedures and direct the patient toward nonoperative measures (65).

Preoperative Expectation

Patient selection can be, perhaps, the most difficult part of spine surgery and is well beyond the scope of this chapter (33,50). It is well known that patients with back pain with degenerative findings on their radiographic and imaging studies may have other psychosocial issues that result in symptoms of pain in the back (14,25,26,48,60,65). This has been described mostly regarding the lumbar and cervical regions of the spine. A typical case is a patient with back or neck pain after involvement in a motor vehicle accident resulting in a workup that reveals a degenerative disk. These patients often have gone from doctor to doctor and have learned appropriate answers and signs. Surgical procedures on these patients invariably result in a failed back and may only worsen the patient's chronic pain complaints (11,26,50,61).

If symptoms persist to be nonorganic, a determination is made that the patient is not a surgical candidate, and he or she is referred to a comprehensive pain clinic, including physical therapy, psychology, and pain relief modalities (21,24–28,65). The spinal surgeon and especially the revision spinal surgeon must realize that not all patients can be helped through surgery, and, often, repetitive surgeries can only do more harm than benefit (11,50,61). This is more significant in the spinal cord region, as the risks during revision surgery are greater than in the lumbar area.

INADEQUATE DECOMPRESSION

Degenerative compressive etiologies of the thoracic spine that require surgery are rare (2,17). By far, the most common pathoetiology requiring decompression in the thoracic spine is TDH (4,6,8,52,53). The majority of symptomatic thoracic degenerative conditions involve the lower thoracic spine (29,59). The surgical approach used in decompressive procedures of degenerative conditions of the thoracic spine is the most common reason for inadequate decompression of the thoracic spine (28,31,53). Unlike the lumbar spine, the spinal cord makes the surgical approach more limiting in its scope of decompression as well as the significance of postoperative morbidity resulting from the choice of approach (i.e., thoracotomy). Often, lack of familiarity with a certain approach may lead the surgeon to a less optimal but more familiar surgical approach (8). Simply, if the pathology lies

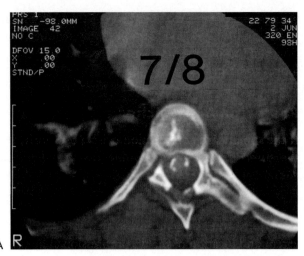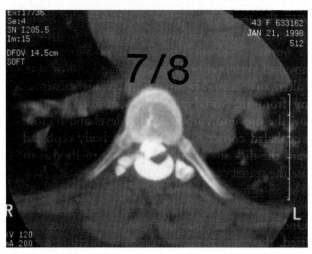

FIGURE 2. **A:** Computed tomography (CT) scan of a patient with a large central herniated disk at T7-8. The patient complained of trunk pain and lower extremity numbness with myelopathic signs. **B:** Six years after right-sided posterolateral decompression and disk excision, the patient continues to complain of trunk pain and "numbness" in the legs. The CT myelogram shows that the large central disk herniation remains without evidence of excision.

anteriorly, then an anterior-transthoracic approach is probably the best option. If spinal compression is posterior, a posterior decompression can be used. In Figure 2, a posterolateral approach was used to excise a central TDH. Postoperatively, the patient continues to complain of similar symptoms of trunk and lower extremity pain. Clearly, the majority of the anterior disk remains postoperatively, displacing the cord posteriorly. The degree of risk is much higher now to remove this scarred and calcified disk anteriorly in this nonmyelopathic patient. An anterior transthoracic decompression initially could have completely decompressed the disk herniation, avoiding the increased risk of a revision spinal cord decompression.

In the revision situation, to determine if the symptoms match the spinal pathology, we have again found the CTM to be more helpful than the postoperative thoracic MRI (63). Even using gadolinium infusion MRI can give a confusing and exaggerated picture when evaluating for completeness of decompression in a postoperative patient (8,35,39,45,54).

Anterior Approaches

Many TDHs are excised anteriorly (transthoracically). Often, herniated thoracic disks are calcified and occasionally migrate superiorly or inferiorly (52,53). Revision surgery of a TDH decompression performed anteriorly via a thoracotomy is unusual (1,3,6,8,19,37,41). The anterior approach provides excellent direct exposure of the herniated disk without manipulation of the nerve root or spinal cord (3). However, many patients have continued chest/rib

(thoracotomy) pain after a thoracotomy for anterior decompression. In some patients, the well-described thoracotomy syndrome develops (15,22,43). Thoracoscopic decompressions appear to have significantly reduced the morbidity associated with anterior disk excisions (15). Results of thoracoscopic spinal procedures are still early but are quite encouraging. For most revision TDHs, the surgeon must ensure appropriate decompression of the specific nerve root and spinal cord when reviewing the postoperative imaging studies. If a retained disk fragment or large vertebral body osteophyte is present, the surgeon must consider the risks of repeat thoracotomy and excision of the remaining extradural defect (2,56). Often, thoracotomy pain can mimic the radicular pain associated with the original TDH. In either case, an intercostal nerve block should be performed if other nonoperative treatments have failed (22,27).

Continued pain following an anterior thoracic decompression (TDH) requiring an anterior revision is typically recognized early in the postoperative period (65). If the revision decompression is performed within 6 months after operation, it can be accomplished through the previous diskectomy site. Even if a fusion had been performed, the fusion bone is usually softer than its adjacent normal bone and can be carefully curetted back to the previous decompression site. Occasionally, a partial or complete corpectomy can provide a safer decompression if the previous intercorporeal fusion has matured or the previous scar makes intervertebral revision decompression more difficult. Removing part or all of the previous fusion starting from normal tissue back toward the previous surgical site allows the spinal surgeon to find the spinal canal proximally or distally at a normal adjacent disk level and allows safer removal of vertebral body, fusion mass, and/or scar. An alternative would be to perform a partial corpectomy from the distal adjacent neuroforamen just below the previously operated disk level and remove the cephalad corner of the vertebral body cephalad toward the disk site. The key in either method is to locate the spinal canal and visualize the dura. A plane can be identified anterior to the dural sac, and the revision decompression can be completed safely.

Once the canal has been successfully decompressed, the spine is reconstructed with either a rib inlay strut across the decompressed intervertebral site or a corpectomy strut graft (i.e., allograft, autogenous iliac crest, or titanium cage) from endplate to endplate if a corpectomy was performed (32). A small anterior rod or plate can be used to support the strut graft to prevent dislodgment. The spinal cord should be monitored using at least somatosensory evoked potentials as well as motor-evoked potentials during revision spinal cord procedures (57). It should be remembered, when considering a revision decompression of a TDH, that the only absolute indication for excision of a primary or a retained TDH is a myelopathic patient.

If an initial posterior decompressive procedure had been performed—that is, a posterior laminectomy—an anterior transthoracic approach would be an obvious choice for revision decompression of an anterior extradural compression. In this case, the anterior spinal canal is virgin, as well as being the causative compressive pathology. Here, the only addition to routine transthoracic diskectomy is the previous loss of the posterior elements. Not only should the anterior interspace be fused in this situation, but anterior instrumentation is needed to provide spinal stability. A short posterior tension band construct and fusion should be included to provide a more stable construct if there is any question concerning the bone quality or anterior column stability. Although a combined anterior-posterior surgical procedure may seem aggressive, in revision spine surgery cases, a minimalist approach may only perpetuate the potential for additional surgery, thus leading toward a failed back syndrome. In the revision spinal surgery situation, the goal is to provide a successful outcome safely and securely and to prevent the ongoing scenario of multiple revision surgeries. Additional surgical failures only heighten the degree of difficulty for salvage. If there is any question regarding the stability of the spinal column, a more aggressive approach should be strongly considered, as

multiple failed surgeries make successful outcome less likely (50,61). Not uncommonly, this requires anterior and posterior spinal surgeries and the use of longer constructs.

Posterior Approaches

If the spinal cord compression exists posteriorly, it is the surgeon's task to determine exactly where the compressive pathology is located. Again, the CTM is our study of choice as the definitive surgical planner. If a previous attempt at decompression was done posteriorly, the surgeon must first determine the extent and location of the decompression. The CTM defines the causative pathology, specifically the bony anatomy of the facets and lateral recesses. Often, the posterior elements have been previously removed in revision posterior decompression cases, leaving the dura exposed during the revision surgical approach. In this case, it is necessary to identify the remaining spinous processes above and below the previous laminectomy site. The remaining spinous processes and lamina provide landmarks for the location of the spinal canal. After identifying the proximal and distal extent of previous decompression, dissection should be carried out laterally toward the transverse processes and facet joints of the previous laminectomy site, leaving a thin mass of scar protecting the spinal cord (57,61,65). Identifying the transverse processes can be helpful in deciphering the often confusing anatomy of revision cases. If the lamina was not excised, the remaining bony posterior elements provide additional anatomic landmarks and protection while exposing the posterior spine. The bony edges of the previous decompression site are carefully exposed using microcurettes. Completion of a previous decompressed site or decompression of an adjacent level can be safely completed once the bony margins of the previous decompression have been clearly exposed. Identification of the bony anatomy cannot be understated. If a remaining lamina or additional lamina is to be excised, the spinal surgeon can enter the spinal canal in virgin tissue above or below the scarred area and, using a small neurosurgical Kerrison, remove bone toward the previous surgical site. This provides visualization of the dura and thus added neurologic safety during the revision decompression. The remaining scar tissue adherent to the dura does not have to be removed, although it may need to be sharply debulked (57,61,65).

If a previous anterior diskectomy has been performed and a CTM or MRI, or both, has identified additional posterior compression—that is, hypertrophic facets—a virgin posterior decompression can be performed in the usual manner (2,56). Again, if both columns, anterior and posterior, have been weakened via decompression, the surgeon should strongly consider posterior fusion and instrumentation, especially if an anterior construct was used. It is much easier to instrument the spine at this juncture than at another revision.

INSTABILITY

Unrecognized

If a degenerative process has led to spinal cord compression, it is imperative that the spinal surgeon evaluate the biomechanical stability of both columns of the spinal segment before proceeding with a decompressive procedure anteriorly or posteriorly. Standing weight-bearing x-rays provide preliminary information regarding the sagittal stability, such as the presence of a junctional kyphosis. This is especially important in the lower thoracic spine at the thoracolumbar junction. Dysplastic posterior elements, for example, may provide little posterior stability to the spine. Anterior column surgery in this case would require secure anterior column support with anterior instrumentation. Flexion/extension sagittal x-rays provide additional information regarding the stability of an intervertebral motion segment but are more informative at the thoracolumbar junction, as the mid- and upper thoracic spine are less mobile due to the anatomic differences, resulting in the stiffer and less mobile thoracic spine described earlier (57).

Instability following anterior thoracic spinal surgery usually results in increased segmental kyphosis, pseudarthrosis, and mechanical pain. Instability following an anterior spinal procedure could potentially lead to dislodgment of an anterior strut graft and to paralysis. Posterior instrumentation using claws or pedicle screws provides stabilization to most anterior spinal constructs, providing that the anterior spinal column is still structurally stable (20). Revision of the anterior column may also be required if its stability has been altered anteriorly. Anterior column support is one of the keys to spinal stability. The spinal surgeon needs to ensure that the anterior column is intact and competent before proceeding with either a primary or revision posterior decompressive procedure. If the anterior column is deficient *mechanically*, a posterior stabilization procedure using segmental fixation is required if a posterior decompressive procedure is planned. If a *structural* anterior column deficit is

present, anterior column strut support is required in addition to the posterior construct.

Acquired Instability

Posterior Column Instability

In degenerative conditions in which posterior laminectomy has been performed at a degenerative level, especially at the thoracolumbar junction or the normal thoracic kyphosis apex, continued pain due to abnormal motion across this level may occur (5,6,38,57,65). Currier et al. (6) noted that their results of transthoracic decompression of TDH were compromised in patients who had undergone previous laminectomy. Curcin (5) described iatrogenic spondylolisthesis occurring after TDH decompression via a posterolateral approach. Workup to assess for posterior spinal instability following decompression includes a careful history and radiographic evaluation, as early radiographic signs may be quite subtle. Increased disk degeneration, hypertrophic spurring, subchondral sclerosis, and listhesis may only be noted late in the postoperative course. If the anterior column is structurally intact, a simple posterior construct is used to achieve proper spinal stability. If the anterior column is structurally deficient (as could be seen with osteoporotic patients), either a longer posterior instrumented construct or anterior strut support may be required.

Anterior Column Instability

In the same manner, a previous anterior decompression across a motion segment due to a TDH that is determined to have an anterior instability and continued pain due to the segmental instability may only require simple posterior instrumentation to stabilize this motion segment. Typically, minor shifts in position or minor subsidence of an intercorporal strut do not require a revision anteriorly and can also be easily salvaged by posterior instrumentation and fusion alone (10). Only in complete dislodgment of an anterior strut anteriorly or in the disastrous case of a posterior dislodgment into the spinal canal would an anterior revision intervertebral fusion be required (57).

Most degenerative cases of the thoracic spine with unrecognized instability at the decompressive site or acquired instability postoperatively require only a posterior revision to provide stability via an instrumented fusion across the unstable level. Of course, the normal thoracic spine sagittal anatomy must be kept in mind, and the spinal surgeon should avoid stopping the posterior construct at the normal thoracic kyphotic apex (T7-8). Pedicle screw posterior constructs may save levels of fusion but should be protected with infralaminar hooks and adjacent cephalad supralaminar hooks or preferably pedicular-transverse process claws. However, many patients have very small thoracic pedicles, and thus the benefits of using pedicle screws in the reduced mobility of the thoracic spine are less obvious than when used in the lumbar spine. The importance of saving motion segments from being incorporated in a fusion construct is more important in the lower thoracic spine and most important in the thoracolumbar spine. Fortunately, the pedicles in the thoracolumbar spine are also larger and better suited for pedicle screws than the remainder of the thoracic spine.

Most posterior spinal constructs are able to be managed via a simple hook configuration in the thoracic spine using claws to obtain maximum fixation stability. Claws can be single vertebral level or spread between two adjacent vertebrae within the thoracic spine from T-2 to T-10. We prefer single level claws, pedicular-transverse process, or pedicular-supralaminar claws. Again, the surgeon should be cognitive of ending the construct sufficiently above or below the patient's normal thoracic kyphotic apex. Extending the construct up T-4 for a T8-9 instability is relatively easy and provides additional stability via additional claws.

POST THORACOTOMY SYNDROME

A common cause of continued pain postoperatively from an anterior decompression of the thoracic spine is a result of the thoracotomy approach (22). With the improved knowledge and techniques regarding minimally invasive procedures, the incidence of this common postoperative problem will significantly decrease (16,22,43).

Currently, if a standard anterior thoracic diskectomy is performed, a standard thoracotomy is done using a rib spreader to provide adequate visualization. Often, patients with radiating pain from a disk herniation are left with a constant radiating pain due to this surgical approach. Thoracotomy pain can be significant, equal to the severity of the preoperative pain. If the postoperative pain continues greater than 3 months postoperatively, a nerve block can be performed at the thoracotomy site. Many continued pain symptoms after thoracotomy can be attributed to this problem. Again, endoscopic spinal surgery has its greatest potential is this area (22).

CONCLUSION

Not many procedures are performed on the degenerative thoracic spine compared to the lumbar or cervical spines, but the same considerations of continued pain after decompressive procedures need to be addressed. The advantage that the thoracic spine has over its adjacent spinal regions is its inherent stability associated with the ribcage, rib articulations, kyphotic alignment, and narrow disks. Many pseudarthroses of thoracic spinal fusions, for instance, are asymptomatic. Continued pain following surgery for the degenerative thoracic spine results from postoperative infection/diskitis, segmental instability, inadequate decompression (or wrong anatomic level), thoracotomy syndrome, wrong diagnosis, or a patient's secondary gain issues. A careful analysis is required once a patient has undergone any previous spinal procedure. It becomes a great source of stress for patient and surgeon to treat a multioperated patient. These patients become marked as a "failed spine" and often become addicted to narcotics and bounce from pain clinic to pain clinic and from surgeon to surgeon. If revision surgery is decided on, it is in the patient's best interest that short cuts are not taken in the procedure. Often, "more is better" as long as the patients' medical status is appropriate. Although occasionally combined anterior and posterior spinal surgery along with fusion and instrumentation is required in revision cases, it is important to "do it right" to stop the cycle of continued pain after inadequate or incomplete spinal procedures followed by additional spinal surgeries.

REFERENCES

1. Albrand OW, Corkill G. Thoracic disc herniation. Treatment and prognosis. *Spine* 1979;4(1):41–46.
2. Barnett GH, Hardy RW Jr, et al. Thoracic spinal canal stenosis. *J Neurosurg* 1987;66(3):338–344.
3. Boriani S, Biagini R, De Iure F, et al. Two-level thoracic disc herniation. *Spine* 1994;19(21):2461–2466.
4. Brown CW, Deffer PA Jr, Akmakjian J, et al. The natural history of thoracic disc herniation. *Spine* 1992;17(6):S97–S102.
5. Curcin A, Lucas PR. Spondylolisthesis after posterolateral thoracic discectomy. Case report and literature review. *Spine* 1992;17(10):1254–1256.
6. Currier BL, Eismont FJ, Green BA. Transthoracic disc excision and fusion for herniated thoracic discs. *Spine* 1994;19(3):323–328.
7. DePalma AF, Rothman RH. The nature of pseudarthrosis. *Clin Orthop* 1968;59:113–118.

8. Dietze DD Jr, Fessler RG. Thoracic disc herniations. *Neurosurg Clin North Am* 1993;4(1):75–90.

9. Fager CA, Freidberg SR. Analysis of failures and poor results of lumbar spine surgery. *Spine* 1980;5(1):87–94.

10. Farey ID, McAfee PC, Davis RF, et al. Pseudarthrosis of the cervical spine after anterior arthrodesis. Treatment by posterior nerve-root decompression, stabilization, and arthrodesis. *J Bone Joint Surg Am* 1990;72(8):1171–1177.

11. Finnegan W, Fenlin J, Marvel J, et al. Results of surgical intervention in the symptomatic multioperated back patient. *J Bone Joint Surg Am* 1979;61:1077–1082.

12. Frymoyer JW, Cats-Baril W. Predictors of low back pain disability. *Clin Orthop* 1987;221:89–98.

13. Frymoyer JW, Hanley EN Jr, Howe J, et al. A comparison of radiographic findings in fusion and non-fusion patients, ten or more years following disc surgery. *Spine* 1979;4:435–440.

14. Frymoyer JW, Rosen JC, Clements J, et al. Psychologic factors in low-back pain disability. *Clin Orthop* 1985; 195:178–184.

15. Hashizumi Y. Pathologic studies on the ossification of the posterior longitudinal ligament. *Acta Pathol Japn* 1980;30:255–273.

16. Horowitz MB, Moossy JJ, Julian T, et al. Thoracic discectomy using video assisted thoracoscopy. *Spine* 1994; 19(9):1082–1086.

17. Hueftle MG, Modic MT, Ross JS, et al. Lumbar spine: postoperative MR imaging with Gd-DTPA. *Radiology* 1988;167:817–824.

18. Kikuchi S, Watanabe E, Hasue M. Spinal intermittent claudication due to cervical and thoracic degenerative spine disease. *Spine* 1996;21(3):313–318.

19. Kojima T, Waga S, Kubo Y, et al. Surgical treatment of ossification of the posterior longitudinal ligament in the thoracic spine. *Neurosurgery* 1994;34(5):854–858.

20. Korovessis PG, Stamatakis MV, Baikousis A, et al. Transthoracic disc excision with interbody fusion. 12 patients with symptomatic disc herniation followed for 2–8 years. *Acta Orthop Scand Suppl* 1997;275:12–16.

21. Krempen JF, Smith BS. Nerve root injection: a method for evaluating the etiology of sciatica. *J Bone Joint Surg Am* 1974;56A:1435–1444.

22. Landreneau RJ, Hazelrigg SR, Mack MJ, et al. Postoperative pain-related morbidity: video-assisted thoracic surgery versus thoracotomy. *Ann Thorac Surg* 1993;56:1285–1289.

23. Le Roux PD, Haglund MM, Harris AB. Thoracic disc disease: experience with the transpedicular approach in twenty consecutive patients. *Neurosurgery* 1993;33(1):58–66.

24. Long DM, Filtzer DL, BenDebba M, et al. Clinical features of the failed back syndrome. *J Neurosurg* 1988;69: 61–71.

25. Long DM. Decision making in lumbar disc disease. *Clin Neurosurg* 1992;39:36–51.

26. Long DM. Failed back surgery syndrome. *Neurosurg Clin North Am* 1991;2:899–919.

27. Long DM. Nonsurgical therapy for low back pain and sciatica. *Clin Neurosurg* 1989;35:351–359.

28. MacNab I. Negative disc exploration: an analysis of the causes of nerve root involvement in 68 patients. *J Bone Joint Surg Am* 1971;53A:891–903.

29. Malmivaara A, Videman T, Kuosma E, et al. Facet joint orientation, facet and costovertebral joint osteoarthrosis, disc degeneration, vertebral body osteophytosis, and Schmorl's nodes in the thoracolumbar junctional region of cadaveric spines. *Spine* 1987;12(5):458–463.

30. Marzluff JM, Hungerford GD, Kempe LG, et al. Thoracic myelopathy caused by osteophytes of the articular processes: thoracic spondylosis. *J Neurosurg* 1979;50(6):779–783.

31. McCulloch JA, Young PH. Complications (adverse effects) in lumbar microsurgery. In: McCulloch JA, Young PH, eds. *Essentials of spinal microsurgery.* Philadelphia: Lippincott–Raven Publishers, 1998:503–529.

32. Meding JB, Stambough JL. Critical analysis of strut grafts in anterior spinal fusions. *J Spinal Disord* 1993; 6(2):166–174.

33. North RB, Campbell JN, James CS, et al. Failed back surgery syndrome: 5-year follow-up in 102 patients undergoing repeated operation. *Neurosurgery* 1991;28:685–690.

34. Ohtsuka K, Terayama K, Yanagihara M, et al. A radiological population study on the ossification of the posterior longitudinal ligament in the spine. *Arch Orthop Trauma Surg* 1987;106(2):89–93.

35. Omojola MF, Cardoso ER, Fox AJ, et al. Thoracic myelopathy secondary to ossified ligamentum flavum. *J Neurosurg* 1982;56(3):448–450.

36. Oppenheimer A. Diseases of the apophyseal (intervertebral) articulations. *J Bone Joint Surg* 1938;20:285–313.

37. Otani K, Yoshida M, Fujii E, et al. Thoracic disc herniation. Surgical treatment in 23 patients. *Spine* 1988;13 (11):1262–1267.

38. Papagelopoulos PJ, Peterson HA, Ebersold MJ, et al. Spinal column deformity and instability after lumbar or thoracolumbar laminectomy for intraspinal tumors in children and young adults. *Spine* 1997;22(4):442–451.

39. Raininko R, Manninen H, Battie MC, et al. Observer variability in the assessment of disc degeneration on magnetic resonance images of the lumbar and thoracic spine. *Spine* 1995;20(9):1029–1035.

40. Resnick D, Guerra J, Robinson CA, et al. Associations of diffuse idiopathic skeletal hyperostosis (DISH) and calcification and ossification of the posterior and longitudinal ligament. *AJR Am J Roentgenol* 1978;131:1049–1053.

41. Rogers MA, Crockard HA. Surgical treatment of the symptomatic herniated thoracic disk. *Clin Orthop* 1994; 300:70–78.

42. Rosenbloom SA. Thoracic disc disease and stenosis. *Radiol Clin North Am* 1991;29(4):765–775.

43. Rosenthal D, Rosenthal R, de Simone A. Removal of a protruded thoracic disc using microsurgical endoscopy. A new technique. *Spine* 1994;19(9):1087–1091.

44. Ross JS, Masaryk TJ, Schrader M, et al. MR imaging of the postoperative lumbar spine: assessment with gadopentetate dimeglumine. *AJR Am J Roentgenol* 1990;155:867–872.

45. Ross JS, Modic MT, Masaryk TJ, et al. Assessment of extradural degenerative disease with Gd-DTPA enhanced MR imaging: correlation with surgical and pathologic findings. *AJNR Am J Neuroradiol* 1989;10(6):1243–1249.

46. Simpson JM, Silveri CP, Simeone FA, et al. Thoracic disc herniation. Re-evaluation of the posterior approach using a modified costotransversectomy. *Spine* 1993;18(13):1872–1877.

47. Smith DE, Godersky JC. Thoracic spondylosis: an unusual cause of myelopathy. *Neurosurgery* 1987;20(4):589–593.

48. Sorenson LV, Mors O, Skovlund O. A prospective study of the importance of psychological and social factors for the outcome after surgery in patients with slipped lumbar disc operated on for the first time. *Acta Neurochir* 1987;88:119–125.

49. Sotiropoulos S, Chaftez N, Lang P, et al. Differentiation between postoperative scar and recurrent disc herniation: prospective comparison of MR, CT, and contrast enhanced CT. *AJNR Am J Neuroradiol* 1989;10:639–643.

50. Spengler DM, Freeman C, Westbrook R, et al. Low back pain following multiple lumbar spine procedures: failure of initial selection? *Spine* 1980;5:356–360.

51. Stillerman CB, Chen TC, Day JD, et al. The transfacet pedicle-sparing approach for thoracic disc removal: cadaveric morphometric analysis and preliminary clinical experience. *J Neurosurg* 1995;83(6):971–976.

52. Stillerman CB, Weiss MH. Management of thoracic disc disease. *Clin Neurosurg* 1992;38:325–352.

53. Stillerman CB, Weiss MH. Surgical management of thoracic disc herniations and spondylosis. In: Menezes AH, Sonntag VKH, eds. *Principles of spinal surgery.* New York: McGraw-Hill, 1996:581–601.

54. Stollman A, Pinto R, Benjamin V, et al. Radiologic imaging of symptomatic ligamentum flavum thickening with and without ossification. *AJNR Am J Neuroradiol* 1987;8(6):991–994.

55. Tomita K, Kaawahara N, Baba H, et al. Circumspinal decompression for thoracic myelopathy due to combined ossification of the posterior longitudinal ligament and ligamentum flavum. *Spine* 1990;15(11):1114–1120.

56. Ungersbock K, Perneczky A, Korn A. Thoracic vertebrostenosis combined with thoracic disc herniation. Case report and review of literature. *Spine* 1987;12(6):612–615.

57. Vaccaro AR, Mirkovic S, Bauer RD, et al. Revision lumbar and cervical degenerative spine surgery—indications and techniques. In: Bridwell KW, DeWald RL, eds. *The textbook of spinal surgery*, 2nd ed. Philadelphia: Lippincott–Raven Publishers, 1997:1457–1493.

58. Vanderburgh DF, Kelly WM. Radiographic assessment of discogenic disease of the spine. *Neurosurg Clin North Am* 1993;4(1):13–33.

59. Videman T, Battie MC, Gill K, et al. Magnetic resonance imaging findings and their relationships in the thoracic and lumbar spine. Insights into the etiopathogenesis of spinal degeneration. *Spine* 1995;20(8):928–935.

60. Waddell G, Somerville D, Henderson I, et al. Objective clinical evaluation of physical impairment in chronic low back pain. *Spine* 1991;17:617–628.

61. Wiesel SW. The multiply operated lumbar spine. *Instr Course Lect* 1985;34:68–77.

62. Wood KB, Garvey TA, Gundry C, et al. Magnetic resonance imaging of the thoracic spine. Evaluation of asymptomatic individuals. *J Bone Joint Surg Am* 1995;77A(11):1631–1638.

63. Yamamoto I, Matsumae M, Ikeda A, et al. Thoracic spinal stenosis: experience with seven cases. *J Neurosurg* 1988;68(1):37–40.

64. Yoshino MT, Seeger JF, Carmody RF. MRI diagnosis of thoracic ossification of posterior longitudinal ligament with concomitant disc herniation. *Neuroradiology* 1991;33(5):455–457.

65. Zeidman SM, Long DM. Failed back surgery syndrome. In: Menezes AH, Sonntag VKH, eds. *Principles of spinal surgery.* New York: McGraw-Hill, 1996:657–679.

THORACIC SPINE: DEFORMITY

LAWRENCE G. LENKE

Primary surgical treatment of various thoracic spinal deformities can be highly successful in obtaining the desired result. However, early and late complications may occur that require consideration for revision thoracic spinal deformity surgery. Although it is difficult to know the exact scope of the problem, there are certainly risk factors that create an environment for failed primary thoracic spinal deformity surgery. Probably the greatest preoperative risk factor is thoracic hyperkyphosis, which can cause several complications, including early instrumentation failure, neurologic injury, and late pseudarthrosis (13–16,42,56). Another common risk factor is attempted excessive correction in the coronal and especially the sagittal planes (28,42,48). In the treatment of hyperkyphosis, instrumentation failure and loss of correction more commonly occur in patients with osteoporotic bone, which is another risk factor (22,56). In addition, failed thoracic scoliosis surgery may also result from postoperative imbalance (17,34,45), pseudarthrosis (4,7,18,32,43,54,55), crankshaft, and other etiologies (50). The goal of this chapter is to highlight common mechanisms of failed thoracic spinal deformity surgery and present treatment options for those who require revision spinal surgery. Topics are discussed in a chronological fashion as to when they appear from early postoperative (e.g., early coronal imbalance or instrumentation failure) to late postoperative (e.g., pseudarthrosis with late instrumentation failure).

POSTOPERATIVE IMBALANCE

Coronal Plane

Postoperative imbalance following thoracic scoliosis correction has been widely reported after the introduction of segmental spinal instrumentation systems (9,17,34,35,49,51,54,55). Most commonly, this has followed the selective posterior thoracic fusion of a King type II or false double major curve (34,49). The common pattern of postoperative coronal decompensation noted has been progression of the unfused lumbar curve to the left,

below the selectively fused thoracic region. A King type II curve is a primary thoracic curve, with a compensatory lumbar curve that crosses the midline but is not structural enough to warrant inclusion in the thoracic instrumentation and fusion (30). Ideally, fusing the thoracic curve alone maintains coronal balance and also maximizes lumbar mobility. Although postoperative decompensation of the lumbar curve has occurred after application of posterior segmental spinal instrumentation, it was virtually unheard of with previous nonsegmental instrumentation systems such as the Harrington rod system (1,24).

Many theories have been espoused as to the cause of coronal decompensation for the treatment of King type II curves with posterior segmental spinal instrumentation, including inadequate selection of those type II curves that are amenable to the technique (34), overcorrection of the main thoracic curve via a 90-degree rod rotation maneuver (17,34), less flexibility of the lumbar spine below to accommodate the thoracic curve correction obtained (49), inappropriate choice of the distal level of instrumentation and fusion that extends partly into the upper portion of the lumbar curve (17), and failure to recognize a junctional thoracolumbar kyphosis in the sagittal plane on the preoperative radiographs (34). Regardless of the etiology, the incidence of postoperative coronal decompensation appears to be decreasing as experience with proper curve identification as well as appropriate posterior segmental spinal instrumentation techniques have been used (35,39).

The treatment of a postoperative lumbar curve decompensation following a selective thoracic instrumentation and fusion depends on several factors, including the degree of decompensation, the degree of skeletal immaturity of the patient, the clinical appearance of the patient, and the sagittal thoracolumbar alignment. A postoperative spinal orthosis may improve alignment in the early postoperative period and promote rebalancing of the spine long term. If the patient is skeletally immature, this should be attempted and discussed with the patient and his or her parents before the initial selective thoracic fusion. Observation of the patient with a decompensated lumbar curve is also an option for the surgeon and patient.

Occasionally, the spine rebalances as the thoracic curve settles into its fused position, with some slight loss of thoracic correction and subsequent repositioning of the lumbar curve below (34). In our experience, this is more apt to happen when the sagittal thoracolumbar alignment is acceptable (i.e., not kyphotic). Occasionally, postoperative lumbar curve decompensation has required extension of the instrumentation and fusion into the mid- to lower lumbar spine (L-3 or L-4) to rebalance the patient and produce acceptable coronal alignment (Fig. 1). This can be performed either with extension of the previous instrumentation and fusion all posteriorly or with a primary anterior thoracolumbar procedure that occasionally allows one distal lumbar level to be saved, versus other procedures in which posterior instrumentation and fusion would be required (e.g., L-3 vs. L-4). Regardless of the approach, the goal is to optimize coronal alignment by having the C-7 plumbline bisect the sacrum and to correct lumbar trunk shift to the midline. As with any instrumentation and fusion into the mid- to lower lumbar spine, the lowest instrumented vertebra ideally should be horizontal to the pelvis, bisected by the center sacral line, as neutral in rotation as possible, and have a harmonious lumbar lordosis.

Another common problem is postoperative shoulder imbalance from overcorrection of the main thoracic curve, with incomplete appreciation of a structural upper thoracic curve (30,37). Occasionally, postoperative shoulder imbalance improves over time to the satisfaction of patients and their families. If not, revision surgery is required to rebalance the shoulders. This often requires extension of previously placed instrumentation and fusion to the upper thoracic spine, usually T-2 (37). Appropriate compression or distraction forces, or both, must be placed on the convexity and concavity, respectively, of the residual upper thoracic curve dependent on the sagittal alignment and the degree of initial shoulder imbalance.

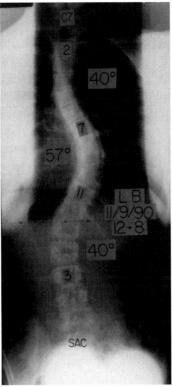
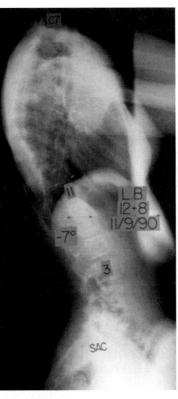
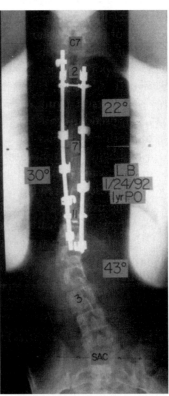

A,B   C

FIGURE 1. **A:** A girl aged 12 years, 8 months, with a 57-degree right thoracic adolescent idiopathic scoliosis and compensatory 40-degree upper thoracic and 40-degree left lumbar curves. **B:** Her preoperative sagittal plane was unremarkable. She underwent a posterior instrumentation and fusion with Cotrel-Dubousset instrumentation from T-2 to T-12, with hooks placed in distraction in the concave aspect of the thoracic spine to the thoracolumbar junction. **C:** When she presented to us at 1 year after operation, she was complaining of a significant trunk shift, with her radiographs demonstrating curve correction at 22 degrees in the upper thoracic region, 30 degrees in the main thoracic region, and progression of the unfused lumbar curve to 43 degrees with significant coronal decompensation to the left. (*continued*)

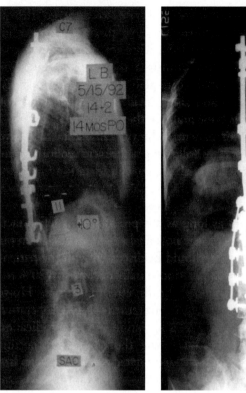
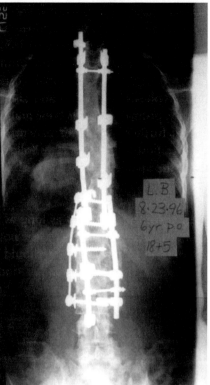
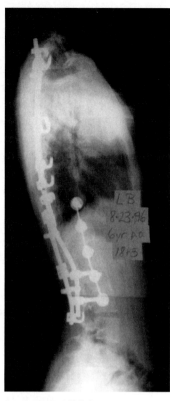

D,E   F

FIGURE 1. (*continued*) **D:** Her postoperative lateral radiograph demonstrates a mild thoracolumbar kyphosis secondary to the distraction forces applied to her thoracolumbar junction. Because of the fixed nature of her deformity, as well as a failed attempt at bracing over the previous year, she underwent a revision anterior and posterior spinal fusion. The anterior procedure was performed from T-11 to L-3 with Zielke instrumentation. She underwent a same-day posterior extension to reinforce the Zielke threaded rod and provide a posterior fusion. This combined approach was performed to attempt to place L-3 in an ideal horizontal and central position. **E:** Her 6-year follow-up radiographs demonstrate maintenance of a well-compensated spine with L-3 horizontal and centered on the sacrum. **F:** Her lateral radiograph demonstrates a harmonious thoracic, thoracolumbar, and lumbar sagittal alignment. (Case performed by Keith H. Bridwell, M.D.)

Sagittal Plane

Acute postoperative sagittal plane imbalance is rarely seen following instrumentation and fusion of thoracic scoliosis with a normalized preoperative sagittal alignment (6). However, it may occur in patients who are hyperkyphotic in the thoracic region or are undergoing spinal deformity surgery for primary thoracic kyphosis problems such as Scheuermann's disease or congenital kyphosis (13,15). In scoliosis surgery, the primary culprit of postoperative sagittal imbalance in the past has been using distraction instrumentation into the mid- to lower lumbar spine (1,2,20,21,24,31). This effectively decreased thoracolumbar and lumbar lordosis and ultimately produced a flatback syndrome consisting of degenerative disk disease below the fusion, forward sagittal imbalance, and degenerative pain syndromes of the lumbosacral region (31). Thus, distraction as a primary force application in the lumbar spine is contraindicated. The primary force application in the lumbar spine should always be posterior compression to preserve or enhance regional and segmental lordosis.

Another common cause of early sagittal imbalance postoperatively is the development of junctional kyphosis directly above a thoracic or thoracolumbar instrumentation and fusion that stops just below or at the thoracic apex (42,48). Normally, the apex of thoracic kyphosis is between T-7 and T-9; thus, it is not advisable to stop the proximal level of a long instrumentation and fusion in the T6-10 region. However, junctional kyphotic transition syndromes can occur in any patient who has instrumentation and fusions in the lower, mid-, and upper thoracic regions (48). Risk factors for the occurrence of a thoracic junctional kyphosis, besides stopping at the apex, include a global sagittal alignment that is forward to the sacrum, ligament disruption at the level directly above the instrumentation and fusion, older patients, female patients, and individuals with multiple medical comorbidities.

The treatment of patients with a thoracic junctional kyphosis includes initial observation to document progression, which can occur either slowly or rapidly. Sequential radiographs document the degree of kyphosis and its progression. Indications for surgical correction of progressive junctional kyphosis include increasing pain, progressive deformity, prominent instrumentation, and the desire to halt further progression. Surgery requires extension of the posterior instrumentation and fusion well above the apex of the thoracic kyphosis, normally to the upper thoracic region at approximately T-3. With significant preoperative thoracic kyphosis, consideration for an anterior release and fusion should be entertained. Often, axial extension devices (i.e., dominoes) can be placed on the previous instrumentation with new rods extending proximally (8). This obviates the need to remove the previously placed instrumentation. A thorough fusion must also then be performed, covering the newly placed instrumentation. Postoperative bracing can be used as an adjuvant reinforcement of the correction and to aid fusion consolidation.

Similarly, for a distal thoracic kyphosis transition syndrome, extending the instrumentation and fusion to the first lordotic segment is required at a minimum. Consideration for anterior structural grafting should also be made in these cases to ensure adequate anterior support and healing of the spine to prevent further sagittal plane problems (10,19). Posteriorly, rigid internal fixation is mandatory to obtain and maintain adequate alignment (11).

Axial Plane

Postoperative imbalance in the thoracic axial plane occurs in two different circumstances: (a) with posterior correction of a scoliosis deformity and inadequate correction of the rib hump (1,33) and (b) with a posterior fusion alone of a skeletally immature patient, with a resultant crankshaft phenomenon producing progressive rotational malalignment to the thoracic rib cage over time. Despite current three-dimensional analysis, detailed preoperative planning, and posterior segmental spinal instrumentation techniques, the ability to derotate the apex of a thoracic scoliosis consistently is still minimal (1,33). Thus, patients should be advised that with a posterior thoracic scoliosis correction, although the convex rib hump usually improves, it may still be clinically prominent. In the adolescent population, consideration for a concomitant thoracoplasty rib resection procedure with the initial instrumentation and fusion should be discussed with patients, providing that their preoperative pulmonary

functions are adequate to undergo the procedure safely (≥60% to 70% predicted flow and volume parameters) (38). Thus, in patients with a sizable rib hump, performing a thoracoplasty resection during the initial correction immediately corrects the rib hump and also provides an ample source of autogenous bone graft for the fusion (38).

For patients who present more than 2 years after operation following a thoracic scoliosis fusion with a prominent rib hump, consideration for a late thoracoplasty procedure can be discussed. The rib segments will regrow (by approximately 6 months after operation) as long as the periosteum is left intact. Besides cosmesis, the potential adverse sequelae on pulmonary function should be discussed with the patient, as pulmonary function usually declines by 20% to 25% for the first 3 months after operation. However, the majority of patients return to the preoperative baseline by 2 years after operation. Another indication to consider having a late thoracoplasty procedure is for chronic scapular-thoracic pain that occurs from posterior protrusion of the scapula on the rib cage. This is especially bothersome when patients sit in hardback chairs and also with extensive use of the ipsilateral upper extremity and shoulder girdle for activities. However, the primary reason for a late thoracoplasty procedure is unacceptable cosmesis, as residual large rib humps can be cosmetically displeasing to the patient and justify a late rib resection procedure.

AVOIDANCE OF POSTOPERATIVE IMBALANCE

It is extremely important to evaluate carefully the preoperative radiographs and clinical examination of a patient who is undergoing a thoracic deformity correction to avoid postoperative imbalance. In the coronal plane, the long cassette upright posteroanterior and lateral x-rays, along with supine long cassette right and left maximum side-bending radiographs, are the minimum number of radiographs required for analysis to evaluate the entire spinal column and the planned correction. A dynamic push-prone radiograph can be obtained to demonstrate the effect that a forceful push on the main curvature has and the resultant spontaneous correction of any curvatures above and below. This often demonstrates accentuation of a structural upper thoracic curve with correction of the main thoracic scoliosis, as well as balance of a compensatory lumbar curve below a more structural thoracic curve above. Evaluation of flexibility of any regional kyphosis can be performed by having the patient obtain a hyperextension lateral x-ray at the apex of the deformity centered over a bolster.

The physical examination is also helpful in postoperative planning. It is essential to evaluate the clinical appearance of the shoulders, especially the height of the shoulders, any trapezial fullness that is present indicating structural rotation of the upper thoracic region, and flexibility when the patient bends into the convexity of the upper thoracic curve (37). In a similar fashion, the thoracic and lumbar regions are examined for asymmetry, trunk shift, and rotational prominence on forward bending as quantified by a scoliometer measurement (36). The clinical examination often demonstrates the amount of clinical deformity present in combined thoracic and lumbar curves and thus helps to decide whether only one of these curves requires fusion or if both curves require fusion. This is especially important in true King type II or false double major curves, which have a more prominent structural thoracic rib prominence than the more compensatory and smaller lumbar hump (34).

The radiographs also give important information to help avoid postoperative coronal and sagittal imbalance of the spine after treatment of the thoracic spinal deformity. In particular, for a scoliosis fusion, spinal balance is of the utmost importance. It is much better to have a balanced spine with mild to moderate residual curvatures than a spine with an overcorrected segment that has produced either shoulder or trunk imbalance, or both, postoperatively. The spinal deformity surgeon should always ponder the resultant effects of compensatory curves that exist above and below the intended region to be corrected with instrumentation and fusion. It is imperative not only to choose the correct proximal and distal levels of instrumentation and fusion but also the amount of correction to be obtained for the instrumented segments (47).

Intraoperative radiographs can help determine the amount of correction obtained with instrumentation. However, the surgeon must also have a reasonable estimate of the anticipated correction planned preoperatively to maintain overall shoulder and spinal balance (12).

ACUTE WOUND INFECTIONS

Postoperative wound drainage following thoracic spinal deformity surgery should not be taken lightly. Any type of wound drainage postoperatively should have a dressing placed over the area to quantify the amount and type of drainage. Any type of purulent drainage should immediately undergo an operative irrigation and débridement with exploration of the wound. More commonly, mild serosanguineous drainage occurs postoperatively that dries up quickly and does not require further attention as long as the patient is otherwise asymptomatic. Wound drainage after 5 to 7 days should raise more significant concerns. If the wound edges are not healed, skin sutures should be removed and the wound probed to document extension below the fascia. If fascial dehiscence is present, operative irrigation and débridement and closure over a drain should be performed (41). Wound cultures should be obtained and appropriate prophylactic antibiotics provided, with length of treatment dependent on the results of the wound culture. Normally, these early postoperative deep wound drainage problems can be cured with an operative irrigation débridement and closure over large bore drains that are kept in for several days until the drainage is minimal (<20 mL per 8 hours). It has been our practice to surgically approach persistent postoperative wound drainage aggressively in patients with spinal deformity so as not to create a chronic wound problem in the future. In addition, attention should be placed on postoperative nutrition, as this is a significant risk factor for early postoperative wound drainage as well as infections (23,52).

In a patient with an obviously infected draining wound, treatment is again urgent—irrigation and débridement, removal of necrotic and devitalized tissue, closure of the wound if possible over large drains, retaining the instrumentation, and bone graft (41). If the infection is overwhelming (which is quite rare), the wound can be packed and returned for inspection and possible closure in 24 to 48 hours. If the instrumentation is secure, it should be left in place. Consultation with infectious disease service should be made to optimize appropriate antibiotic treatment, which usually is provided for at least 6 weeks in the face of acute, deep postoperative wound infection.

The treatment of delayed postoperative wound drainage is somewhat different. In the patient who is at least 1 to 2 years postoperative and has a solid spinal arthrodesis, postoperative wound drainage may either occur from a chronic indolent infection or possibly even from fretting corrosion from the metal debris of the spinal instrumentation (49). In either case, the instrumentation should all be removed, with the fusion explored to confirm a solid arthrodesis. If the spine fusion is solid, treating the wound with appropriate treatment, closure, and antibiotics normally solves the problem. If pseudarthroses are present, the wound should be addressed first, and the repair of pseudarthroses addressed secondarily if required; then consideration for a circumferential fusion is made (29,46).

INSTRUMENTATION FAILURE/LOSS OF CORRECTION

Early postoperative instrumentation failure with subsequent loss of correction may occur after correction of a thoracic coronal or sagittal plane deformity (13,14). It is much commoner when a kyphotic deformity has been corrected with or without an associated scoliosis deformity. Most early (the first 3 months) instrumentation failures occur at the bone-metal interface, such as a hook pull-off from a fractured lamina or a screw pullout from a pedicle. In addition, metal-metal failure may occur, such as dislodgment of a rod from a coupling mechanism attached to either a hook, screw, or wire. In addition, wires or cables may dislodge from the bone by either fracturing (wires) or by actually cutting through the bone because of high tension forces (cables).

Many risk factors are associated with acute instrumentation failure with loss of correction and include significantly those patients with soft osteoporotic bone. Another risk factor is an inadequate number of fixation points applied to the anterior or posterior spine, or both, during correction of a deformity. With the current use of posterior segmental spinal instrumentation, it is possible to immobilize the spine rigidly on a segment-by-segment basis with a combination of hooks, wires, and/or screws. The choice of type and location of fixation points should be planned preoperatively, with alterations available depending on the anatomy encountered and any variations necessitated during the surgical procedure. In general, hooks and wires (either sublaminar or spinous processes, or both) are standard for the thoracic spine, whereas pedicle screws have become quite popular for the thoracolumbar junction and especially the lumbar spine but must be placed accurately to avoid complications (3,26,27,40,53). Adequate equal lever arms above and below the main deformity being corrected must be obtained to balance the instrumentation. As a general rule, six fixation points both above and below the apex of a deformity are the minimum required to stabilize the spine and obviate postoperative immobilization. Another risk factor for instrumentation failure and loss of correction includes hyperkyphosis of the thoracic spine. This places increased tension forces on the posterior construct, with a higher probability of instrumentation failure and correction loss. It is

always wise to consider an anterior spinal fusion in hyperkyphotic patients, not only to increase curve flexibility but also to improve the fusion rate (14,15,19) (Fig. 2). It is best to attempt to save the segmental vessels during the anterior procedure to optimize spinal cord vascularity (5,44).

Preoperative, intraoperative, and postoperative factors may limit the occurrence of early instrumentation failure postoperatively. Preoperatively, the flexibility of the curvatures must be determined with flexibility radiographs. Excessive correction obtained far beyond what normal flexibility x-rays allow may predispose to early instrumentation failure with correction loss. If an excessive amount of correction is contemplated, especially with a kyphosis deformity, adequate secure fixation of the spinal column must be obtained to prevent hook or screw pull-off. Specifically, the use of transverse process hooks should be avoided below the T-4 or T-5 levels, because the transverse processes tend to be quite fragile in the mid- and lower thoracic region. The use of thoracic supralaminar hooks provides much sturdier fixation. Using claw constructs at the top and bottom of instrumentation sequences is also advantageous. A claw is two ipsilateral hooks going in opposite directions that grip the posterior elements in a solid fashion. They can be applied on either one or two levels and most commonly involve a pedicle and transverse process (or supralaminar) hook configuration proximally and a supralaminar-infralaminar construct distally. The hooks are seated toward each other in compression and should rigidly immobilize the segment(s) over which they are applied.

Basic rules of scoliosis correction must be adhered to such that distraction forces are applied on concave closed disks, with compression forces applied on convex open disks (35). Similarly, for sagittal plane considerations, distraction forces applied posteriorly are kyphogenic, whereas compression forces applied posteriorly are lordogenic. These biomechanical forces must be considered during the operative correction of various thoracic deformities. Last, screw fixation in the thoracolumbar and lumbar spine must be secure at the lower end of constructs. Reinforcing a screw with an infralaminar hook at the same level improves the pullout strength of that screw and thus improves purchase of the distal construct. Using the largest diameter screw that fits the isthmus of the pedicle also improves pullout strength, more so than the length of the screw and subsequent purchase in the anterior vertebral body. In severely osteoporotic bone, consideration for using multiple hook fixation points may provide bet-

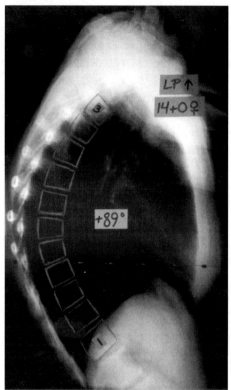
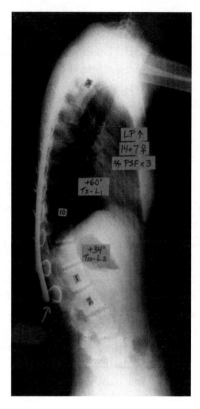
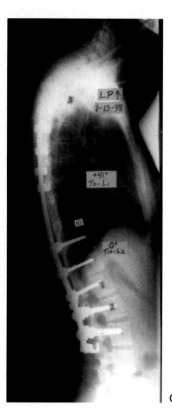

A,B   C

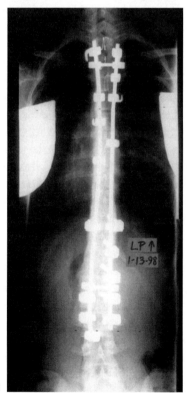

D

FIGURE 2. **A:** A 14-year-old girl with an 89-degree thoracic hyperkyphosis with significant back pain and clinical deformity. She underwent a posterior-only instrumentation from T-2 to L-1 with Luque rods and sublaminar wires at another institution. She only had allograft bone for her posterior fusion and had no anterior fusion performed. When she presented to us approximately 10 months after her initial procedure, she had undergone two additional procedures for distal instrumentation failure, with loss of correction and development of a thoracolumbar kyphosis. She presented with continued pain and a dorsal hump located at her thoracolumbar region; the tip of the rods could be palpated in this patient, who was quite thin. **B:** Lateral long cassette radiograph showed 54 degrees of thoracolumbar kyphosis from T-10 to L-2, with a broken wire at the L-1 level with posterior migration of the distal rods and suspected pseudarthrosis. She underwent a revision posterior procedure, including instrumentation removal, pseudarthrosis exploration, and revision instrumentation and fusion with autogenous bone graft. Intraoperatively, she was noted to have pseudarthroses at the lowest two levels, with a solid spine fusion noted elsewhere. She thus was reinstrumented with segmental spinal instrumentation with fusion mass hooks used in the upper thoracic spine and pedicle screw instrumentation in the thoracolumbar and lumbar region to L-3. She had abundant autogenous bone grafting performed over her posterior elements from T-11 to L-3. **C:** Postoperative lateral radiographs demonstrate normalization of the thoracolumbar sagittal alignment and acceptable overall sagittal balance with secure instrumentation down to L-3. **D:** Revision postoperative long cassette coronal view shows revision instrumentation and a solid fusion mass visible down in the lumbar spine to the transverse processes at L-3.

ter fixation than screw purchase unless the screws are supplemented with methylmethacrylate or other substances that increase pullout strength.

The postoperative avoidance of early instrumentation failure revolves around two important components: the use of supplemental external support such as a brace and patient compliance with activity restrictions. Patients who are treated for a hyperkyphotic thoracic deformity often benefit from supplemental orthotic wear postoperatively to decrease some of the tension forces that are present on the posterior instrumentation. For patients who are undergoing a high thoracic deformity correction, use of a neck extension to the orthosis may also be beneficial to control the cervical-thoracic region. In extremely difficult circumstances, the placement of a halo attached rigidly to either a cast or brace may also be required to maintain alignment during the healing phases of the fusion. Bracewear for hyperkyphotic patients is usually required for 6 to 9 months postoperatively until a fusion is adequately consolidating.

TREATMENT OF EARLY INSTRUMENTATION FAILURE WITH LOSS OF CORRECTION

Most patients with early instrumentation failure invariably notice when a problem develops. Often a pop or snap is felt by the patient, with or without accompanying pain. A bump or prominence may be palpable either in the lower or upper region of the wound due to proximal or distal instrumentation, or both dislodgment and pullout. In addition, patients or their friends or families may notice loss of the previously obtained correction of the spinal deformity. However, occasionally, early instrumentation failures are only noted as subtle changes on postoperative radiographs that should be obtained on a regular basis for the first year. It is imperative to compare follow-up radiographs with the first postoperative radiograph to ensure that all fixation points are unchanged in position, correction is being maintained, and the overall position of the spine is similar. Often the only suggestion of an acute instrumentation failure is mild posterior positioning of a proximal or distal hook in relation to the posterior elements of the spine. If uncertain, a computed tomographic scan may further evaluate the region in question to determine if any adverse events have occurred. However, the majority of early instrumentation failures are visible on careful evaluation of the upright posteroanterior and lateral long cassette radiographs of the spine.

The treatment for early instrumentation failure is to resecure the instrumentation via a revision surgery and provide abundant autogenous bone for a fusion. The goal is to reinstrument the same levels of the spine, if possible, as long as the initial levels are still deemed appropriate. This may require altering fixation points, especially if laminar fractures or screw pullouts have occurred. Occasionally, extending the levels of instrumentation either more proximally or more distally is required to gain adequate purchase on the spine during treatment of the instrumentation failure. On occasion, consideration for supplemental anterior fusion or instrumentation, or both, is advisable (28,29). Maintaining as many mobile segments above and below the corrected deformity must also be kept in mind and should be a goal even in these salvage surgeries. Consideration for external immobilization with a brace should also be made to lessen the anxiety after the revision surgery and also to minimize patient activity during the early healing phase.

It is often tempting to avoid early revision surgery in these patients with acute instrumentation failure. However, the patient normally continues to lose correction and eventually requires surgery, often with more fusion levels required for the revision procedure. Thus, we advocate early surgery in these patients to correct the current problem and prevent it from getting worse.

TREATMENT OF LATE INSTRUMENTATION FAILURES

The occurrence of a late (after 6 months) instrumentation failure is almost always a *sine qua non* for a pseudarthrosis (4,24,32). This may occur with the patient being asymptomatic, but commonly the patient is symptomatic, usually from pain as well as the developing instability at the level(s) involved. Almost invariably, revision surgery is required to treat the pseudarthrosis and revise the instrumentation.

Many factors need to be decided on when revising a late instrumentation failure and concomitant pseudarthrosis, including the following: Will a circumferential fusion be required at the level of the pseudarthrosis? How will the spine be rigidly immobilized with revision instrumentation? Do the revision instrumentation and fusion need to be extended either proximally or distally to maintain a well-balanced and compensated spine? Can the surgery be performed all in 1 day, or do two stages have to be divided over 2 separate operative days? Finally, is enough autogenous bone graft available to harvest to provide a solid arthrodesis (4,23,52)?

Pseudarthrosis and instrumentation failure in the thoracic spine can often be treated with a posterior revision and instrumentation fusion surgery alone. However, in patients with known risk factors for pseudarthrosis, including smoking, advanced age, significant spinal deformity, and multiple previous pseudarthroses, a circumferential fusion should be performed over the pseudarthrotic level(s) using abundant autogenous bone graft (32,43,46). The spine must be rigidly immobilized with revision

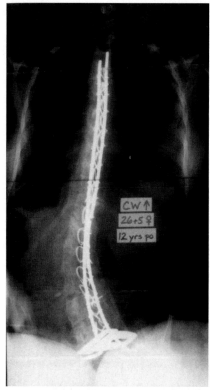

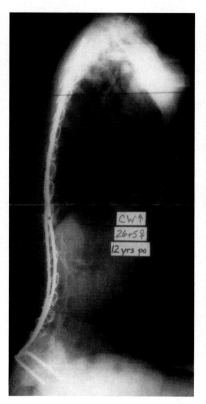

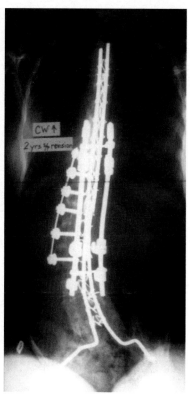

A,B

C

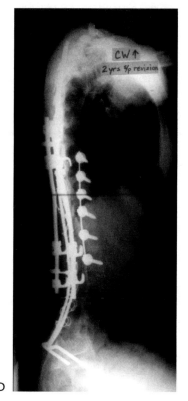

D

FIGURE 3. A 26-year-old woman with a fairly severe quadriplegic cerebral palsy and normal mentation. She presented 12 years after a posterior-only instrumentation and fusion for a long sweeping neuromuscular spinal deformity. She was a nonambulator who used a wheelchair for her mobility. She presented with significant thoracolumbar pain that was recalcitrant to conservative treatments. She had a bone scan that lit up sharply at the thoracolumbar junction in the area where her broken rod was located. **A:** Long cassette coronal view 12 years after operation demonstrated a broken rod and suspected pseudarthrosis at the thoracolumbar junction. **B:** Long cassette lateral radiograph demonstrated a fractured rod with acceptable overall alignment. To maximize her chance for obtaining a solid fusion, she was prepared for a revision anterior and posterior spinal fusion. Posteriorly, the spine was explored, and a two-level pseudarthrosis located at the thoracolumbar junction was confirmed that was re-fused and reinstrumented with compression instrumentation attached into her fusion mass. On the same day, she underwent a supplemental anterior fusion with instrumentation covering levels above and below her instrumentation for additional support and healing. **C:** Two years status post her revision procedure, she was noted to have a solid spine fusion with complete relief of her pain. **D:** Long cassette lateral radiograph demonstrates her acceptable sitting alignment.

instrumentation, often using fusion mass hooks in areas above and below the pseudarthroses that are adequately healed (Fig. 3). If it is decided that extension of the previous fusion will be required either proximally or distally, primary fusion of those regions must be performed, along with secure spinal

instrumentation. Normally, these surgeries can all be performed in a single stage even if done circumferentially. However, under extreme circumstances with significant amounts of surgery required, a two-stage procedure should be performed, often with supplemental circumferential hyperalimentation provided

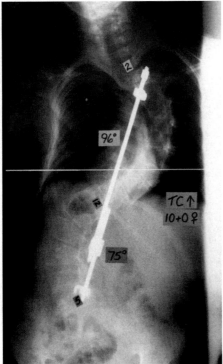
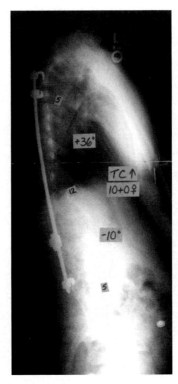
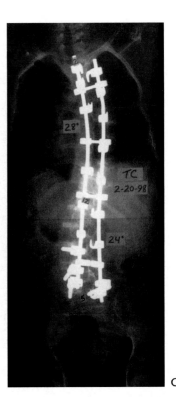

A,B

C

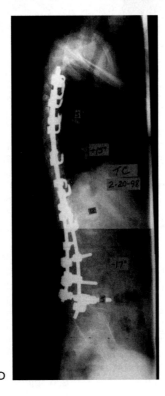

D

FIGURE 4. A 10-year-old girl with Marfan's syndrome. At the age of 4 years, she had a posterior subcutaneous rod placed from T-3 to L-4 to control a progressive double major scoliosis. Unfortunately, she had no future rod lengthenings or procedures. She presented to us with a significant spinal deformity in the coronal and the sagittal planes. **A:** Long cassette coronal x-ray showed a 96-degree right thoracic, 75-degree left lumbar deformity with significant truncal imbalance to the right. **B:** Long cassette lateral radiograph demonstrated a flat lumbar spine from the distraction instrumentation with only 10 degrees of lordosis between T-12 and L-5. At this point, she was still quite skeletally immature and had early cardiac abnormalities caused by her Marfan's syndrome. She also had mild pulmonary compromise from her deformity and poor exercise tolerance. For these reasons, she underwent a staged procedure with intervening halo traction. Her first stage consisted of posterior rod removal, wound exploration, and facet and interspinous ligament release. On the same day, she also underwent a right thoracic anterior spinal fusion from T-3 to T-12 to loosen up her thoracic spine and prevent any crankshaft occurring in the future. She then underwent 8 weeks of halo gravity traction and was returned to the operating room, where she underwent a first-stage anterior lumbar release and fusion with structural grafting from T-12 to L-5 to create a more flexible lumbar curve as well as improve her sagittal alignment and secure a solid fusion. On the same day, she underwent a revision posterior fusion from T-3 to L-5 with segmental spinal instrumentation. **C:** Postoperative coronal x-ray shows significant correction of her coronal imbalance as well as her thoracic and lumbar curves. **D:** Lateral radiograph demonstrates structural grafting in the lumbar disk spaces as well as acceptable overall sagittal alignment. This young girl underwent a notable amount of surgery; however, her significant deformity as well as crankshaft risk warranted this.

to minimize the nutritional depletion that occurs during these staged spinal surgeries (23,52) (Fig. 4).

CRANKSHAFT

Progressive thoracic spinal deformity may occur in skeletally immature patients who are undergoing a posterior-only instrumentation and fusion for a scoliosis deformity. The constellation of radiographic and clinical deformity progression is termed the *crankshaft phenomenon*. It occurs when treating skeletally immature patients who have not reached their peak height velocity before the performance of a posterior instrumentation and fusion. With continued anterior spinal growth, the spine crankshafts around

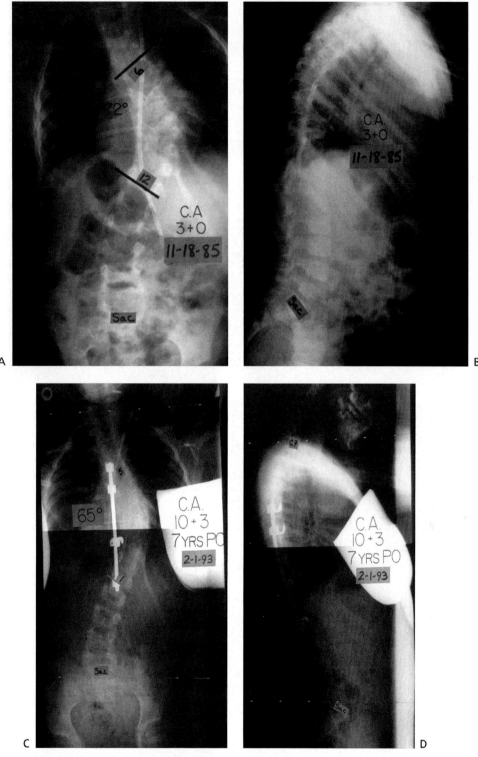

FIGURE 5. A girl aged 3 years, 0 months, when she presented with a congenital scoliosis. **A:** Coronal x-ray shows a 72-degree right thoracic curvature with a hemivertebra at the apex. **B:** Lateral view was fairly unremarkable. At that time, she underwent a posterior-only instrumentation from T-4 to L-1 with a single rod-and-hook system and a posterior-only fusion. Seven years after the operation, she had undergone significant crankshafting to present with a **(C)** 65-degree right thoracic curvature with adding on above and below, creating a significant truncal imbalance. **D:** The lateral radiograph demonstrates acceptable overall alignment continuing. At this point she was still skeletally immature and premenarchal, with open triradiate cartilages noted on her coronal radiograph. She thus underwent a staged anterior and posterior spinal reconstruction. Anteriorly, she had anterior release and fusion of the thoracic spine from T-5 to L-1. Posteriorly, she had instrumentation removal, posterior osteotomies at the T-6 to T-7 and T-12 to L-1 levels, as well as reinstrumentation and fusion from T-2 to L-3. (*continued*)

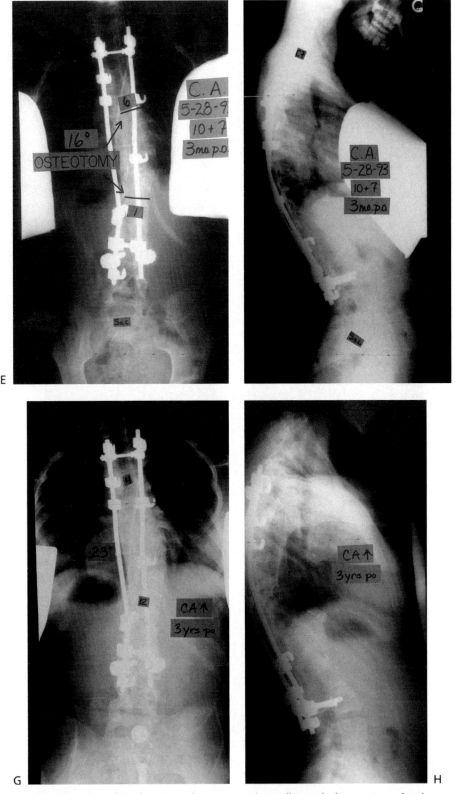

FIGURE 5. (*continued*) **E:** Three-month postoperative radiograph demonstrates her improved coronal alignment to 16 degrees and good balance of the spine. **F:** Early revision postoperative lateral radiograph demonstrated acceptable regional and global sagittal balance. Three-year postoperative radiographs demonstrate overall maintenance of her correction in the coronal **(G)** and sagittal **(H)** planes.

the solid posterior instrumentation and fusion. This leads not only to progression of the coronal Cobb measurement but, more importantly, progression of apical and spinal rotation and rib cage abnormalities (1,33). Clinically, patients are noted to have increasing chest cage and rib hump deformity and, occasionally, progressive spinal imbalance. Prevention is the key to this phenomenon, with appropriate preventative anterior spinal fusions performed in those patients who are at high risk for crankshaft phenomena, including all infantile and juvenile patients and adolescents who are extremely skeletally immature (Risser 0, premenarchal, open triradiate cartilages, and before the adolescent growth spurt).

When faced with a postoperative patient with a crankshaft phenomenon who has gone beyond the initial surgery and has a healed posterior fusion, a significant spinal reconstruction is required. Often not only anterior release and fusion but also posterior osteotomies are needed to reposition the previously fused posterior column into a more acceptable alignment (25). This is followed by a revision posterior instrumentation and fusion, often extending more proximally and distally to cover the levels above and below that have decompensated with time. Although a major undertaking, it can be quite beneficial to young patients with a significant residual deformity despite previous posterior-only operative correction (Fig. 5).

CONCLUSION

The surgical management of failed thoracic spinal deformity surgery is often a significant undertaking. As in all forms of spinal deformity surgery, it is imperative to perform a detailed preoperative assessment, followed by meticulous and thorough operative techniques, as well as to provide adequate postoperative activity restrictions to ensure a successful outcome. When revision thoracic spinal deformity surgery is required, even more attention to these important details is required to produce a successful result. Nonetheless, for appropriate indications, revision thoracic spinal deformity surgery can be quite successful in the eyes of the patient and the surgeon.

REFERENCES

1. Aaro S, Dahlborn M. The effect of Harrington instrumentation on the longitudinal axis rotation of the apical vertebra and on the spinal and rib cage deformity in idiopathic scoliosis studied by computer tomography. *Spine* 1982;7:456–462.
2. Aaro S, Dahlborn M. The effect of Harrington instrumentation on the sagittal configuration and mobility of the spine in scoliosis. *Spine* 1983;8:570–575.
3. Akbarnia B, Asher M, Hess F, et al. Safety of pedicle screw in pediatric patients with scoliosis and kyphosis. Thirty-first Annual Meeting, Scoliosis Research Society, Ottawa, Canada, 1996.
4. Aurori BF, Weierman RJ, Lowell HA, et al. Pseudarthrosis after spinal fusion for scoliosis (a comparison of autogeneic and allogeneic bone grafts). *Clin Orthop* 1985;199:153–158.
5. Ben-David B, Haller G, Taylor P. Anterior spinal fusion complicated by paraplegia. A case report of a false-negative somatosensory-evoked potential. *Spine* 1987;12:536–539.
6. Benson DR. Idiopathic scoliosis. The last ten years and state of the art. *Orthopedics* 1987;10:1691–1698.
7. Bialik V, Piggott H. Pseudarthrosis following treatment of idiopathic scoliosis by Harrington instrumentation and fusion without added bone. *J Pediatr Orthop* 1987;7:152–154.
8. Birch JG, Herring JA, Roach JW, et al. Cotrel-Dubousset instrumentation in idiopathic scoliosis. A preliminary report. *Clin Orthop* 1988;224:24–29.
9. Boachie-Adjei O, Bradford DS. The Cotrel-Dubousset system—results in spinal reconstruction (early experience in 47 patients). *Spine* 1991;16:1155–1160.
10. Boachie-Adjei O, Dendrinos GK, Ogilvie JW, et al. Management of adult spinal deformity with combined anterior-posterior arthrodesis and Luque-Galveston instrumentation. *J Spinal Disord* 1991;4:131–141.
11. Boos N, Webb JK. Pedicle screw fixation in spinal disorders: a European view. *Eur Spine J* 1997;6:2–18.
12. Bradford DS. Adult scoliosis: current concepts of treatment. *Clin Orthop* 1988;229:70–87.
13. Bradford DS, Ahmed KB, Moe JH, et al. The surgical management of patients with Scheuermann's disease. *J Bone Joint Surg Am* 1980;62A:705–712.
14. Bradford DS, Daher YH. Vascularized rib grafts for stabilization of kyphosis. *J Bone Joint Surg Br* 1986;68B:357–361.
15. Bradford DS, Moe JH, Montalvo FJ, et al. Scheuermann's kyphosis. Results of surgical treatment by posterior spine arthrodesis in twenty-two patients. *J Bone Joint Surg Am* 1975;57A:439–448.
16. Bridwell KH, Lenke LG, Baldus C, et al. Major intraoperative neurologic deficits in pediatric and adult spinal deformity patients: incidence and etiology at one institution. *Spine* 1998;23:324–331.
17. Bridwell KH, McAllister JW, Betz RR, et al. Coronal decompensation produced by Cotrel-Dubousset "derotation" maneuver for idiopathic right thoracic scoliosis. *Spine* 1991;16:769–777.
18. Brown CW, Orme TJ, Richardson HD. The rate of pseudarthrosis (surgical nonunion) in patients who are smokers and patients who are nonsmokers: a comparison study. *Spine* 1986;11:942–943.

19. Byrd JA, Scoles PV, Winter RB, et al. Adult idiopathic scoliosis treated by anterior and posterior spinal fusion. *J Bone Joint Surg Am* 1987;69A:843–850.

20. Cochran T, Irstam L, Nachemson A. Long-term anatomic and functional changes in patients with adolescent idiopathic scoliosis treated by Harrington rod fusion. *Spine* 1983;8:576–584.

21. Connolly PJ, Von Schroeder HP, Johnson GE, et al. Adolescent idiopathic scoliosis. Long term effect of instrumentation extending to the lumbar spine. *J Bone Joint Surg Am* 1995;77A:1210–1216.

22. Cummine JL, Lonstein JE, Moe JH, et al. Reconstructive surgery in the adult for failed scoliosis fusion. *J Bone Joint Surg Am* 1979;61A:1151–1161.

23. Dick J, Boachie-Adjei O, Wilson M. One stage vs. two stage anterior and posterior spinal reconstruction in adults. *Spine* 1992;17:S310–S316.

24. Erwin WD, Dickson JH, Harrington PR. Clinical review of patients with broken Harrington rods. *J Bone Joint Surg Am* 1980;62A:1302–1307.

25. Floman Y, Penny JN, Micheli LJ, et al. Osteotomy of the fusion mass in scoliosis. *J Bone Joint Surg Am* 1982;64A:1307–1316.

26. Glassman S, Dimar JR, Puno RM, et al. A prospective analysis of intraoperative electromyographic monitoring of pedicle screw placement with computed tomographic scan confirmation. *Spine* 1995;20:1375–1379.

27. Hamill CL, Lenke LG, Bridwell KH, et al. The use of pedicle screws to improve correction in the lumbar spine of adolescent idiopathic scoliosis: is it warranted? *Spine* 1996;21:1241–1249.

28. Herndon WA, Emans JB, Micheli LJ, et al. Combined anterior and posterior fusion for Scheuermann's kyphosis. *Spine* 1981;6:125–130.

29. Johnson JR, Holt RT. Combined use of anterior and posterior surgery for adult scoliosis. *Orthop Clin North Am* 1988;19:361–370.

30. King HA, Moe JH, Bradford DS, et al. The selection of fusion levels in thoracic idiopathic scoliosis. *J Bone Joint Surg Am* 1983;65A:1302–1313.

31. LaGrone MO, Bradford DS, Moe JH, et al. Treatment of symptomatic flatback after spinal fusion. *J Bone Joint Surg Am* 1988;70A:569–580.

32. Lauerman WC, Bradford DS, Transfeldt EE, et al. Management of pseudarthrosis after arthrodesis of the spine for idiopathic scoliosis. *J Bone Joint Surg Am* 1991;73A:222–236.

33. Lenke LG, Bridwell KH, Baldus C, et al. Analysis of pulmonary function and axis rotation in adolescent and young adult idiopathic scoliosis patients treated with Cotrel-Dubousset instrumentation. *J Spinal Disord* 1992;5:16–25.

34. Lenke LG, Bridwell KH, Baldus C, et al. Preventing decompensation in King type II curves treated with Cotrel-Dubousset instrumentation: strict guidelines for selective thoracic fusion. *Spine* 1992;17:274–281.

35. Lenke LG, Bridwell KH, Baldus C, et al. Cotrel-Dubousset instrumentation for adolescent idiopathic scoliosis. *J Bone Joint Surg Am* 1992;74-A:1056–1067.

36. Lenke LG, Bridwell KH, Baldus C, et al. Ability of Cotrel-Dubousset instrumentation to preserve distal lumbar motion segments in adolescent idiopathic scoliosis. *J Spinal Disord* 1993;6:339–350.

37. Lenke LG, Bridwell KH, O'Brien MF, et al. Recognition and treatment of the proximal thoracic curve in adolescent idiopathic scoliosis treated with Cotrel-Dubousset instrumentation. *Spine* 1994;19:1589–1597.

38. Lenke LG, Bridwell KH, Blanke K, et al. Analysis of pulmonary function and chest cage dimension changes following thoracoplasty in idiopathic scoliosis. *Spine* 1995;20:1343–1350.

39. Lenke LG, Bridwell KH, Blanke K, et al. Radiographic results of Cotrel-Dubousset instrumentation for the treatment of adolescent idiopathic scoliosis: a five- to ten-year follow-up study. *J Bone Joint Surg Am* 1998;80:807–814.

40. Lenke L, Padberg AM, Russo MH, et al. Triggered electromyographic threshold for accuracy of pedicle screw placement: an animal model and clinical correlation. *Spine* 1995;20:1585–1591.

41. Lonstein JE, Winter R, Moe J, et al. Wound infection with Harrington instrumentation and spine fusion for scoliosis. *Clin Orthop* 1973;96:222–233.

42. Lowe TG. Scheuermann's disease. Current concept review. *J Bone Joint Surg Am* 1990;72A:940–945.

43. May VR, Mauck WR. Exploration of the spine for pseudarthrosis following spinal fusion in the treatment of scoliosis. *Clin Orthop* 1967;53:115–122.

44. McElvein RB, Nasca RJ, Dunham WK, et al. Transthoracic exposure for anterior spinal surgery. *Ann Thorac Surg* 1988;45:278–283.

45. Moore MR, Baynham GC, Brown CW, et al. Analysis of factors related to truncal decompensation following Cotrel-Dubousset instrumentation. *J Spinal Disord* 1991;4:188–192.

46. O'Brien JP, Dason MH, Heard CW, et al. Simultaneous combined anterior and posterior fusion. A surgical solution for failed spinal surgery with a brief review of the first 50 patients. *Clin Orthop* 1986;203:191–195.

47. Ogilvie JW. Anterior spine fusion with Zielke instrumentation for idiopathic scoliosis in adolescents. *Orthop Clin North Am* 1987;10:1691–1698.

48. Reinhardt P, Bassett GS. Short segmental kyphosis following fusion for Scheuermann's disease. *J Spinal Disord* 1990;3:162–168.

49. Richards BS, Birch JG, Herring JA, et al. Frontal plane and sagittal plane balance following Cotrel-Dubousset instrumentation for idiopathic scoliosis. *Spine* 1989;14:733–737.

50. Richards BS. Delayed infections following posterior spinal instrumentation for idiopathic scoliosis. Twenty-ninth Annual Meeting, Scoliosis Research Society, Portland, Oregon, 1994.

51. Roye DP Jr, Farcy JP, Rickert JB, et al. Results of spinal instrumentation of adolescent idiopathic scoliosis by King type. *Spine* 1992;17:S270–S273.

52. Shufflebarger HL, Grimm JO, Bui V, et al. Anterior and posterior spinal fusion: staged versus same-day surgery. *Spine* 1991;16:930–933.

53. Suk S, Choon KL, Won-Joong K, et al. Segmental pedicle screw fixation in the treatment of thoracic idiopathic scoliosis. *Spine* 1995;20:1399–1405.

54. Thompson JP, Transfeldt EE, Bradford DS, et al. Decompensation after Cotrel-Dubousset instrumentation of idiopathic scoliosis. *Spine* 1990;15:927–931.

55. West JL, Boachie-Adjei O, Bradford DS, et al. Decompensation following CD instrumentation: a worrisome complication. *Orthop Trans* 1989;13:78–79.

56. Winter RB, Moe JH, Bradford DS, et al. Spine deformity in neurofibromatosis. *J Bone Joint Surg Am* 1979; 61A:677–694.

THORACIC SPINE: TRAUMA

ELDIN E. KARAIKOVIC, WICHARN YINGSAKMONGKOL, AND ROBERT W. GAINES, JR.

The thoracic spine, with the attached thoracic cage, is (except for the sacrum) the stiffest part of the spinal column. Because of the inflexibility of this segment, much greater or more focused stresses are necessary to create violent injuries of the thoracic spine than in the other major spinal segments. Injuries that do occur are much more likely to be fracture dislocations (injuries with translation) and then commonly involve injuries of many ribs or transverse processes, or both. These patients frequently have a spinal cord injury, with or without an injury to the aorta (transection or intimal tears) (3,26,34).

PATIENT SELECTION

As in other areas of the spine, the decision to treat a given spine fracture nonoperatively or operatively is a comprehensive patient-related decision that is based to a great degree on the anatomy of the fracture site (17) but also is conditioned by patient-related variables. These variables include the age and weight of the patient, the level of injury, the presence or absence of neurologic deficit, associated injuries, morbidities and the surgical risk, and the patient's occupation and expectations.

The majority of thoracic spine fractures can be successfully treated nonsurgically with adequate length of bed rest. However, surgical treatment is generally recommended for grotesquely displaced fracture dislocations and three-column injuries and in patients with neurologic deficit. In technologically advanced countries, surgical treatment of thoracic spine fractures is also performed to mobilize patients sooner. This permits prompt treatment of pulmonary contusion. Early surgery may also help prevent complications such as deep venous thrombosis and pneumonia that are associated with prolonged bed rest.

SURGICAL ALTERNATIVES

Because the thoracic spine is a less mobile area, posterior long segment instrumentation is generally the treatment of choice for surgical instrumentation, as the addition of a few segments generally does not limit functional motion. Posterior short segment or anterior instrumentation, or both, is therefore rarely done in the thoracic spine.

Primary and revision surgical treatment of thoracic spine fractures is performed for several reasons: first, to prevent or reverse neural deficit; second, to prevent or correct spinal deformity; and third, to prevent or relieve mechanical pain caused by prominent implants, pseudarthrosis, or loosening of a construct. The presence of infection can require drainage. Spinal cord or nerve root compression that is not relieved at the time of the initial procedure can cause dysesthesia or pain, or both, in the involved segment or lead to failure of an incomplete neurologic deficit to resolve completely. Syringomyelia at the level of the injury can be a source of nonmechanical symptoms as well.

PEDICLE SCREWS IN TREATMENT OF THORACIC SPINE FRACTURES

Pedicle screw fixation has improved the stability of spinal fusion constructs, produced better correction, made more generous posterior spinal decompression possible, produced shorter fusions (limiting posterior long segment instrumentation and fusion in the majority of cases to two levels above and two levels below the injury), produced better retention of intraoperative correction of spinal deformity, and almost eliminated nonunion as a complication (10,13,21,24). It also enables a surgeon to perform a pedicle subtraction osteotomy for spinal deformity when one is indicated. Although pedicle screws have been generally accepted for lumbar use, many surgeons have doubted that they could be safely used in the thoracic spine.

The most feared complication of this application of the thoracic pedicle screw is nerve root injury. Although this has been reported (6,33), the incidence is very low, even when misplacement is clearly documented. Besides spinal cord or nerve root injury, mis-

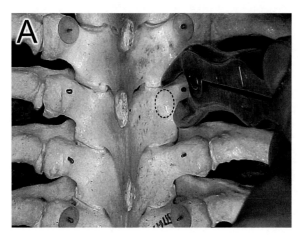
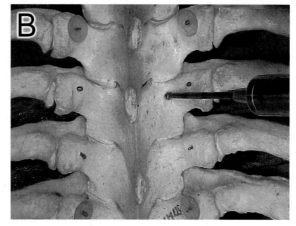

FIGURE 1. Visualization of the posterior vertebral bony anatomy is critical. The cortex over the thoracic pedicle entrance (an intersection of the lateral half of the inferior facet joint and at the center of the transverse process) is removed using a rongeur (our preference) **(A)** or a high-speed burr **(B)** (in this example, right T-4 pedicle).

placed screws in the thoracic spine may endanger the intercostal vessels or nerves, the esophagus, the azygous vein, the inferior vena cava, the thoracic duct, the lungs, and the sympathetic chain. Several cadaveric studies (2,15,16,18,20,25,27,31,35) have reported pedicle diameters at all thoracic spinal levels and showed their variability, as well as accessibility, for currently available pedicle screw sizes in different population groups (11,14).

Although several studies demonstrated a high incidence of pedicle screws that breached the pedicular cortex (29,30), our experimental and clinical experience has been different. Expensive computer-generated imaging technology has been proposed to minimize the rate of improper screw placement (9,19). We believe that this is cumbersome, expensive, and unnecessary.

We directly visualize the pedicle entrance intraoperatively and use the posterior portion of the pedicle (the part posterior to the isthmus) as a "funnel" to place the pedicle probe correctly through the pedicle isthmus. We then tap and place an appropriate-diameter screw. Although here we describe the "funnel" technique for the thoracic spine, it can easily be applied to cervical (12) and lumbar pedicles as well.

"PEDICLE AS A FUNNEL" TECHNIQUE

A general estimate of pedicle size is obtained from anteroposterior and lateral plain radiographs or computed tomography (CT) scans (we do not routinely perform CT scan through every pedicle to be instrumented). The posterior cortex of the lamina overlying area of the posterior projection of the pedicle axis is removed by a rongeur or burr (Fig. 1). We remove a 6- to 10-mm circle of cortical bone overlying the entire top of the pedicle (Fig. 2). The isthmus of the pedicle is directly visualized by removing the cancellous bone from the upper part of the pedicle with a

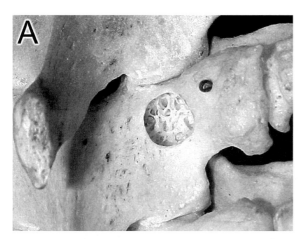
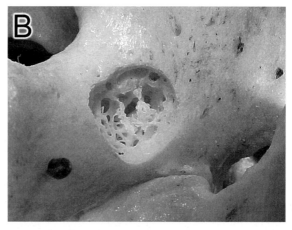

FIGURE 2. A: A 6- to 10-mm circumferential cortical defect over the top of the pedicle exposes the cancellous bone above the isthmus of the pedicle. **B:** A close look at the trabecular bone at the entrance of the thoracic pedicle.

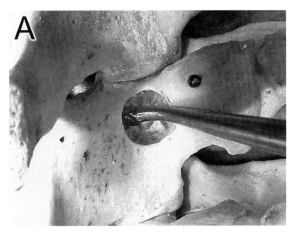

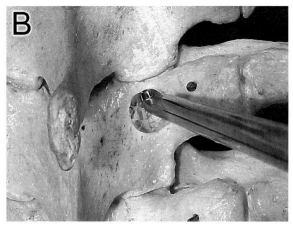

FIGURE 3. **A:** The cancellous bone is removed with a curette, which is advanced deeper through the wider posterior part of the pedicle "funnel" into its isthmus. **B:** Sometimes, hard overhanging cortical edges have to be removed with a Kerrison rongeur or a curette, allowing the surgeon to see into the upper portion of the pedicle isthmus.

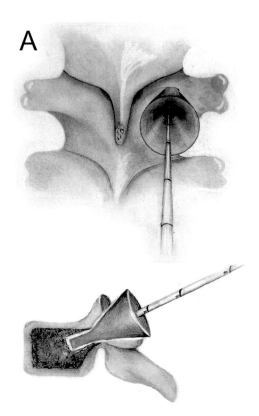

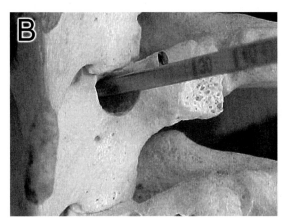

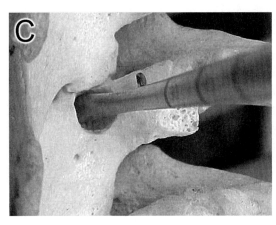

FIGURE 4. **A:** Diagram shows the funnel created in the upper part of the pedicle to guide the pedicle probe down through the isthmus. Once the isthmus of the pedicle is demonstrated, converging toward midline, first a pediatric pedicle probe **(B)** followed, if possible, by a standard pedicle probe **(C)** is introduced down through the isthmus of the pedicle medullary canal into the vertebral body.

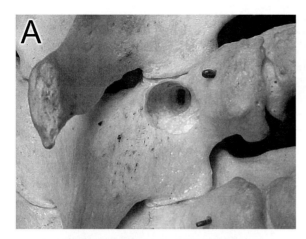

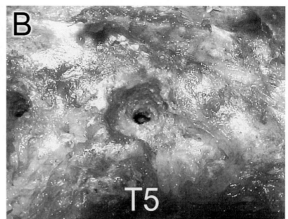

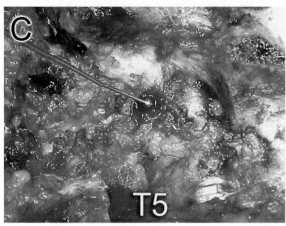

FIGURE 5. A right thoracic pedicle funnel can be clearly seen on a dry **(A)** and a fresh frozen **(B)** specimen. The funnel is created in the upper part of the pedicle to guide the pedicle probe down through the isthmus. **C:** An intraoperative photo–T-5 pedicle: The accurate placement of the pedicle probe is clinically confirmed by a venous return from the vertebral body, a so-called bleeding sign. Also, the integrity of the pedicle is confirmed clinically by palpating its walls using a ball-tipped probe (feeler; see Fig. 7B).

small curette. With further removal of cancellous bone, enlargement of the pedicle funnel leads the curette into the posterior part of the pedicle isthmus (Fig. 3). The use of the cortical margins of the upper part of the pedicle acts as a funnel. This funnel permits safe insertion of the pedicle probe across the pedicle isthmus. Careful probing of the pedicle is performed with the 2-mm pediatric probe and then, if the pedicle inner diameter allows it, with the stan-

dard Steffee pedicle probe (Fig. 4). A pedicle ball-tipped probe is used to inspect the depth of the opening as well as all four walls of the pedicle for a perforation (Fig. 5).

Metallic markers (Steinmann pin segments) are then inserted into the pedicles, and the orientation and depth of the pins are checked using an image intensifier (Fig. 6). The pedicles are then tapped with taps of gradually increasing diameter to achieve corti-

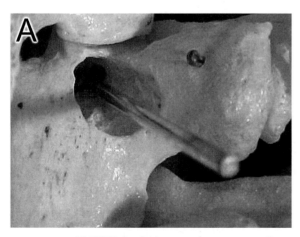

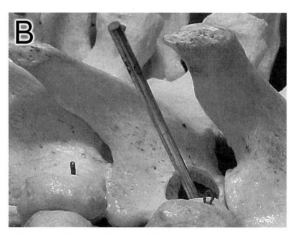

FIGURE 6. Steinman pin segments, 2 mm in diameter (55 mm in length), are introduced down through the pedicle into the vertebral body **(A, B)** and used as intraoperative radiographic markers to confirm a proper direction of the pedicle probe in anteroposterior **(C)** and lateral **(D)** views. (*continued*)

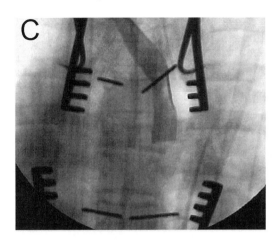

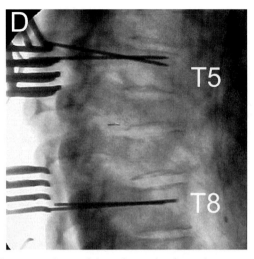

FIGURE 6. (*continued*) Pedicle screw lengths are estimated based on the lateral radiographs **(D)**.

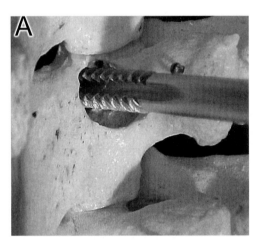

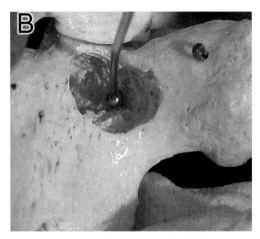

FIGURE 7. **A:** Progressively larger taps are used to cut threads into the pedicle isthmus until firm cortical purchase is achieved. *In vivo*, we used the diameters of thoracic pedicle screws that varied from 4.00 to 7.75 mm (see text). **B:** A ball-tipped probe is used to feel the threads cut into the isthmus of the pedicle inner cortex to confirm the integrity of all four (medial, lateral, superior, and inferior) cortical walls of the pedicle and the integrity of the bottom of the pedicle tunnel in the vertebral body.

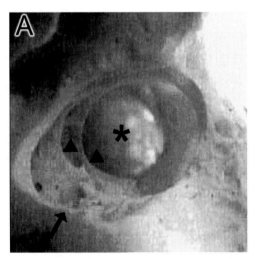

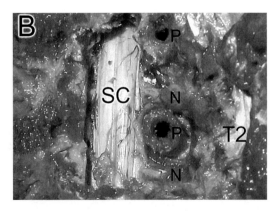

FIGURE 8. **A:** Anatomy of the pedicle funnel (*arrow*: the outer rim of the pedicle entrance; *arrowheads*: a cortical thread in the pedicle isthmus for screw purchase; *star*: a cancellous bone of the vertebral body). **B:** Anatomy around the isthmus of the right T-2 pedicle of a fresh frozen specimen. SC, spinal cord; N, nerve root; P, pedicle.

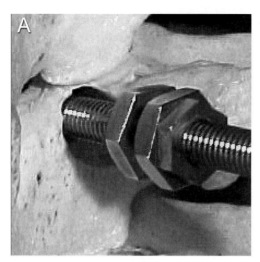
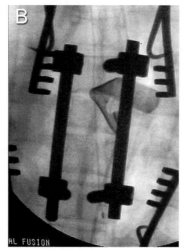
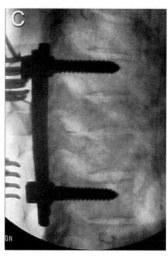

FIGURE 9. Screws of appropriate lengths and diameters are applied **(A)**, and their position and length are checked intraoperatively on anteroposterior **(B)** and lateral **(C)** radiographs using an image intensifier.

cal contact and determine the proper screw diameter for each individual pedicle. The screw diameter is only estimated by preoperative plain radiography, but the screw diameter is ultimately chosen by the feel of a tight fit of a tap used to create threads for screws in the inner cortex of the pedicle isthmus. The feeling of firm cortical purchase of the tap in the isthmus of the pedicle is the most accurate way to determine the appropriate outer diameter of the screw. The pedicle walls are checked again with a ball-tipped probe to feel the threads for perforation before an appropriate-sized screw is placed into each pedicle (Figs. 7 and 8). The final position and the length of each screw are again confirmed by the image intensifier (Fig. 9).

CADAVERIC STUDY ON THE ACCURACY OF THORACIC PEDICLE SCREW PLACEMENT USING THE FUNNEL TECHNIQUE

The reliability of the funnel technique in placement of the thoracic pedicle screws was proved in our cadaveric study (Yingsakmongkol W, Karaikovic EE, Gaines RW Jr. The reliability of the pedicle screw placement using the "funnel technique"; a cadaveric study. Personal communication, March 2000). The study was conducted by three spine surgeons with significantly different levels of experience: one spine fellow who, before the study, had no experience in thoracic pedicle screw placement; a junior spine surgeon experienced in thoracic pedicle screw placement in the past; and a senior spine surgeon who originated the technique.

Nine consecutive Euro-American cadavers from the Department of Pathology of the University of Missouri-Columbia School of Medicine were identified by age, sex, and height. They included three males and six females. The average age at the time of death was 81 (range, 75–97) years, and the average height was 165 (range, 155–175) cm. None of the individuals had evidence at postmortem examination of infectious or neoplastic diseases, and we found no evidence of congenital or developmental spinal malformation in any of the specimens. All cadavers had an various degrees of osteoporosis and degenerative changes expected for age, and one specimen had an unreported healed T11-12 fracture dislocation that was found intraoperatively.

No radiographs or other imaging of the thoracic spine was used before probing the pedicles. All pedicles were probed based on the examiner's clinical judgment of their size. If pedicles were clinically too small to be used and would be in an *in vivo* intraoperative situation abandoned as anchors for pedicle screws, that was recorded during probing. After that, these pedicles were probed to assess the accuracy of our clinical judgment.

The cadavers were positioned prone, and a standard posterior approach was used. A total of 216 pedicles (T1-12) were used (three cadavers or 72 pedicles per surgeon). A pediatric and a standard pedicle probe were used for pedicle medullary canal localization. After that, the pedicle was tapped with a 5.5-mm tap (DePuy AcroMed, Raynham, MA). All the pedicles were then evaluated for perforation using a ball-tipped probe by one of the authors who was not involved in probing of the particular pedicles. If a perforation was found, a 5.5-mm Isola pedicle screw was introduced, the lamina and transverse process were removed, and the degree of perforation of the outer pedicle cortex was assessed. Perforations of the outer cortex of the pedicles were divided into noncritical (perforations without contact of the pedicle screw with an adjacent nerve root or the dura) and critical (contact of the screw with the root or dura) perforations.

Two pedicles (T-12 on the same cadaver and not in the patient with fracture dislocation) were clinically rated as "too small" for pedicle screws. They would have been abandoned in a real situation as well. These pedicles were excluded from the study. When these pedicles were probed to prove the accuracy of our clinical estimate, critical perforations were found along both pedicle screws (injury to the dura due to medial pedicle cortex perforation).

The rest of the 214 pedicles were included in the study. A total of 14 (14 of 214, or 6.5%) screws perforated the outer pedicle cortex. Only one (1 of 214, or 0.5%) of these perforations was rated as critical due to the contact of the pedicle screw with the dura after T-8 medial cortex perforation (obvious signs of the dural laceration were not found). This perforation was made on the first cadaver operated on by the spine fellow. The rest of the perforations were rated as noncritical (13 of 214, or 6.1%): 1 at T-5, T-7, and T-10; 2 at T-2 and T-6; and 3 at T-3 and T-4. The majority of perforations were found on the lateral wall of the pedicle (5 of 214, or 2.3%: 2 at T-2 and T-3 and 1 at T-10). The medial (4 of 214, or 1.8%: 2 at T-4 and 1 at T-5 and T-8), inferior (3 of 214, or 1.4%: 2 at T-6 and 1 at T-4), and inferolateral perforations (2 of 214, or 0.9%: 1 at T-3 and T-4) were less common. No perforations of the superior wall of the pedicles were found.

The incidence of pedicle perforation of the spine fellow (9 of 72 pedicles, or 12.5%) compared with the junior staff member (4 of 72, or 5.5%) and the senior staff surgeon (1 of 70, or 1.4%) clearly demonstrated a learning curve and evidence that more clinical experience improved performance. Nevertheless, all but one of the perforations were noncritical (no contact of a screw with a nerve root or dura). This study showed that the funnel technique is a simple and safe technique for thoracic pedicle screw placement.

OUR CLINICAL EXPERIENCE WITH PLACEMENT OF THORACIC PEDICLE SCREWS

One hundred twenty-nine patients were retrospectively identified to have had at least one thoracic pedicle instrumented with a screw. Of these patients, 12 were lost to follow-up and 2 died before the review, leaving 115 patients who are the basis of this report (Viau M, Tarbox B, Wonglertsiri S, et al. Thoracic pedicle instrumentation. A review of the "pedicle as a funnel" technique. Personal communication, 1999).

All patients were treated at a single medical center under the supervision of the senior author (RWG) between January 1987 and November 1995. Diagnoses included 41 scoliosis (idiopathic: 30, neuromuscular: 9, congenital: 2), 63 fractures (neurologically intact: 35, neurologic deficit: 28), six degenerative conditions, two tumors, one Scheuermann's kyphosis, one neurofibromatosis, and one gunshot wound to the spine.

After completing training in pedicle screw placement on sawbones and calf and cadaver spines, 25 different residents on their first or second spine surgery rotation were responsible for placing 50% to 60% of pedicle screws. The attending and five different fellows placed the remainder. The decision to use pedicles as anchors for screws was made preoperatively by the attending surgeon based on their size on anteroposterior radiographs of the spine.

The medical charts were reviewed for intraoperative, perioperative, and long-term complications. The plain film radiographs were evaluated for screw placement, implant failure, and fusion mass. CT scans and myelograms were also evaluated for screw placement when available.

Evaluation of Accurate Thoracic Pedicle Screw Placement

Besides clinical intraoperative visual and tactile evaluation, there is no available perfect radiographic intraoperative method for evaluation of accuracy of pedicle screw placement. Radiographs produce a high rate of false-positive and false-negative evaluations of pedicle screw placed from T-11 to S-1, with interrated adjusted percent agreement for radiograph ratings of 0.74 (between two observers false-positive rates were 8.1% and 6.5%, and false-negative were 14.5% and 12.9%) (7,32).

Because most of the screws in this series were made of stainless steel, which interferes with CT imaging (5), we do not believe that additional postoperative CT radiation and expense are necessary. CT done postoperatively has been shown not to be very accurate either. Although more misplaced screws were clearly seen on CT scans than on plain radiographs, no statistically significant difference was found in a clinical study. Intraobserver differences

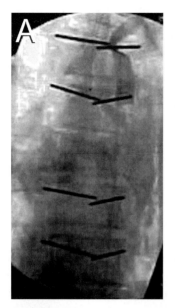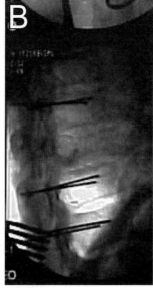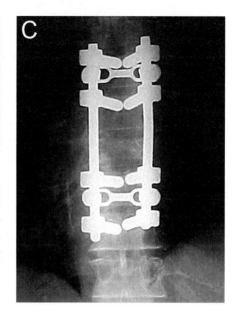

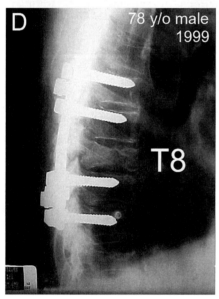

FIGURE 10. The anteroposterior and lateral radiographs of the T-8 fracture dislocation with metallic markers **(A, B)** and screws **(C, D)** placed in the T-6, T-7, T-9, and T-10 pedicles. The transverse connectors were placed to increase rotational stability of the construct.

approached statistical significance when the results of the two tests were compared (23).

No author has advocated routine use of CT in postoperative evaluation of pedicle screw placement in clinically asymptomatic patients because of the risk of additional radiation, discomfort to the freshly operated patient, and increased costs. Although in our study no screws were obviously out of the pedicle on plain radiography, we recognize the limitations of this method for determining screw position, the accuracy of which, according to some authors (7,8), varied from 73% to 83% depending on the experience of the surgeon grading the radiograms. We agree that the surgeon must not rely solely on the radiographs but instead continue to use tactile sensory skills, anatomic knowledge, and additional modalities (7). Thus, if screws were misdirected by

us, it was not demonstrated on our detailed clinical and radiographic examination.

Intraoperatively, the evaluation of pedicle screw placement was done by the surgeons in the operating team (one attending and one fellow or senior resident) and was based on the pedicle screw location on anteroposterior, lateral, and oblique radiographs on the image intensifier (Fig. 10). Postoperatively, the proper placement and localization of the pedicle screws were evaluated clinically for the level of function, pain, and presence or absence of neurologic symptoms (pain in a radicular distribution, new onset of neurologic deficit, deterioration of the postinjury neurologic deficit) and radiographically on the anteroposterior and lateral radiographs (by a fellow and a senior resident on rotation) as described by Weinstein et al. (32).

Intraobserver reproducibility and interobserver reliability were not evaluated, because the failure of pedicle screw fixation was made by consensus of this group of orthopedic surgeons. A failure was defined as the evidence of any cortical perforation on any side of the pedicle in or outside of the spinal canal or the presence of any signs of neurologic irritation or deficit even without obvious cortical violation of the pedicle. Screws maintained within the pedicle without any cortical disruption were considered successful (32).

Clinical Data Regarding Thoracic Pedicle Screw Placement

Included were 65 females and 50 males with ages ranging from 9 to 82 years. The average follow-up was 17 months (range 6–81 months). The total number of screws inserted was 348 (T-5: 1, T-6: 4, T-7: 3, T-8: 10, T-9: 21, T-10: 49, T-11: 106, T-12: 154). The screw diameter ranged from 4.00 mm to 7.75 mm. No patients had vascular or pulmonary complications. Postoperatively, one patient had transient anterior thigh numbness; otherwise, no new neurologic deficit was noted postoperatively. In fracture patients with a neurologic deficit, ten of 28 (35%) had documented neurologic improvement postoperatively, and none was made worse by the procedure. No screws were found to have penetrated the pedicle cortex. Four broken screws, one broken rod, two loose screws, and three connector disengagements occurred. Eleven patients had implants removed because of tenderness over implants. In four patients, a pseudarthrosis developed that required additional surgery. No patients needed implant removal for misplaced screws. Two deep wound infections occurred. The two perioperative deaths were unrelated to the spinal instrumentation (one patient died from metastatic cancer, and the other died from pulmonary failure from the initial injury).

CLINICAL ADVANTAGES OF THORACIC PEDICLE SCREW FIXATION

Although the use of thoracic pedicle screws is controversial, several clinical studies have reported their successful application (1,4,22,28). In a study of 78 idiopathic thoracic scoliotic curves, segmental correction with pedicle screws was superior in all three planes when compared to hooks or sublaminar wires. In the coronal plane, significantly better correction of the major curve (72%) and compensatory curve (70%) and smallest loss of correction (1%) were reported in the group with pedicle screws compared to segmental correction with Cotrel-Dubousset hooks (55%, 57%, and 6%, respectively). The sagittal plane curve correction was also better (18 degrees vs. 14 degrees). The authors achieved better rotational correction with pedicle screws (59%) than with hooks (19%). Postoperative CT scans showed that 3% of screws were malpositioned (of 13 screws, 6 were positioned superiorly, 5 laterally, 2 inferiorly, and 0 medially in regard to the pedicle). No neurologic deficits or decrease in curve correction was noticed due to malpositioned screws (28).

Use of thoracic pedicle screws allowed successful use of posterior short segment instrumentation and fusion in low-point total thoracolumbar fractures [based on the load-sharing classification (17)]. No complications due to use of the thoracic pedicle screws were reported (10,21).

CONCLUSION

The thoracic pedicles can be safely instrumented provided that the entry point is precisely located, pedicle morphology is well known, and the "funnel" technique is used to feel the isthmus of the pedicle. Pedicle screws in the thoracic spine have the same advantages as in the lumbar spine, providing immediately stable and rigid fixation, allowing shorter constructs that preserve motion segments. The fixation that they provide is biomechanically superior to that of any other currently used posterior spinal instrumentation. Also, they can be used when posterior elements are deficient.

Violation of the thoracic pedicle integrity and serious injuries to the adjacent structures with a pedicle probe, tap, and/or screw are possible due to smaller pedicle diameters and proximity of the adjacent neural structures (the nerve root or spinal cord). Intraoperatively, there are a limited number of ways to evaluate the accuracy of pedicle screw placement. Preoperative evaluation of the pedicle size on anteroposterior and lateral plain radiographs of the spine and accurate intraoperative surgical judgment of screw placement are the keys to successful pedicle screw placement. Awareness of individual variations in pedicle sizes is also very important. However, based on our experience, a detailed knowledge of pedicle anatomy, sound surgical technique, and thorough radiographic intraoperative monitoring make placement of thoracic pedicle screws a safe procedure.

Our intentions are not to recommend thoracic pedicle screw instrumentation for any specific use but rather to show its safe application when using the funnel technique. Our technique is simple and safe. It provided, in our series, even entry-level surgeons with a safe way to identify and place thoracic pedicle screws with no clinical problems. We believe that this technique is a much safer and cost-effective alternative to any other currently recommended techniques for pedicle screw placement.

REFERENCES

1. Aebi M, Etter C, Kehl T, et al. Stabilization of the lower thoracic and lumbar spine with the internal spinal skeletal fixation system: indication, techniques, and first results of treatment. *Spine* 1987;12:544–551.
2. Berry JL, Moran TM, Berg WS, et al. A morphometric study of human lumbar and selected thoracic vertebrae. *Spine* 1987;12:362–367.
3. Bolesta MJ, Bohlman HH. Mediastinal widening associated with fractures of the upper thoracic spine. *J Bone Joint Surg Am* 1991;73(3):447–450.
4. Dick W. The "Fixatuer Interne" as a versatile implant for spine surgery. *Spine* 1987;12:882–900.
5. Ebraheim NA, Rupp RE, Savolaine ER, et al. Use of titanium implants in pedicular screw fixation. *J Spinal Disord* 1994;7(6):478–486.
6. Esses SI, Sachs BL, Breysin V. Complications associated with the technique of pedicle screw fixation. *Spine* 1993;18:2231–2239.
7. Ferrick MR, Kowalski JM, Simmons ED Jr. Reliability of roentgenogram evaluation of pedicle screw position. *Spine* 1997;22(11):1249–1252.
8. Gertzbein SD, Robbins SE. Accuracy of pedicular screw placement in vivo. *Spine* 1990;15:11–14.
9. Glossop ND, Hu RW, Randle JA. Computer-aided pedicle screw placement using frameless stereotaxis. *Spine* 1996;21(17):2026–2034.
10. Holt BT, McCormack T, Gaines RW. Short segment fusion-anterior or posterior approach—the load-sharing classification of spine fractures. *Spine: State of Art Reviews* 1993;7(2):277–285.
11. Hou S, Hu R, Shi Y. Pedicle morphology of the lower thoracic and lumbar spine in Chinese population. *Spine* 1993;18:1850–1855.
12. Karaikovic EE, Daubs M, Matsen R, et al. Morphologic characteristics of human cervical pedicles. *Spine* 1994;19(12):1390–1394.
13. Karaikovic EE, Gaines RW. Short segment fixation using VSP plates and pedicle screws for trauma. In: Brown CW, McCarthy RE, eds. *Spinal instrumentation techniques.* Rosemont, IL: Scoliosis Research Society, 1994.
14. Kim NH, Lee HM, Chung IH, et al. Morphometric study of the pedicles of thoracic and lumbar vertebrae in Koreans. *Spine* 1994;19(12):1390–1394.
15. Kothe R, O'Halleran J, Liu W, et al. Internal architecture of the thoracic pedicle—an anatomic study. *Spine* 1996;21:264–270.
16. Krag MH, Weaver DL, Beynnon BD, et al. Morphometry of the thoracic and lumbar spine related to transpedicular screw placement for surgical spinal fixation. *Spine* 1988;13:27–32.
17. McCormack T, Karaikovic EE, Gaines RW. The load-sharing classification of spine fractures. *Spine* 1994;19(15):1741–1744.
18. Misenhimer GR, Peek RD, Wiltse LL, et al. Anatomic analysis of pedicle cortical and cancellous diameter as related to screw size. *Spine* 1989;16:888–901.
19. Nolte LP, Zamora LJ, Jiang Z, et al. Image guided insertion of transpedicular screws: a laboratory setup. *Spine* 1995;20:497–500.
20. Panjabi MM, Takata K, Goel V, et al. Thoracic human vertebrae; quantitative three-dimensional anatomy. *Spine* 1991;16:888–901.
21. Parker JW, Lane J, Karaikovic EE, et al. Successful short-segment instrumentation and fusion for thoracolumbar spine fractures; a consecutive 4 1/2-year series. *Spine* 2000;25:1157–1170.
22. Roy-Camille R, Saillant G, Mazel C. Plating of thoracic, thoracolumbar, and lumbar injuries with pedicle screw plates. *Orthop Clin North Am* 1986;17:147–159.
23. Sapkas GS, Papadakis SA, Stathakopoulos DP, et al. Evaluation of pedicle screw position in thoracic and lumbar spine fixation using plain radiographs and computed tomography. A prospective study of 35 patients. *Spine* 1999;24(18):1926–1929.
24. Sasso RC, Colter HB. Posterior instrumentation and fusion for unstable fractures and fracture-dislocations of the thoracic and lumbar spine. A comparative study of three fixation devices in 70 patients. *Spine* 1993;18(4):450–460.
25. Scoles RV, Linton AE, Latimer B, et al. Vertebral body and posterior element morphology: the normal spine in middle life. *Spine* 1988;10:1082–1086.
26. Stambough JL, Ferree BA, Fowl RJ. Aortic injuries in thoracolumbar spine fracture-dislocations: report of three cases. *J Orthop Trauma* 1989;3(3):245–249.
27. Suk SI, Lee JH. A study of the diameter and change of the vertebral pedicle after screw insertion. Presented at the Third Intermeeting, SIROT, Boston, 1994.
28. Suk SI, Lee CK, Kim W, et al. Segmental pedicle screw fixation in the treatment of thoracic idiopathic scoliosis. *Spine* 1995;20:1399–1405.
29. Vaccaro AR, Rizzolo SJ, Allardyce TJ, et al. Placement of pedicle screws in the thoracic spine. Pt I: Morphometric analysis of the thoracic vertebrae. *J Bone Joint Surg* 1995;77A(8):1193–1199.
30. Vaccaro AR, Rizzolo SJ, Balderston RA, et al. Placement of pedicle screws in the thoracic spine. Pt II: An anatomical and radiographic assessment. *J Bone Joint Surg* 1995;77A(8):1200–1206.

31. Weinstein JN, Rydevik BL, Rauschming W. Anatomic and technical considerations of pedicle screw fixation. *Clin Orthop* 1992;284:34–46.

32. Weinstein JN, Spratt KF, Spengler D, et al. Spinal pedicle fixation reliability and validity of roentgenogram-based assessment and surgical factors on successful screw placement. *Spine* 1988;13:1012–1018.

33. West JL III, Ogilvie JW, Bradford DS. Complications of the variable screw plate pedicle screw fixation. *Spine* 1987;12:160–166.

34. Williams JS, Graff JA, Uku JM, et al. Aortic injury in vehicular trauma. *Ann Thorac Surg* 1994;57(3):726–730.

35. Zindrick MR, Wiltse LL, Doornik A, et al. Analysis of the morphometric characteristics of the thoracic and lumbar pedicles. *Spine* 1987;12:160–166.

THORACIC SPINE: TUMOR

FAIQ MAHMUD, STEVEN D. GLASSMAN, AND JOHN R. DIMAR II

An aging population has led to a greater number of patients seen with metastatic cancer (53,53a). In fact, cancer has become the second leading cause of death in the United States (44), and metastatic disease affects two-thirds of the patients with cancer (7). The skeletal system is third only to the lung and liver in terms of metastatic disease (6), and the vertebral column is most frequently involved within the skeletal system (2). The true incidence of vertebral metastasis is difficult to determine radiographically, as radiographic evidence of metastasis becomes apparent only after destruction of 30% to 50% of the bone (23). However, autopsy studies have revealed that up to 90% of patients who die from cancer have evidence of spinal metastases (39). Seventy-five percent of vertebral metastases originate from carcinoma of the breast, prostate, kidney, thyroid, lymphoma, or myeloma (17), and no primary lesion is identified in up to 20% of the patients reported in some series (3).

Along with an increasing prevalence of metastatic disease in the population, the concomitant advances in radiation therapy, chemotherapy, and surgical management have led to prolonged survival rates (15). Thus, whereas palliative therapy was the mainstay of treatment for metastatic spine lesions in the past, today's goal is often stabilization with anticipation of a prolonged survival. Moreover, it is not unusual to see patients who have previously undergone surgery, radiotherapy, and/or chemotherapy survive long enough to require additional surgical intervention. Revision tumor spine surgery not only carries all the hazards of revision surgery performed for other indications, but there are also special considerations involved in tumor cases. The need for revision surgery is often secondary to complications of chemo- or radiotherapy, complications of previous surgery, inadequacy of prior surgery, or recurrence of disease. The purpose of this chapter is to address some of these issues.

COMPLICATIONS OF RADIATION THERAPY

The advent of radiation therapy has dramatically improved the prognosis of many tumors that affect the spine. Several tumor types that could only be managed with surgical excision in the past can now be treated with either radiation alone or a combination of radiation and surgery. Among tumors that metastasize to the spine, the myeloproliferative lesions, such as myeloma and lymphoma, are highly radiosensitive. Lung, breast, colon, and prostate tumors are moderately radiosensitive; melanoma, renal cell carcinoma, and thyroid tumors are relatively resistant to radiation therapy (18).

Thus, when a patient presents with a metastatic radiosensitive spine lesion, radiation and bracing are often a viable option. Surgical intervention can be avoided in many patients with widespread metastatic disease or in a situation in which the lesion is too intimate to vital organs to allow *en bloc* surgical excision. However, surgery may become necessary despite primary radiation therapy if the tumor is not totally eradicated and continues to pose a threat to the neural elements or structural stability of the spine. Furthermore, surgery may become necessary even if radiation is successful in completely eradicating the pathologic tissue. This failure of radiotherapy results if remnants of bone, either normal remaining bone or reactive bone, are left impinging neural tissue.

In certain situations, surgical treatment may be more efficacious than radiotherapy despite the fact that the lesion is radiosensitive. If the tumor mass involves significant stabilizing structures of the spine, its eradication may result in spinal instability. Another special situation that may lead to failure of primary radiation therapy is the case in which tumor tissue has encircled the spinal cord or cauda equina. Eradication would then result in scar tissue that acts as a constrictive lesion (Mark Bilsky, Sloane-Kettering Memorial Hospital, New York. Personal communication, 1996). Surgical decompression is preferable in this case, regardless of the radiosensitivity of the lesion.

Due to the proximity of neurovascular and osseous structures in the spine, high doses of radiation may not be tolerated. Radical ablative surgery is often not possible because of similar considerations. Thus, a combination of radiation and surgery is often used to treat metastatic spine lesions. In such cases, it is best to perform the surgical excision first and delay radio-

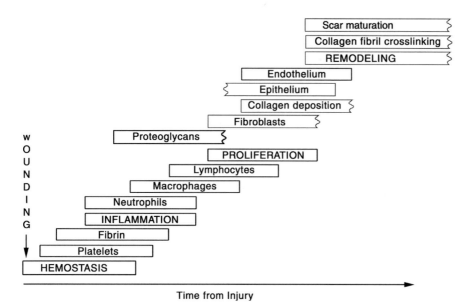

FIGURE 1. Timeline of wound healing. (From Mast BA. The skin. In: Cohen K, Diegelmann RF, Linblad WJ, eds. *Wound healing: biochemical and clinical aspects.* Philadelphia: WB Saunders, 1992, with permission.)

therapy for 6 to 8 weeks (52). The delay allows for early wound healing and minimizes the risk of wound breakdown or infection.

Although wound healing progresses through a complex continuum of events, the cascade has been divided into three stages (30) (Fig. 1). During the initial stage of inflammation, an influx of macrophages and monocytes occurs at the wound site. These cells release humoral factors and trigger local fibroblasts to proliferate. The inflammatory stage occurs during the first 24 to 48 hours after injury and is thought to be the most sensitive to radiation and chemotherapy.

The second stage of wound healing is described as the *proliferative stage*. During this time, which can last up to a week after injury, fibroblasts reproduce and begin forming collagen and proteoglycans. The final stage of wound healing is described as the *maturation stage*, but its time frame is not clearly delineated. During this time, newly produced collagen fibers become cross-linked and the wound gains tensile strength. Although a surgical wound will continue to increase in tensile strength for up to 2 years, the greatest gains occur in the first 6 to 8 weeks. A delay of this duration after surgery is thus advisable.

In some situations, one may decide to use radiation before surgery. For instance, preoperative radiation can be used to decrease the size of a lesion to resectable dimensions. In cases in which surgery follows radiation, a delay of 6 to 8 weeks between the two is also desirable. During the first 6 weeks after radiation, the skin structures are in the acute and subacute phase of injury and repair. During this period, not only does the cellular layer of the dermis (the basal layer) regenerate, but secondary structures

such as hair follicles and sweat glands also recover. Beyond this time, the remaining damage is likely to be permanent. Thus, to allow the skin to recover maximally and maximize its ability to withstand surgical intervention, at least a 6-week period between radiation and surgery is recommended (30) (Fig. 2).

Several studies have shown high wound healing complication rates when surgery is performed within 3 weeks of radiation therapy. Bujko et al. (8) studied more than 200 patients with soft tissue sarcomas who underwent surgical resection within 3 weeks of preoperative radiotherapy. The overall wound complication rate was 37% (8). In another study, a group of 42 patients underwent resection of Ewing's sarcoma after preoperative radiation. Fourteen of these patients experienced complications of wound heal-

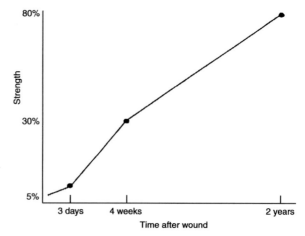

FIGURE 2. Relationship between wound strength and the duration of healing. (From Springfield DS. Surgical wound healing. In: Verwell J, Pinedo HM, Suit HE, eds. *Multidisciplinary treatment of soft tissue sarcomas.* Boston: Kluwer Academic Publishers, 1993, with permission.)

ing. In a comparable group of 28 patients who did not receive radiation, wound healing complications developed in only two patients (20).

Prior irradiation may affect or even lead to revision surgery in a variety of ways. In a patient with one metastasis to the spinal column, a recurrence or a new lesion may develop within a previously irradiated field. Alternatively, secondary sarcomas of the spine may arise if the vertebral column has been included in the radiation field that is used to treat nonvertebral tumors. Hodgkin's disease, breast cancer, and cervical cancer are the three commonest primary neoplasms for which the spine is included in the radiation portals (45). In addition to these tumors, radiotherapy is used in cases of incomplete resection of primary spine lesions, such as giant cell tumor or Paget's disease, that may also result in osteosarcoma. In fact, one-third of all osteosarcomas of the spine are secondary to radiotherapy (18). These lesions grow rapidly and respond poorly to conventional radio- and chemotherapy protocols.

In one of the largest studies on postradiation sarcomas of the spine, Sundaresan et al. (47) reported on 15 patients in whom spine lesions developed at a median of 10 years after they received radiotherapy for non-spine tumors. Interestingly, skin and subcutaneous changes of prior radiation, such as telangiectasia, atrophy, and fibrosis, were present in up to one-third of the patients even one decade after initial radiation treatment. No patient in this series survived longer than 8 months. In fact, no cures have been reported in the literature for postradiation spine sarcomas. Two reasons suggested for such a dismal prognosis are the lack of early diagnosis and insufficiently aggressive treatment. Therefore, a complete tumor workup, including a magnetic resonance imaging (MRI) scan, computed tomography scanning, and myelography, must be carried out relatively quickly in patients who complain of spinal pain or neurogenic symptoms and have a history of distant treatment for Hodgkin's disease, breast, and cervical cancer. In addition, aggressive resection, which often entails a combined anterior-posterior approach with strut grafting or methylmethacrylate use, is preferred over a simple laminectomy for tumor debulking. The authors noted that such radical resection resulted in longer survival rates, averaging 2 years in three patients.

COMPLICATIONS OF CHEMOTHERAPY

Although most of the literature on the subject has focused on complications of revision surgery follow-ing radiation treatment, significant difficulties may also arise during revision surgery after chemotherapy. New chemotherapeutic regimens are being developed rapidly, and the interaction of each agent with surgical intervention must be individualized. However, there are a few generalizations regarding the effect of these agents on wound healing. In general, drug dose is correlated directly to the effect on wound healing, but the critical dose for most drugs has not been established. Time of administration is also critical. The most detrimental effect on wound healing is observed when the agent is given within 2 weeks preceding surgery or within 1 week after surgery.

In contrast to radiation, the effect of chemotherapy is systemic yet transient. Because of its systemic nature, it is not possible to place surgical incisions away from the field of treatment, as can be done with radiation therapy. For instance, using an anterior approach to the spine, a retroperitoneal or thoracic incision can be placed at a distance from an irradiated vertebral body (9). After chemotherapy, wound healing in the entire body is affected.

Although a distant incision may not be able to decrease the effect of chemotherapy, elapsed time can take advantage of its transient nature. Incisions made more than 3 weeks after chemotherapy appear to heal with nearly normal tissue tensile strength (25). At the same time, it has become clear that all effects of chemotherapeutic agents may not be transient.

The prolonged effect of chemotherapy on wound healing may be indirect through neutropenia and nutritional deficiency (11). A nadir in the white cell count occurs after chemotherapy. The nadir is critical to wound healing because neutrophils and monocytes appear to be the most critical cellular elements of the wound healing cascade. Monocytes transform into macrophages and release local humoral factors that are responsible for stimulating cell division and new capillary formation. The monocyte also has a significant effect on fibroblast stimulation and the rate of new collagen production at the wound site. Although never studied prospectively, it has been well recognized clinically that an absolute neutrophil count below 500 predictably results in wound healing complications. Unfortunately, the timing of the nadir cannot be predicted from patient to patient, or even from one administration of a particular drug to its second administration. Laboratory examination must be performed after each therapeutic cycle.

Patients undergoing chemotherapy often experience significant nutritional depletion. Several agents adversely affect appetite in addition to causing nausea and vomiting. Chemotherapeutic agents can also interfere with normal gastrointestinal absorption and function. In addition, patients undergoing any surgical procedure are well known to be in a catabolic state. If the procedure is staged, the catabolic state is extended and further nutritional depletion results.

Although there is little literature on patients undergoing a procedure for spinal metastasis in particular, Mandelbaum et al. (28) have clearly shown the detrimental effect of nutritional deficiency on wound healing of spine patients. In a group of spinal patients undergoing a staged procedure, 67% developed nutritional deficiency as manifested by a decrease in albumin and total lymphocyte count into a clearly abnormal range. More alarmingly, 87% of the malnourished patients experienced at least one infectious complication, and postoperative wound infections developed in nearly 13%. Other infectious complications included urinary tract infection, pneumonia, and sepsis.

Stambough and Beringer (48) studied spine patients who had an established postoperative infection. They found that nearly 43% of their 19 patients were nutritionally depleted before the development of the infection. These authors have suggested aggressive prophylactic therapy with nutritional supplementation and total parenteral nutrition. These recommendations appear to be even more relevant in the spine tumor patient undergoing surgery combined with chemotherapy because not only is the patient likely to be in a catabolic state, but malnutrition is further aggravated by a decrease in appetite and gastrointestinal function.

COMPLICATIONS OF PREVIOUS SURGERY

Primary surgical resection may fail because of inadequate tumor resection, inadequate stabilization, development of iatrogenic instability, or recurrence of tumor. Inadequate initial tumor resection can be a result of underestimation of tumor extent due to inaccurate imaging, inappropriate choice of surgical approach, or limitation to resection due to the proximity of essential neurovascular structures (4,14).

Preoperative planning based on accurate imaging of the entire spine is critical in avoiding incomplete resection of tumor. Plain radiographs are inadequate in visualizing the extent of the lesion in the marrow spaces (23) and therefore must be supplemented with an MRI scan. In addition, up to 20% of patients with spinal metastasis present with multiple lesions, often several vertebral levels below the lesion that is under study (9). Thus, the entire vertebral column should be imaged before a surgical procedure is planned.

Once the procedure has been defined based on appropriate imaging, the requirements of future imaging must be kept in mind. One may wish to follow the patient for completeness of resection or for recurrence using an MRI scan after surgery. Titanium implants should be used in such cases, not only for spinal instrumentation but also for embolization procedures or vascular clips, or both.

Inadequate tumor resection can result not only from inaccurate imaging but also from incomplete access to the lesion. Thus, the surgical approach for spinal lesions needs to be considered carefully. Before selection of the surgical approach, the position of the lesion relative to the spinal cord must be clearly established. Laminectomy—the traditional approach to tumor resection—is indicated for tumors that are located posterior to the dura, for neural decompression, for pain relief caused by secondary hypertrophic stenosis, and if intradural exploration is necessary (46). For tumors located anterior to the dura, an anterior decompression provides greater access to the lesion.

In the revision situation, the selection of an approach becomes even more important. Traditionally, the posterior approach has been used for most primary resections, often leaving some tumors anteriorly. Thus, an anterior or a combined anterior-posterior approach is often the approach of choice for the revision. In addition, use of the anterior approach allows greater fusion area, especially after laminectomy, and in cases in which a pseudarthrosis is suspected from the prior operation. For patients who cannot tolerate an anterior approach, a posterolateral approach may allow access to the anterior spine.

Primary tumor surgery may fail despite successful resection if stabilization of the spine is not adequate (27). Multisegmental fixation is advisable, and some authors have suggested segmental wiring fixation as performed for metabolic and neuromuscular disease. In addition, the tumor mass visualized before surgery can often be completely removed, but if undetected tumor foci are present at sites to which fixation is performed, loss of implant fixation can occur. An MRI scan can help in limiting this possibility, but microscopic tumor foci may nevertheless be present in bone that appears normal even on an MRI scan. Thus, consideration should be given to fixation across a greater number of segments than that required for other causes of instability.

Iatrogenic instability is another cause for failure of primary tumor surgery. In the past, laminectomy without fusion has been routinely used for tumor "decompression." In addition to providing inadequate resection of a tumor located anterior to the dura, a laminectomy can destabilize the spine if the anterior or middle columns have already been compromised (46).

Findlay (13) reviewed the literature to determine outcomes for nearly 2,000 patients to compare laminectomy alone with laminectomy and radiotherapy and radiotherapy alone. Of the patients treated with radiation alone, 51% were able to walk at the end of treatment, compared with 38% treated with a combination, and 32% of those who were treated with laminectomy alone. However, 11% of the patients who had surgery sustained a major complication, and the mortality from surgery was 9%.

In a randomized prospective study, Young et al. (55) compared the results of laminectomy plus radiation with those of radiotherapy alone. Patients were randomly assigned to each group, and all patients had significant block caused by extradural tumor compression on a preoperative myelogram. The authors found no statistically significant difference in terms of pain relief or neurologic improvement. They suggested that laminectomy, as a surgical procedure, may not improve the overall outcome of the tumor patient because tumor located anterior to the dura cannot be excised and because laminectomy can produce iatrogenic instability, a further cause of pain and neurologic deterioration.

Postlaminectomy instability is often manifested as kyphosis and has been well documented in the literature, especially in children. Factors that may contribute to the kyphosis, in addition to the laminectomy, include implant cutout from bone, development of tumor above or below the fixation, or development of a pseudarthrosis. Pain and deficits resulting from the kyphosis often necessitate a revision procedure. Finally, despite an optimum decision-making approach and fixation technique for an individual patient, recurrent tumor may lead to failure of fixation, recurrence of pain, and/or neurologic symptoms.

PATIENT EVALUATION

Indications for revision tumor surgery in the spine depend heavily on prognosis and life expectancy. The spine surgeon must work closely with the oncologist in balancing overall patient care. With increasing emphasis on quality-of-life issues, appropriate surgical intervention on accessible lesions has gained support. However, this decision-making process is highly variable.

Tokuhashi (50) attempted to quantify this process using six parameters: (a) the general condition of the patient, (b) the number of extraspinal metastases, (c) the number of spinal metastases, (d) the resectability of metastases to the major internal organs, (e) the primary site of the tumor, and (f) the severity of spinal cord palsy. Zero to two points were assigned for each parameter. Patients with a total score of higher than 9 (from a maximum of 12) survived an average of 12 months or more; those with a total score of less than 5 survived for less than 12 weeks. The authors concluded that excisional surgery with intent to cure should be performed for patients with a score of greater than 9 and that palliative surgery should be reserved for those with a score of less than 5. In this regard, if palliative measures such as radiation, steroids, bracing, and analgesia are not expected to provide relief for the patient during his or her remaining life expectancy, revision surgery should be considered.

In general, life expectancy in patients with skeletal metastases has been noted to be less than 5 years for those with thyroid or prostate carcinoma, approximately 3 years in multiple myeloma, 2 years in breast carcinoma, 1 year in renal cell carcinoma, and poor in patients with lung and gastrointestinal carcinomas. Survival time for patients with malignant myeloma is less than 14 weeks after the onset of neurologic symptoms (18).

In addition to expected survival time, one must consider other factors that take into account the general health of the patient. Tokuhashi's system, described above, is one method of doing so.

TECHNIQUES OF REVISION TUMOR SPINE SURGERY

Prior Radiation and Chemotherapy

In revision tumor cases in which surgery is performed through a previously irradiated field, poor wound healing is well documented (1,18,41). Histologically, the skin is composed of three layers: the epidermis, the dermis, and the subcutaneous tissue. The deepest portion of the epidermis—the basal layer—contains continuously dividing cells that are responsible for skin turnover. Because sensitivity to radiation is proportional to mitotic activity, this regenerative layer of skin is severely affected. In addition, the middle layer of the skin, the dermis, contains capillaries, sweat glands, and connective tissues that give skin its suppleness. Damage to this layer results in a shiny, dry skin that is quite brittle.

Radiation changes to the skin can be divided into acute, subacute, and chronic. The acute phase occurs within the first 3 weeks and consists of edema and local tenderness. Histologically, vascular damage and an inflammatory exudate are found. Recovery from this phase occurs if the germinal layer is able to replace the epidermis, but the damage to the microvasculature is often permanent (22). If the germinal layer itself is too severely damaged to recover, ulceration may occur.

The subacute phase of radiation damage lasts from 6 to 12 months after treatment. This phase is characterized by obstructive endarteritis and replacement of the supple structure of the dermis by dense, rigid fibrous tissue (29,49).

The chronic phase is merely the residue of damage that could not be repaired during the acute and subacute phases. This damage is permanent. Because of the loss of sweat and sebaceous glands, the skin becomes dry. Hair is lost secondary to follicular damage, and the subcutaneous fat and collagen are replaced by a dense, leathery fibrous tissue. In addition, due to loss and damage to the microcirculation, the skin's ability to respond to infection and trauma (e.g., surgical) is severely compromised (12).

With this cascade of damage in mind, the following recommendations have been made in the literature (12):

Variable	Recommendation
Timing	Surgery should be delayed until the subacute phase has passed to allow the maximum recovery by the regenerative cells of the germinal layer.
Portals	An attempt should be made to place skin and fascial incisions either away from portals or portals receiving the least dose of radiation.
Surgical technique	1. Incisions should be planned through fascia (e.g., in the midline, if anterior).
	2. Strict subperiosteal dissection must be carried out.
	3. Retraction should be minimized; tension on compromised vasculature can result in loss of blood supply to the elevated flap.
	4. A multilayered watertight closure is essential.
	5. Wound débridement should not be out to bleeding edges, as this may entail excessive excision because of the chronic vascular damage.
	6. If the irradiated skin does not tolerate primary reapproximation, provisions should be made for free-flap closure.

Extensive research has been done in the last 5 years to develop new surgical techniques and chemical modulators that may assist in the care of surgical wounds in irradiated tissue. In cases in which discrete portals have been used, tissue expansion techniques have shown great promise in raising flaps of normal tissue adjacent to the irradiated areas (35). Although with less predictable results, tissue expansion has actually been used to expand irradiated skin (24). With the advent of molecular and genetic techniques, various factors are being isolated that may enhance neovascularization (21), collagen regeneration (1), and tissue repair (5,33,37), thus reversing tissue damage caused by radiation.

When considering revision tumor surgery in the context of prior radiation therapy, one must address the delayed healing of bone graft as well as the skin. Although the most noticeable changes in tissue structure due to radiation damage are in the healing of skin and soft tissues, several authors have shown that auto- and allograft are very slow to incorporate if placed in tissue that has been previously irradiated (16,36). Delayed healing, the fact that large gaps often need to be bridged after resection, and the fact that the life expectancy of patients undergoing revision tumor surgery may be uncertain can lead to an unincorporated biological graft during the lifetime of the patient. This pseudarthrosis may become symptomatic.

Thus, in primary tumor surgery, an acceptable alternative to biological grafts has been methylmethacrylate. Its use makes even more sense in a revision environment. When combined with metallic implants, very successful results have been obtained after significant vertebral resection, and patients can usually be mobilized immediately, often without bracing (16,36). At present, several investigators are reporting on alternatives to acrylic that provide its advantages without side effects (10,32), such as generation of heat close to neural tissues and weakness in tension and shear (54). Ono et al. (34) and Matsui et al. (31) have shown excellent results with ceramics used as spacers for tumor surgery.

With regard to prior chemotherapy, the issues are very similar to those seen with radiation therapy. In addition, chemotherapy cannot be coned down to a specific field. However, problems encountered after chemotherapy have not been as evident as those after radiotherapy because, almost always, adjuvant chemotherapy can be delayed until after the surgical intervention. In such cases, the delay in starting chemotherapy should be at least 2 weeks, if the patient's condition permits, to allow early wound healing and initial graft vascularization. Otherwise, recommendations for wound management are similar to those described for the postradiation patient.

Previous Spine Surgery

As a result of studies that document the complications associated with laminectomy, alternative treatment options for failed radiotherapy, chemotherapy, or prior surgical intervention have been investigated (Fig. 3). Noting that nearly 85% of metastases that cause spinal instability or canal compromise arise anteriorly, Harrington (16) has advocated anterior resection of tumor with stabilization of the spine using Knodt rods and methylmethacrylate. In a series of 77 patients, 42 of the 62 patients who had significant neurologic compromise recovered significantly, and more than half recovered completely. Only six patients required further surgery, with a follow-up of at least 42 months. Harrington states that posterior exposure for a laminectomy destabilizes the posterior structures in patients who already have compromised anterior structures. In addition, the author believes that postradiation patients experience hyperemic softening of bone that further compromises posterior fixation. Thus, although newer segmental fixation is not addressed in this paper, Harrington cautions against posterior-only approaches.

In another study, the authors reviewed the results of anterior stabilization and instrumentation carried out as a revision procedure after failure of initial radiotherapy (42). Unlike Harrington's series, these patients did not manifest obvious instability, but all patients had significant neurologic deficit and pain secondary to myelographically documented cord compression. Eighty percent of 44 patients were able to ambulate after anterior decompression and fusion, as compared to 26% before surgery. Only 7% of the patients had incapacitating pain after surgery, as compared to 96% before surgery, and 61% had complete resolution of their pain. The average follow-up in this study was 10 months.

In one of the few prospective studies in the literature, Siegal and Siegal (43) compared anterior decompression and stabilization in patients with tumor anterior to the cord, laminectomy for patients with tumor entirely posterior to the cord, and radiotherapy alone. Only 30% of the patients treated with radiation alone regained the ability to ambulate, as compared to 40% of the patients with laminectomy and 80% of the anteriorly decompressed patients.

Despite these studies, posterior decompression may still have a role in revision tumor surgery. If metastases involve more than two adjacent levels, with extensive posterior epidural spread, anterior decompression may be nearly impossible. In such a situation, along with cases of instability without significant neurologic compromise, posterior decompression with segmental fixation offers the best surgical option (26). Galasko (56) reported 55 patients who underwent posterior decompression and fusion for pain alone or for very mild posterior compression. Complete pain relief was reported for 49 of the patients.

Rompe et al. (38) published a review of 50 patients treated with posterior decompression and segmental fixation with Cotrel-Dubousset instrumentation. More than half of the patients were found to have multiple vertebral metastases that would have required an extensive procedure if addressed anteriorly. The patients in this study had more involved disease than those reported in the previous series: Only 23 of the 50 patients were alive after 12 months, and only 7 were alive at 2 years. However, 45 of the 50 patients experienced significant pain relief after the posterior-only surgery, and 10 of 15 patients improved at least one Frankel grade. Six of eight patients who were unable to ambulate preoperatively were able to walk after surgery.

In both of these series, two cases of instrumentation cutout were reported. In addition, Galasko (56) reported two cases of rod breakage. Heller and Zdeblick (19) addressed the question raised by these studies and the criticism of several authors who have questioned the strength of posterior-only instrumentation as compared to anterior instrumentation. They used a calf model to mimic spinal instrumentation for metastatic disease (19). They reasoned that, because 85% of spinal metastases occur in the body, a partial anterior vertebrectomy model would mimic the tumor situation. Subsequently, the specimens were fixed either anteriorly or posteriorly to compare the ability of anterior and posterior instrumentation to reliably restore and stabilize the spine with weakened anterior structures. They found that, unless anterior instrumentation (a Harms cage and anterior Texas Scottish Rite Hospital instrumentation in this study) was used alone or in combination with posterior instrumentation, axial, sagittal, and torsional stiffness could not be restored.

Thus, anterior decompression and fusion are favored by many authors for lesions that are located anterior to the dura. However, some patients may not be able to withstand the physical stress associated with an anterior procedure. In such cases, a posterolateral approach for decompression has been combined with posterior fusion. Sheth et al. (41) described four patients with anterior vertebral metastases who

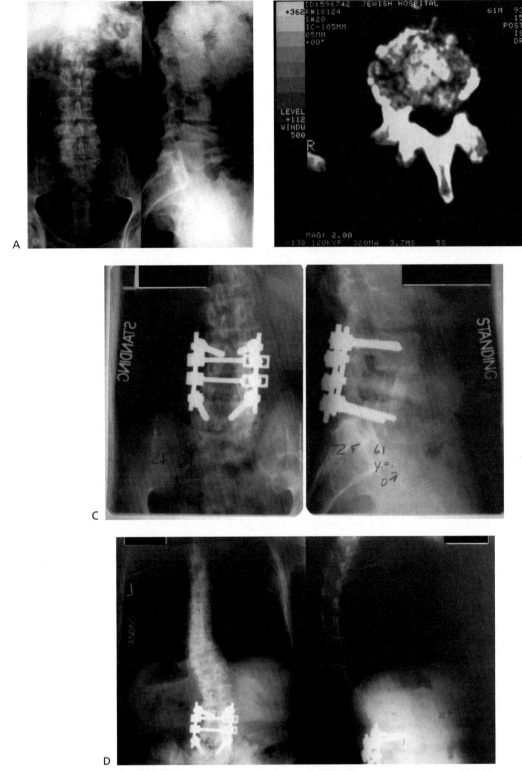

FIGURE 3. Course and treatment of a 61-year-old man who presented with a history of low back pain 3 years after an L4-5 diskectomy. Plain x-ray **(A)** demonstrates destruction and collapse at the level of the L-4 vertebral body. Postmyelographic computed tomography (CT) scan **(B)** demonstrates destruction of the vertebral body, suggestive of underlying tumor. Initial staging studies were negative, and the patient underwent an anterior vertebral body resection with fibular strut grafting and posterior pedicle screw stabilization from L-3 to L-5 **(C)**. Pathologic studies revealed the lesion to be metastatic thyroid carcinoma. Over the next 4 years, the patient was successfully managed with a combination of chemotherapy and radiotherapy. He then presented with progressive mechanical back pain and kyphosis despite bracing and radiation **(D)**. (*continued*)

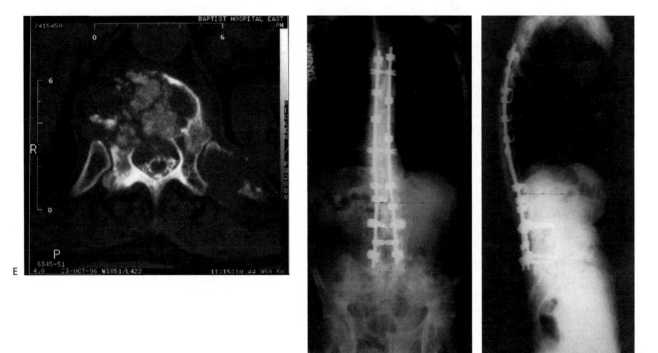

FIGURE 3. (*continued*) Postmyelographic CT scan demonstrates destruction of the vertebral body at T-12 **(E)**. Palliative management at this point required extension of the fusion to the thoracic spine **(F)**.

underwent "total or almost total" vertebral resection. Immediate stabilization was performed using methylmethacrylate anteriorly and instrumentation posteriorly (41). Unfortunately, follow-up was not reported in this series.

In a larger series, Bridwell et al. (4) reported on 25 patients who underwent a similar procedure. Part of this study group included patients with multilevel disease, cases in which an anterior decompression and fusion is not an ideal option (4). The difference between this study and the report of Sheth et al. was that no reconstruction was performed anteriorly. Nineteen of the 25 patients experienced significant pain relief, but the remaining six had a tumor that was inaccessible by this approach, and they continued to be symptomatic. Five patients required revision secondary to instrumentation failure, perhaps reflecting the biomechanical instability due to lack of anterior reconstruction, as had been pointed out in the *in vitro* study by Heller and Zdeblick (19).

patients surviving long enough to undergo tumor surgery of the spine, but many patients also have a prognosis that is good enough to warrant revision spine surgery.

A revision situation can be encountered in the context of prior radiation, chemotherapy, or surgery. Prior radiation and chemotherapy significantly affect wound healing and dictate not only certain changes in surgical technique but also the time frame of the revision surgery. Prior surgical intervention can affect the imaging capabilities of the spine as well as the approach and fixation used for the revision surgery.

The goal of spine surgery for metastatic disease is not usually cure but rather to improve quality of life. If the prognosis warrants intervention, and if the patient is able to tolerate a second procedure, imaging, approach selection, resection, and multisegmental fixation to healthy bone should be carried out as discussed in this chapter.

CONCLUSION

As our patient population ages, we are seeing an increase in patients with metastatic disease of the spine. In addition, with improvements in surgical and radiotherapy techniques and the development of more potent chemotherapeutic agents, not only are

REFERENCES

1. Bernstein EF, Salomon GD, Harisiadis L, et al. Collagen gene expression and wound tensile strength in normal and radiation-impaired wounds. *J Dermatol Surg Oncol* 1993;19(6):564–570.
2. Bhalla SK. Metastatic disease of the spine. *CORR* 1970; 73:52–60.

3. Takakura K. *Metastatic tumors of the central nervous system.* New York: Igaku-Shoin, 1982.

4. Bridwell KH, Jenny AB, Saul T. Posterior segmental spinal instrumentation with posterolateral decompression and debulking for metastatic thoracic and lumbar spine disease. *Spine* 1988;1383–1394.

5. Bridwell KH, DeWald RL, eds. *The textbook of spinal surgery.* Philadelphia: JB Lippincott Co, 1991.

6. Boland PJ, Lane JM, Sundaresan N. Metastatic disease of the spine. *CORR* 1982;169:95–102.

7. Borg SA, Rubin P, DeWys VVD. Metastases and disseminated disease. In: Rubin P, ed. *Clinical oncology for medical students and physicians—a multidisciplinary approach,* 6th ed. New York: American Cancer Society, 1983:498–499.

8. Bujko K, Suit HD, Springfield DS, et al. Wound healing after pre-operative radiation for sarcomas of soft tissues. *Surg Gynecol Obstet* 1993;176(2):124–134.

9. Deckey JE, Mahmud F, Weidenbaum MA. Metastatic tumors of the spine. In Haher TR, ed. *State of the Art Reviews* 1996;10(3):455–465.

10. Dolin MG. Acute massive dural compression secondary to methylmethacrylate replacement of a tumorous lumbar vertebral body. *Spine* 1989;14:108–110.

11. Drake BD, Scott NO. Wound healing considerations in chemotherapy and radiation therapy. *Clin Plast Surg* 1995;22:31–37.

12. El-Tamer MB, Chaglassian T. Wound management in spinal surgery. In: Sundaresan N, Schmidek HH, Schiller AL, et al., eds. *Tumors of the spine: diagnosis and clinical management.* Philadelphia: WB Saunders, 1990:86–91.

13. Findlay GF. Adverse effects of the management of malignant spinal cord compression. *J Neurol Neurosurg Psychiatry* 1984;47:761–768.

14. Gilbert RW, Kim JH, Posner JB. Epidural spinal cord compression from metastatic tumor: diagnosis and treatment. *Ann Neurol* 1978;3:40–51.

15. Harrington KD. Management of unstable pathologic fractures—dislocations of the spine and acetabulum secondary to metastatic malignancy. *Inst Course Lect* 1980;24:51–61.

16. Harrington KD. Anterior decompression and stabilization of the spine as a treatment of vertebral collapse and spinal cord compression from metastatic malignancy. *Clin Orthop* 1988;233:177–197.

17. Harrington KD. Metastatic disease of the spine. *J Bone Joint Surg Am* 1986;68A:1110–1115.

18. Heller JG, Pedlow FX. Tumors of the spine. In: Garfin SR, Vaccaro AR, eds. *Orthopaedic knowledge update: spine.* Chicago: AAOS, 1997:235–256.

19. Heller JG, Zdeblick A, Kunz DA, et al. Spinal instrumentation for metastatic disease: in vitro biomechanical analysis. *J Spinal Disord* 1993;6:17–22.

20. Hillmann A, Ozaki T, Rube C, et al. Surgical complications after preoperative irradiation of Ewing's sarcoma. *J Cancer Res Clin Oncol* 1997;123(1):57–62.

21. Hom DB, Assefa G, Song CW. Endothelial cell growth factor (ECDGF) application to irradiated soft tissue. *Laryngoscope* 1993;103(2):165–170.

22. Hopewell JW, Calvo W, Jaenke R, et al. Microvasculature and radiation damage. *Recent Results Cancer Res* 1993;130:1–16.

23. Jaffe HL. Tumors metastatic to the skeleton. In: Jaffe HL, ed. *Tumors and tumorous conditions of the bones and joints.* Philadelphia: Lea & Febiger, 1959:589–618.

24. Kane WJ, McCafferey TV, Wang TD, et al. The effect of tissue expansion on the random flap viability and wound tensile strength of previously irradiated rabbit. *Skin Arch Otor* 1993:119(4):417–422.

25. Kolb BA, Buller RE, Connor JP, et al. Effects of early postoperative chemotherapy on wound healing. *Obstet Gynecol* 1992;79:988–992.

26. Kostiuk JP, Weinstein JN. Differential diagnosis and surgical treatment of metastatic spine tumors. In: Frymoyer JW, ed. *The adult spine: principles and practice.* New York: Raven Press, 1991:861–888.

27. Kostiuk JP, Errico TJ, Gleason TF, et al. Spinal stabilization of vertebral column tumors. *Spine* 1988;13:250–256.

28. Mandelbaum BR, Tolo VT, McAfee PC, et al. Nutritional deficiencies after staged anterior and posterior spinal reconstructive surgery. *CORR* 1988;234:5–11.

29. Marino H. Biologic excision. *Plast Reconstr Surg* 1967; 40:180.

30. Mast BA. The skin. In: Cohen K, Diegelmann RF, Linblad WJ, eds. *Wound healing: biochemical and clinical aspects.* Philadelphia: WB Saunders, 1992:37.

31. Matsui H, Tatezaki S, Tsuji H. Ceramic vertebral body replacement for metastatic spine tumors. *J Spinal Disord* 1994;7:248–254.

32. McAfee PC, Bohlman HH, Ducker T, et al. Failure of stabilization of the spine with methylmethacrylate. *J Bone Joint Surg Am* 1986;68A:1145–1157.

33. Nall AV, Brownlee RE, Colvin CP, et al. Transforming growth factor beta 1 improves wound healing and random flap survival in normal and irradiated rats. *Arch Otolaryngol Head Neck Surg* 1996;122(2):171–177.

34. Ono K, Yonenobu K, Ebara S, et al. Prosthetic replacement surgery for cervical spine metastasis. *Spine* 1988; 817–822.

35. Paonessa KJ, Hostnik WJ, Zide BM. Use of tissue expanders for wound closure of spinal infections or dehiscence. *Orthop Clin* 1996;27(1):155–170.

36. Panjabi MM, Hopper W, White AA, et al. Posterior spinal stabilization with methylmethacrylate. *Spine* 1977; (2):241–247.

37. Randall K, Coggle JE. Expression of TGFB I in mouse skin during the acute phase of radiation damage. *Int J Radiat Biol* 1995;68(3):301–309.

38. Rompe JD, Eysel P, Hopf C, et al. Decompression/stabilization of the metastatic spine. *Acta Orthop Scand* 1993;64:3–8.

39. Rompe JD, Eysel P, Hopf CH, et al. Metastatic spinal cord compression—options for surgical treatment. *Acta Neurochir* 1993;123:135–140.

40. Reference deleted.

41. Sheth D, Albuqurque K, Suraiya JN. Circumdural decompression by posterior vertebrectomy for relief

of cord compression due to metastatic disease of tho-racic and lumbar spine. *Ind J Cancer* 1992;29:43–48.

42. Siegal Tiqva P, Siegal T. Vertebral body resection for epidural compression by malignant tumors. *J Bone Joint Surg Am* 1985;67-A:375–381.

43. Siegal T, Siegal T. Surgical decompression of anterior and posterior malignant epidural tumors compressing the spinal cord. *Neurosurgery* 1985;17:424–430.

44. Silverberg E. Cancer statistics. *CA Cancer J Clin* 1984; 34:7–23.

45. Suit HD, Austin-Seymour M. The role of radiation therapy. In: Sundaresan N, Schmidek HH, Schiller AL, et al., eds. *Tumors of the spine: diagnosis and clini-cal management.* Philadelphia: WB Saunders, 1990: 86–91.

46. Sundaresan N, Krol G, Digiacinto GV, et al. Metastatic tumors of the spine. In: Sundaresan N, Schmidek HH, Schiller AL, et al., eds. *Tumors of the spine: diagnosis and clinical management.* Philadelphia: WB Saunders, 1990: 279–304.

47. Sundaresan N, Rosenthal DI, Schiller AL, et al. Postra-diation sarcomas involving the spine. In: Sundaresan N, Schmidek HH, Schiller AL, et al., eds. *Tumors of the spine: diagnosis and clinical management.* Philadelphia: WB Saunders, 1990:240–244.

48. Stambough JL, Beringer D. Postoperative wound infec-tions complicating adult spine surgery. *J Spinal Disord* 1992;5:277–285.

49. Telok HA, Mason NIL, Wheelock MD. Histopathol-ogy study of radiation injuries of the skin. *Surg Gynecol Obstet* 1950;90:335.

50. Tokuhashi Y, Matsuzaki H, Toriyama S, et al. Scoring system for the preoperative evaluation of metastatic spine tumor prognosis. *Spine* 1990;15:1110–1113.

51. Reference deleted.

52. Vegesna V, McBride WFL, Withers HR. Postoperative irradiation impairs or enhances wound strength depend-ing on time of administration. *Radiat Res* 1995;143(2): 224–228.

53. Weinstein JN, McLain RF. Primary tumors of the spine. *Spine* 1987;12:843–851.

53a. Dreghorn CR, Newman RJ, Hardy GJ, et al. Primary tumors of the axial skeleton. Experience of the Leeds Regional Bone Tumor Registry. *Spine* 1990;15:137–140.

54. Whitehall R, Reger LI, Fox E, et al. The use of methyl-methacrylate cement as an instantaneous fusion mass in posterior cervical fusions. *Spine* 1984;9:246–255.

55. Young RF, Post EM, King GA. Treatment of spinal epi-dural metastasis. Randomized prospective comparison of laminectomy and radiotherapy. *J Neurosurg* 1980;53: 741–748.

56. Galasko CSB. Spinal instability secondary to metastatic cancer. *J Bone Joint Surg Br* 1991;73:104–108.

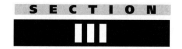

LUMBAR SPINE

13

LUMBAR SPINE: EVALUATION

MICHAEL E. GOLDSMITH, WILLIAM C. LAUERMAN, AND GUNNAR B.J. ANDERSSON

One of the most challenging problems for the spine surgeon is the patient with persistent or recurrent pain after low back surgery. Surgeons in the United States perform approximately 300,000 laminectomies and 70,000 spinal fusions per year. With these numbers on the rise, the patient with failed low back surgery represents a dilemma that will become increasingly common, requiring an organized approach to diagnosis and treatment (42).

Currently, approximately 15% of patients undergoing initial low back operations fail to achieve adequate relief from surgery, helping to generate an increasing number of revision spine surgeries each year. Although 85% of patients improve with the initial operation, only 50% find relief with their second operation, and the odds of improvement continue to drop off with each successive surgery (14). These percentages impart the importance of preventing an unnecessary operation. To improve the results, a logical approach to the failed low back patient must be undertaken. Each evaluation must begin with a thorough history and physical examination and then proceed with a medical evaluation as needed. Imaging studies are performed as indicated, and strict surgical indications must be adhered to in the hope of obtaining good results.

In the initial evaluation of a failed back, the physician should be generating a differential diagnosis. Factors leading to failure may be preoperative, intraoperative, or postoperative. Preoperative errors include choosing the wrong patient, arriving at the wrong diagnosis, and evaluating the patient inadequately, all leading to selection of the wrong operation. Intraoperative complications include technical errors, surgery at the wrong level, and inadequate surgery. Postoperative failure can be due to infection, recurrent compression due to disk material or stenosis, arachnoiditis, epidural fibrosis, or instability.

We revisit each of these areas later in this chapter. They are the types of diagnoses that should be entertained during the workup of each patient. The main distinction that should be made is between mechanical and nonmechanical causes for the pain, because

mechanical causes may be amenable to further surgery, whereas other causes usually are not.

HISTORY

Eighty-five percent of most diagnoses in medicine are made because of a thorough history, and nowhere is this more pertinent than in the complicated area of the failed back. A detailed, thorough history is essential in the process of eliciting the cause behind the patient's failed surgery. The answer usually lies with the patient, the operative reports, and the previous surgeon, and the proper questions are the key to obtaining these answers. Typically, a mass of information exists that the surgeon must sort through and organize. Although all of this information can be useful, three particularly important points should be attended to closely.

First, the original presenting complaint of the patient should be sought, specifically attempting to determine the contribution of back and leg pain, including which side was predominantly involved. Investigation of the initial indications for surgery, including old imaging studies and operative reports, can help to determine the appropriateness of the surgery.

Second, the number of operations performed and the perioperative history of each are important predictors of success. After two low back operations, some authors have found that a patient is statistically more likely to be made worse, rather than better, from further surgery (13,43). Although this does not mean that the proper third, fourth, or even fifth operation may not help the proper patient immensely, it underscores the importance of a cautious approach to the patient with a multiply operated back.

Third, the pain-free interval after each surgery should be evaluated. When no pain-free interval exists, especially in the case of a clear-cut herniated nucleus pulposus (HNP) with proper indications, inadequate surgery is usually the case. In a patient with initial improvement that lasts for less than 6 months, and if the workup does not demonstrate instability, the physician should begin to think about infection, fibrosis, or medical causes. In a patient who has more than 6 months of relief, a recurrent HNP at the same (similar pain pattern) or different (different pain pattern) level may be the cause (46).

In addition, the relative contribution of back pain and leg pain is an important factor, as it helps to place a patient into certain diagnostic categories. Back pain following failed back surgery can emanate from instability, scar tissue, tumor, or infection. In addition, a postoperative patient may have back pain similar to that of patients with no history of surgery due to muscle spasm, ligament or tendon strain, facet joint arthritis, or no obvious cause. Leg pain, on the other hand, indicates other pathology that is usually consistent with nerve root compression, typically disk herniation or stenosis.

Finally, the nature of the pain can indicate the type of pathology. Unremitting pain suggests neuropathic causes or scarring due to fibrosis or arachnoiditis. Intermittent pain is usually consistent with mechanical causes, especially when it is associated with provocative tests or positions that worsen the pain and palliative maneuvers that alleviate the pain. Spinal claudication can present with pain that begins with activity and abates with sitting or stooping. Activities involving extension usually exacerbate the pain, whereas flexion alleviates the symptoms.

Spinal claudication should be differentiated from vascular insufficiency when severe leg pain exists after walking a short distance. In the case of spinal claudication, patients need to sit or bend forward when they stop. In contrast, patients with vascular claudication achieve quick relief in the standing position. Patients with spinal stenosis also have a positive "grocery cart" sign in which they have no difficulty walking in the grocery store because they lean over the cart and obtain relief. These same patients, however, are not able to walk shorter distances without the cart, such as walking in a mall.

PHYSICAL EXAMINATION

The physical examination in a failed back patient should begin in a fashion similar to that for any patient with back pain. Special attention should be paid to neurologic differences from before surgery and any changes from previous postoperative visits. A pattern of neurologic involvement, which is consistent with findings on imaging studies, is highly suggestive of a mechanical problem that can be successfully treated with surgery. A neurologic deficit is usually only significant if it is a finding that was either not present before surgery or had resolved in the postoperative period and is now new or recurrent. A prior footdrop that did not resolve after a laminectomy is, therefore, not a significant finding.

Tension signs such as the straight-leg raise test (for lesions affecting the L-5 and S-1 nerve roots) and the femoral nerve stretch test (L-3 and L-4 nerve roots) should be elicited, although they are not as sensitive an indicator of radiculopathy and disk herniation in the failed back patient. The classic straight-leg raise, Lasègue's sign, is more likely to be positive in the younger patient. The leg must be raised between 30 and 75 degrees. In addition, the crossed straight-leg raise, the crossed Lasègue's, should be elicited by raising the contralateral limb and eliciting the same pain pattern for which the patient complains. A positive contralateral test with a positive Lasègue's sign indicates a high probability of disk herniation. The femoral nerve stretch test is performed with the patient prone; the knee is flexed and the hip extended. This test implicates an L2-3 or L3-4 disk herniation.

Like all tension signs, Lasègue's sign must reproduce the symptoms for which the patient complains and is not positive with the mere production of back pain. Inorganic signs of pain such as a nonanatomic distribution of signs or symptoms or distraction findings have been suggestive of a poor prognosis in repeat spine surgery. Waddell (42) has described a number of functional or nonorganic signs that should be elicited. He showed that the presence of three of five of the following signs indicated a high surgical failure rate: simulation, distraction, skin tenderness, overreaction to stimuli, and regional disturbances (44).

Additional tests should be performed and include Mannkopf's sign, in which deep palpation of a truly painful area raises the pulse, and the flexed hip examination, in which the patient is supine with the examiner's hand under the knee and spine; the knee is raised, and if pain occurs in the back before the knee moves, the pain is not organic. Finally, it should be noted that epidural and perineural fibrosis can cause a positive tension sign in the previously operated low back patient.

Provocative tests should be elicited in the physical examination as well. Range of motion of the back is important to assess. When leg pain is exacerbated by extension of the spine, stenosis may be present because of narrowing due to extension. In the case of HNP, forward flexion of the spine typically provokes leg pain. Finally, segmental instability can be painful in flexion and extension, and a characteristic reversal of normal spinal rhythm in returning from forward flexion may be seen (26).

A detailed neurologic examination is essential in identifying the cause of recurrent low back pain or radicular pain and does not differ from the examination of a patient with the new onset of symptoms. One should always keep in mind the specific findings for each nerve root level. For the L-4 root, the specific muscles are the tibialis anterior and the quadriceps, the reflex is the patellar tendon, and sensation is over the posterolateral aspect of the thigh, below the patella and on the anteromedial aspect of the leg. Extension of the knee may be weak, with quadriceps atrophy.

For the L-5 root, the specific muscles that should be tested are the extensor hallucis longus, the long toe extensions, and the gluteus medius; the sensory distribution is over the posterior aspect of the thigh, the anterolateral leg, and the dorsum of the foot. A Trendelenburg sign may be present, or dorsiflexion of the toes and foot may be weak, and the anterior compartment may demonstrate atrophy. No reflex is specific for L-5.

For the S-1 nerve root, the specific muscle that should be tested is the peroneus longus and brevis, the specific reflex is the Achilles, and sensory distribution is over the posterior thigh, posterior leg, and lateral aspect of the foot and toes. In addition, weakness may exist in plantar flexion of the foot and toes, and atrophy may be seen in the posterior compartment. An important part of the routine examination, in addition to observing normal gait, is observing the patient when attempting to walk on heels and tiptoes; difficulty with heel or toe walking can be a subtle sign of weakness that is not otherwise elicited on manual motor testing.

IMAGING

Previous imaging studies should be reviewed and compared. Before studies are ordered in the failed back patient, a solid differential diagnosis needs to exist, with a highly probable diagnosis being entertained before the study. As with patients without a history of surgery, virtually all imaging studies of the lumbar spine have a high rate of false positives that can lead to improper diagnoses unless the studies are obtained to confirm a clinical diagnosis based on history and physical examination.

X-Ray

The initial study should be plain films that help delineate the extent of the laminectomy defect, the level of

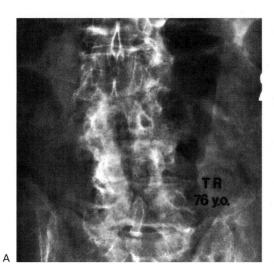

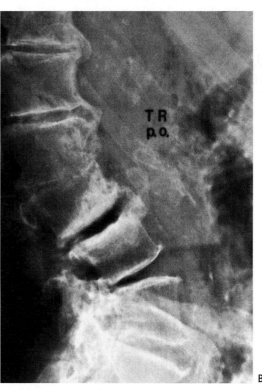

FIGURE 1. Standing anteroposterior (AP) **(A)** and lateral **(B)** radiograph of a 76-year-old man with intractable back pain and difficulty standing erect 1 year after a decompressive laminectomy, with evidence of collapse on the AP and lateral views. The vacuum disks at L3-4 and L4-5 (Knuttson's sign) are suggestive of instability.

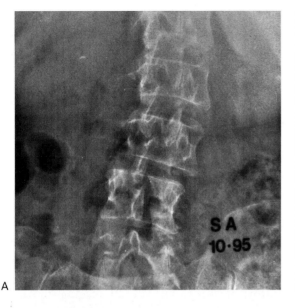

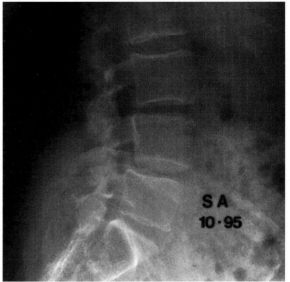

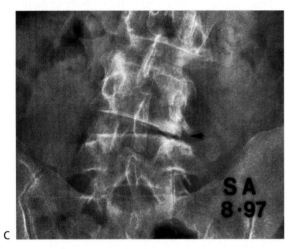

FIGURE 2. Standing anteroposterior (AP) **(A)** and lateral **(B)** radiograph of a 69-year old woman following a right L4-5 hemilaminectomy with no improvement in her right leg pain. **C:** Her AP radiograph following a second right-sided decompression. Excessive resection of the pars can be appreciated, along with increased localized collapse into scoliosis. Foraminal stenosis can be diagnosed based on the plain x-ray.

the previous operation, spinal deformity or collapse (Fig. 1), abnormal anatomy, and instability on flexion and extension films. Films should be weight bearing and should be closely scrutinized to assure that the correct level was decompressed; then they should be systematically examined in the same fashion as all spine films. Spinal alignment should be assessed for scoliosis, which can be idiopathic or degenerative. Postsurgical scoliosis in the adult patient can result in a deformity that causes neural impingement or may be evidence, in and of itself, of instability (Fig. 2). The films should be reviewed for any evidence of isthmic (commonly L-5 to S-1) or degenerative (L4-5) spondylolisthesis. Postsurgical spondylolistheses can occur at any level secondary to an excessive laminectomy, facet resection, or postoperative fracture of the pars.

Flexion and extension lateral radiographs may detect segmental instability, which is suggested by 4 mm or more of slippage, 15% translation, or 20% or more of angulation (25% at L-5 to S-1). Spondylolis-

thesis on x-ray may not always explain the patient's symptoms, although a significantly higher incidence of abnormal spinal motion patterns has been shown to be present in patients with continued symptoms after surgery (29).

Prior fusion should be assessed (Fig. 3). Lateral radiographs can usually demonstrate a successful interbody fusion by noting the continuity of bone between the outer margin of the adjacent vertebral bodies (3). Posterior fusion masses can be more difficult to delineate because overlying structures can obscure the fusion mass on anteroposterior and on lateral views. Further support for the diagnosis of pseudarthrosis, seen on plain films, includes hardware failure such as pullout of a screw, bony erosion (halo effect) around a screw, or breakage of a rod, plate, or screw. The actual correlation of plain films with surgical findings is on the order of 65% to 70%; plain radiographs can be as specific as 90% to 95% in demonstrating that a fusion is solid, but

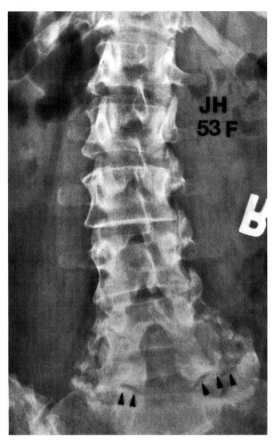

FIGURE 3. Supine anteroposterior radiograph of a 53-year-old woman 1 year after decompression and fusion. A cleft extending through both sides of the fusion mass (*arrowheads*) is seen, suggesting pseudarthrosis. However, the patient had excellent relief of her back and leg pain and was therefore treated with observation.

their sensitivity in detecting a pseudarthrosis has been reported to be as low as 37% to 60% (6). These numbers highlight the important point that x-ray findings need to be correlated with the examination to make them significant and that further studies should be entertained when clinical suspicion is high. The authors routinely use dynamic lateral radiographs in surgical decision making when considering reoperation for nonunion; unless motion can be demonstrated, surgery is less likely to result in successful pain relief.

Computed Tomography

After failure of an appropriate course of conservative management, more expensive or invasive studies should be considered based on the working diagnosis. Although many of its uses have been supplanted by magnetic resonance imaging (MRI), computed tomography (CT) scanning is an excellent study for the evaluation of spinal stenosis, spinal instrumentation, and postoperative fusion masses. In patients for

whom an MRI is contraindicated secondary to pacemakers, claustrophobia, or other reasons, CT, particularly following myelography, is still efficacious in evaluating disk herniation, facet arthrosis, arachnoiditis, epidural fibrosis, infection, dural tears, and epidural hematomas.

In the evaluation of central spinal and intervertebral foraminal stenosis, multiplanar CT scan provides a great amount of information and continues to be favored by some as the diagnostic test of choice. Newer CT scans are very sensitive in detecting facet degenerative changes, hypertrophy, and spurring. Central stenosis can be seen with anteromedial spurs projecting off the facet joints. Lateral recess stenosis can also be detected as anteroposterior narrowing of the subarticular groove.

The evaluation of lateral foraminal stenosis is facilitated by sagittal reconstruction in addition to the axial images and can help to identify three types of stenoses: up-down (cephalocaudad), front-back (anteroposterior), and pinhole (combined) (37). These reformatted images can be integral in preoperative planning for surgical approaches. The images can also be reconstructed in a three-dimensional fashion, which can present a topographic map that defines the position, extent, and morphologic features in one clear image. The drawback is that any error is magnified and any missed finding between cuts remains absent.

CT scanning is also useful in evaluating postoperative hardware placement (Fig. 4). After pedicle screw placement, postoperative CT can accurately detect intraspinal or neural encroachment by a misplaced

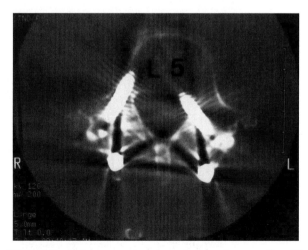

FIGURE 4. Axial computed tomography image of a 67-year-old woman approximately 2 weeks after revision fusion with transpedicular instrumentation. In the hospital she had no significant leg pain but, at the first follow-up visit, complained of severe pain down the left leg with weakness. Intrusion of the left L-5 screw into the lateral recess is seen.

screw. Reports of the accuracy of CT scanning in detecting misplaced screws range from 68% for cobalt chrome screws to 87% for titanium screws (49). It should be noted, however, that as many as 20% to 25% of patients have asymptomatic misplacement after transpedicular instrumentation and, therefore, careful correlation of postoperative symptoms to CT findings is essential (15). Displacement of hardware is also optimally visualized by CT, and strut displacement or strut fracture can also be assessed.

Multiplanar CT scans aid in detecting the status of the fusion mass. Gaps in the fusion or pseudarthrosis can be detected, and fusion overgrowth or fragmentation can also be seen. In addition to close evaluation of the fusion, the first motion segment above or below the fusion mass should be closely investigated because of the increased incidence of spinal degeneration in these adjacent motion segments (25).

Myelography

Plain myelography lacks a high degree of specificity as an isolated study, especially in the postoperative period, and is of limited value in the multiply operated patient because of its inability to differentiate mechanical nerve root compression from epidural scar (22). It is also unable to visualize root entrapment beyond the nerve root sheath and cannot detect lateral or foraminal disk herniations and ste-

nosis. Because missed lateral spinal stenosis is a leading cause of failed back surgery, myelography is as ineffective postoperatively as it is preoperatively. Moreover, CT and MRI have supplanted plain myelography because of superior diagnostic accuracy with less downside: Myelography is invasive and exposes the patient to more radiation than either plain films or CT.

The current indications are few for plain myelography; the diagnosis of arachnoiditis can be confirmed in cases in which MRI is nondiagnostic or in patients with hardware in place (Fig. 5). In addition, in patients with multiple segmental instability or multilevel central stenosis, myelographic depiction of the longitudinal dimension of the canal can be helpful (9,16). Finally, the dynamic aspect of myelography with flexion and extension views can depict the presence and extent of dynamic stenosis in patients with instability.

Although myelography has limited utility alone, when combined with CT the two modalities can be very useful in the multiply operated low back patient. CT myelography (CTM) images are more reliable than plain CT in assessing nerve root and thecal sac compression or arachnoiditis (8,41). Lateral processes are demonstrated very well, including lateral disk herniation, lateral foraminal stenosis, and lateral recess stenosis (25). CTM can be very valuable in demonstrating arachnoiditis, as chronic

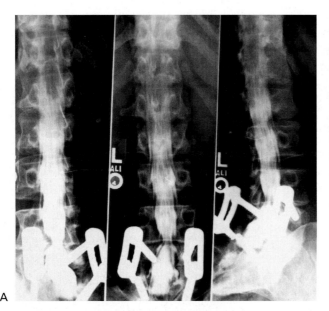 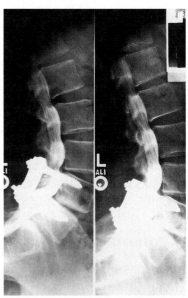

FIGURE 5. Myelogram of a 39-year-old woman 2 years after fusion and instrumentation for degenerative spondylolisthesis. After a pain-free interval of 1 year, the patient complains of back and left leg pain. Magnetic resonance imaging was nondiagnostic secondary to scatter from retained hardware. Computed tomography did not lend significant information. **A:** Myelogram demonstrates a decreased dye flow above the previous fusion at L3-4 centrally and peripherally, consistent with stenosis. **B:** The lateral view demonstrates a retrolisthesis at L3-4 with thecal sac tenting over this area.

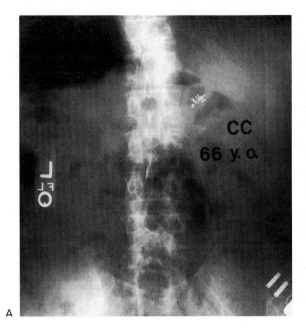

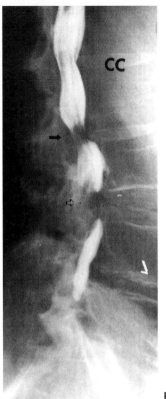

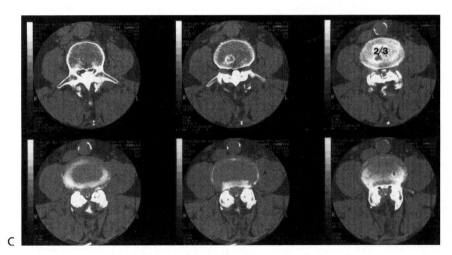

FIGURE 6. A: Anteroposterior radiograph of a 66-year-old man who has had four prior operations, including a posterior fusion from L-3 to S-1, laminectomy at L-3, and placement of a spinal cord stimulator for chronic intractable pain. Magnetic resonance imaging was difficult to interpret below the previous fusion as well as at the next most proximal level. **B:** Myelography demonstrates stenosis at L2-3 (*arrow*) and findings of arachnoiditis at L3-4 (*open arrow*) distal to the stenosis. **C:** Postmyelography computed tomography shows stenosis at L2-3.

inflammatory tissue leads to abnormal clumping, either centrally or peripherally, of the intrathecal nerve roots (Fig. 6).

Magnetic Resonance

MRI is an excellent study to image the low back for radicular and nonradicular pathology (34). MRI is preferable to myelography in that it is noninvasive and is preferable to CT in that it produces no ionizing radiation. In addition, it provides orthogonal views of the spine and directly images neural structures. In nonenhanced studies, the regions of cortical bone and vertebral endplates have a decreased signal intensity on T1- and T2-weighted images. On T1-weighted images, the central portion of the disk has a slightly decreased signal intensity compared with the peripheral portion. The appearance is similar on T2, although the intensities are reversed. Cortical bone is low in intensity, whereas cancellous bone is of high intensity because of the marrow fat.

Three types of signal changes have been described by Ross and Modic (34) in the degenerative spine. Type I changes show decreased T1 intensity and increased T2 intensity in the disk. Histologically, type I changes reflect disruption and fissuring of the endplate and vascularized fibrous tissue within the marrow. Type I changes are indicative of a subacute process. They can look similar to infection, although the intervertebral disk typically shows abnormally high signal intensity on T2 with infection. Type II changes have strong T1 and T2 images. Histologically, type II changes reflect yellow marrow replacement in the vertebral body. Finally, type III changes show decreased intensity on T1 and on T2. This change reflects the relative absence of marrow in the vertebral bodies and correlates with bony sclerosis on plain films (36). One important point to remember is that T2 images are the most sensitive for finding degenerative changes in the disk and decreased intensity due to a loss of hydration.

A herniated disk on MRI is denoted by a smooth focal extension of the disk beyond the margin of the vertebral endplate. The T1 signal intensity of the herniation is usually similar to that of the parent disk. With larger herniations, the T2 image is generally intense, whereas in smaller herniations it is hypointense. Clinical examination must always be correlated to MRI findings to improve the clinical utility of the study. Boden et al. (4) demonstrated HNP by MRI in 20% of asymptomatic patients younger than 60 years of age, and 50% of asymptomatic patients older than 60 years of age had an abnormal MRI, indicating either HNP or spinal stenosis.

In the postoperative period, routine MRI can sometimes be difficult to interpret because confusion can exist over normal postoperative changes versus pathology. Therefore, enhancement with gadolinium–diethylenetriamine pentaacetic acid (Gd-DTPA) is used to improve imaging in the postoperative period. After the application of Gd-DTPA, enhancement can be expected in the epidural venous plexus and the ventral and dorsal nerve root ganglia. The normal cord, nerve roots, and intervertebral disk do not enhance unless certain pathologic changes have occurred. MRI with Gd-DTPA enhancement has been shown to be highly accurate in differentiating recurrent disk herniation from postoperative scar after 6 months following surgery. Epidural scar tissue shows characteristic findings on MRI; early images demonstrate enhancement secondary to the abundant vascularity that persists for 45 minutes.

In recurrent disk herniations, on the other hand, only a thin rim of enhancement occurs, which outlines the granulation tissue surrounding the avascular disk (18,36) (Fig. 7). The Gd enhancement lights up scar tissue because of its vascularity, whereas a recurrent herniated disk does not enhance because it is avascular. Furthermore, HNP is wrapped in scar and may enhance on delayed studies secondary to diffusion of contrast from adjacent scar tissue (35). Gd-DTPA–enhanced MRI has been demonstrated to have a 96% correlation with surgery in its ability to distinguish epidural fibrosis from disk material (21). Enhanced MRI is also useful in the diagnosis of spinal stenosis, infection, and arachnoiditis (4,5).

Within the first 6 months following surgery, Gd MRI can reveal pathologic changes despite a lack of symptoms (35). In the immediate postoperative period, a residual mass effect on the neural elements

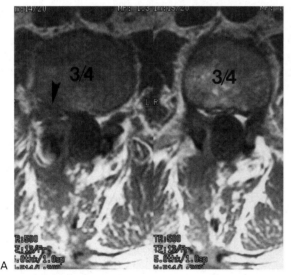 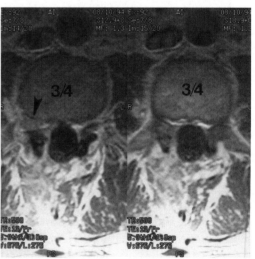

FIGURE 7. A 72-year-old man who, 6 months before this study, underwent his third operation for right anterior thigh pain. Postoperatively, he was no better. **A:** Axial magnetic resonance images, before gadolinium injection, demonstrating a soft tissue mass in the right L3-4 foramen (*arrow*). **B:** After the injection of gadolinium, enhancement is seen only around the rim of the mass, typical of a recurrent disk herniation. Reoperation and diskectomy resulted in complete relief of the patient's thigh pain.

simulates pathology. Care must therefore be shown in relying on this study in the early postoperative period. Boden et al. (5) showed abnormal MRI findings in 6 of 15 asymptomatic postoperative patients that gradually resolved over a period of 6 months.

Nuclear Studies

Bone scanning has a limited role in the postoperative back patient. Scintigraphy uses radiation emitted from injected chemicals to detect pathology through a disturbance in vascularity or osteogenesis. This study has a low specificity; therefore, it is vital to use the information in conjunction with a thorough history and physical examination, as well as other diagnostic modalities. Bone scans can locate an area of suspected pathology, but usually without much ability to differentiate between pathologic entities. The lesion must be metabolically active to be detected, although "cold spots" can be identified in areas of avascularity. Three commonly used radionuclides include technetium, indium, and gallium.

Technetium-99 is the most commonly used agent. This scan can be used as a "scout" to screen the entire skeleton for abnormal activity to localize an area in which a process may be occurring or to pinpoint secondary sites of pathology. It is useful in the assessment of possible metastatic processes in which radiographic changes or physical findings lag behind bone activity. Any process that disturbs the normal balance of bone production and reabsorption can produce a finding on technetium bone scan. Although technetium has limited utility in the postoperative spine patient, the study can still find use in identification of a pseudarthrosis following fusion.

Single-photon emission CT (SPECT) scanning is a newer modality, consisting essentially of tomographic images after radionuclide injection. Normal findings after spinal fusion are a uniform increase in radiotracer uptake in the fusion area because of new bone formation. In areas of nonunion or pseudarthroses, radiotracer is increased in focal spots instead of in a diffuse pattern (31). In the symptomatic postoperative spine, the sensitivity and specificity of SPECT scanning have been reported to be 78% and 83%, respectively. Interestingly, in one report, 6 of 11 asymptomatic patients showed areas of focal uptake that were thought to represent painless pseudarthroses (39).

Gallium-67 citrate is a common adjunct to help increase the specificity in the detection of an inflammatory process. This radionuclide has an affinity for neutrophils and thus accumulates in areas of ongoing infection. Also, it is one of the first diagnostic tests to revert to normal with successful treatment. In imaging the spine, it is usually coupled with SPECT scanning for better spatial localization. The drawbacks are the increased radiation dosage compared to technetium and the accumulation of gallium in hepatomas and lymphomas. Indium scans are the most specific bone scan for infection. White blood cells are labeled with the radionuclide that becomes localized in areas of inflammation. The indium-labeled white cells selectively accumulate in areas of infection, as compared to reactive tissue or new bone formation. This study is very sensitive for acute infections, whereas gallium is more helpful for chronic infections. Drawbacks are that the procedure is very lengthy and that the thoracolumbar junction can be difficult to image because of high amounts of accumulation in the liver and spleen. Neither indium nor gallium scanning is as sensitive or specific as MRI in the diagnosis of infection, and MRI has evolved as the imaging modality of choice when evaluating a patient with a suspected spine infection following surgery.

Electrical Studies

Electrodiagnostic studies are part of the diagnostic armamentarium when the physician is attempting to rule out neuropathy, especially in the case of diabetes, myopathy, or neuritis as a cause of radicular pain. If the finding is to be attributed to postsurgical causes, the timing of the study must be carefully considered, because a study performed too early may give false results (1). The electromyographic (EMG) examination assesses primarily the peripheral, rather than the central, nervous system. The examination includes a nerve conduction study (NCV) and a needle electrode examination.

The benefit of the EMG postsurgically varies tremendously, depending primarily on the time elapsed since surgery, the diagnosis, and the examiner in question. During the first 10 to 14 days after operation, the test only reveals an abnormality that existed before surgery, because any changes seen that early are due to a lesion that occurred earlier.

During the early postoperative period, ranging from 3 weeks to 4 months, EMG can detect a previously unsuspected lesion, including a radiculopathy secondary to impingement from a level different from the operative level. It can also demonstrate a plexopathy, a mononeuropathy, or a motor neuron disease. In a patient with weakness postoperatively, a normal motor amplitude after 1 week excludes motor axon loss. Therefore, in a patient with footdrop post-operatively, EMG studies allow early, accurate prognostication. In the case of weakness in the face of normal motor amplitudes, the differential includes neuropraxia, an upper motor neuron lesion, and functional magnification. The main drawback to EMG is that it cannot answer the most vexing of questions: Was the nerve root adequately decompressed? After root compression is relieved, EMG abnormalities often persist. The fibrillation potentials and chronic neurogenic changes in a myotome distribution slowly regress in a proximal to distal direction over many months. Therefore, an EMG performed at 3 months may show no change or improvement, while one done at 6 to 12 months may still be difficult to interpret. However, the more time that has elapsed from the time of surgery, the more likely it is that the EMG abnormalities are being caused by a persistent or new compressive lesion (47).

Diskography

Historically, the three indications for diskography have been to define the morphology of the disk, radiographic views as augmentation for other studies, and provocation of pain to determine if the pattern is the same as that reported by the patient. CT diskography is a newer adjunct that can be helpful in diagnosing subtle abnormalities.

The use of diskography as an adjuvant to define the morphology of the disk radiographically is no longer a useful test. With the availability of superior studies, such as CT or MRI, this diagnostic test is of limited utility for this purpose.

CT diskography appears to be a sensitive and accurate indicator of intradiskal architecture and pathology. High accuracy, greater than 90%, can be achieved in the confirmation of foraminal or extraforaminal lumbar disk herniations, which is higher than with any other modality (22). In a patient who cannot undergo Gd-enhanced MRI or in whom the MRI study is equivocal, CT diskography can also differentiate recurrent lumbar disk herniations from epidural scar tissue.

The use of diskography for identification of the pain generator in patients with low back pain is a much-debated topic. It has been proposed as a diagnostic tool to identify internal disk disruption that may cause low back pain. Proponents believe that if pain is reproduced during injection into the disk, in similar character and distribution to that of which the patient typically complains, the area of pathology has been localized and can therefore be surgically addressed.

In 1968, Holt (19) reported a false-positive rate of 37% on asymptomatic prisoners, and this modality has been highly controversial ever since. Walsh et al. (45) discredited Holt's study, demonstrating a false-positive rate of 0% in normal subjects. Currently, the North American Spine Society follows the Position Statement on Discography offered by the Executive Committee; diskography is indicated in the evaluation of a patient if unremitting spinal pain, with or without extremity pain, is of greater than 4 months' duration and when the pain has been unresponsive to all appropriate methods of conservative therapy. Furthermore, diskography should only be used when a decision has been made that the clinical problem requires surgical treatment (27).

Diskography should not be the sole diagnostic test to decide on surgery in the multiply operated low back patient. If used at all, it needs to be correlated with other studies including MRI. In addition, its greatest use is in a patient with nonradicular low back pain with questionable MRI findings because of the involvement of multiple levels or equivocal MRI findings at a certain level (Fig. 8). Horton and Daftari (20) identified situations in which diskography was useful after MRI in patients with nonradicular low back pain: intermediate patterns on MRI, including speckled, dark, or bulged disks. In these cases, demonstration of a positive pain response by diskography is recommended before proceeding with surgery. In low-probability findings such as a white or flat disk with no cleft, diskography is of low yield. In single level abnormalities with a high probability for a positive provocation test such as a dark or torn disk, these authors also believe that diskography should be avoided because of a high likelihood of superfluous information at a high expense (20).

Selective Nerve Root Infiltration

Finally, selective nerve root infiltration (irritation) has found renewed interest, especially in the area of the multiply operated low back. In a situation in which MRI and CT with or without myelography is inconclusive, nerve root infiltration can be a helpful adjunct to localize a level or to help to determine the importance of findings on other studies in the setting of a confusing clinical picture. This test is a dynamic assessment of the lumbosacral nerve roots carried out under image intensification. The nerve roots are localized and first irritated. The patient determines whether the pain is identical to the pain that he or she typically experiences or is different. Contrast medium is then injected to assure that the

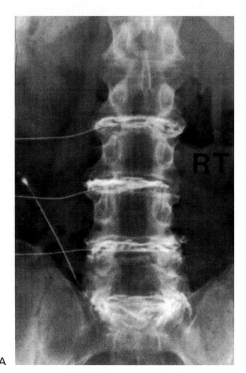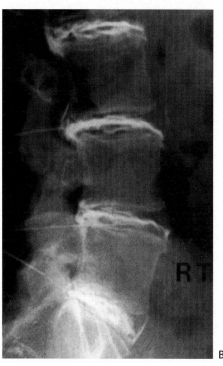

A   B

FIGURE 8. Diskograms of a 53-year-old man with continued back pain after a lumbar laminectomy **(A)** AP and **(B)** lateral. The patient never received relief after decompression. Magnetic resonance imaging revealed dark disk disease at all disk levels below the L-2 vertebral
body. Injections into multiple levels were performed, with reproduction of the same pain at
L4-5 and L-5 to S-1. The levels above did not reproduce the same pattern. The patient
underwent a 360-degree fusion at the involved levels with relief of symptoms.

root is being injected. Finally, if the pain pattern is
identical, lidocaine is injected to assess symptomatic
relief. Dooley and associates have defined four different types of responses: group 1, a single symptomatic
root; group 2, a single level not relieved by injection;
group 3, a single level not reproduced in a typical
pain pattern but with relief following injection; and
group 4, a single level not reproduced in a typical
pain pattern and not relieved by injection. Dooley et
al. (12) showed in their retrospective review of 62
patients that patients with a group 1 response had an
85% accuracy in identifying a single symptomatic
root. Group 2 response patients had findings of multiple root involvement at surgery and benefited from
decompression but did not fare as well as group 1
patients. Finally, group 3 and 4 patients had a poor
response to surgical intervention, with few patients
relieved of radicular pain.

Some of the drawbacks to this diagnostic examination are the dependence of the test on technique and
patient cooperation. Furthermore, nerve root injection does not identify the underlying cause of the
symptomatology and should be used in addition to
other studies, not in their place. If strict criteria are
used, however, and the examination is properly performed, valuable information can result. Stanley et al.

(40), in a prospective analysis of 50 patients, found 1
of 20 false-positive results. This patient fared the
poorest from operative intervention, whereas the
other patients with positive tests all had good outcomes. No patient with negative or equivocal results
underwent an operation (40).

DIFFERENTIAL DIAGNOSIS

The differential diagnosis of a failed back patient can
be approached beginning with the primary complaint:
back pain, leg pain, and extraspinal pain. Many
patients with back pain either have lumbar instability
or diskitis, although the majority of patients with persistent low back pain following surgery have either
diskogenic pain or nonmechanical causes. Leg pain is
usually secondary to an HNP, spinal stenosis, arachnoiditis, or epidural fibrosis. Extraspinal pain can be
caused by an array of afflictions, ranging from visceral
to medical to psychogenic in nature.

Instability

In addition to back pain, the patient with instability
may have deformity and neurologic deficits secon-

dary to the inability of the spine to bear physiologic loads. Three main causes should be sought: preexisting instability due to an unrecognized isthmic or degenerative spondylolisthesis treated by decompression alone; iatrogenic instability due to removal of excessive amounts of the posterior elements, usually greater than 50% of the facet joints; and pseudarthrosis with painful motion at the fusion site (17).

Back pain, especially when arising from a chair or returning from forward bending, is a consistent complaint. Physical examination may demonstrate a reversal of normal spinal rhythm, and tension signs are negative (32). Several radiographic findings may suggest instability, although these must be viewed with caution, because not all patients with instability have back pain. Motion on dynamic lateral radiographs exceeding 4 mm or 15% of translation or 20 degrees of angulation (25 degrees at L-5 to S-1) is widely accepted as diagnostic of instability. Progressive anterolisthesis on a static lateral view or asymmetric collapse, particularly when the concavity of the collapse correlates with the side of leg pain, on a static frontal view may also be evidence of instability. Fusion at the affected level is indicated when instability exists in the setting of unremitting back pain without other obvious causes.

Pseudarthrosis after spine surgery has been reported to occur in 5% to 35% of fusions (33). Patients with instability and pain secondary to a pseudarthrosis may obtain relief from repair, but a clinical and radiographic failure rate of as high as 50% has been reported following nonunion repair (24). Therefore, determining that a pseudarthrosis is the cause of persistent pain following surgery is most difficult, and a very cautious approach to surgery for this indication is recommended. Documenting motion on dynamic radiographs is one way to demonstrate that the ultimate purpose of the fusion, the elimination of motion, has been achieved (Fig. 6). Risk factors for pseudarthrosis are anemia, smoking, gout, excessive postoperative motion, and inadequate decortication (9).

Diskitis

Severe back pain can also be caused by a postoperative disk space infection. After an initial pain-free interval of 2 to 4 weeks, patients present with the spontaneous onset of low-grade fever and back pain that is unremitting, even at rest. Paraspinal muscle spasm causes rigidity, and pain occurs with any motion. A well-healed incision without erythema should not dissuade the physician from the diagnosis of diskitis, as the incision usually heals uneventfully (11). Laboratory workup should include blood cultures, white blood cell count, erythrocyte sedimentation rate, and a C-reactive protein. The erythrocyte sedimentation rate should return to normal by postoperative week six in the uncomplicated patient after spine surgery (2).

Plain radiographs usually do not reveal any change early; late changes demonstrate disk space narrowing and endplate erosions. Gd-enhanced MRI is the test of choice, with disk space enhancement confirming the diagnosis (Fig. 9). Initial treatment should include bed rest, bracing, and antibiotics. Antibiotics can be started empirically and adjusted to the culture results. Failure to respond to these measures within 2 to 3 days warrants a needle biopsy (33). The initial need for biopsy is controversial, but if it is required, CT or fluoroscopically guided biopsy can be safely performed (10,30). Surgery is indicated in cases of sepsis, cauda equina syndrome, or worsening neurologic examination, or in failure of conservative treatment.

Recurrent Herniated Nucleus Pulposus

Leg pain secondary to an HNP can be a new or recurrent herniation or a retained fragment. The history of symptoms is essential in determining the cause. The absence of any pain-free interval suggests a retained fragment, a pain-free interval followed by same-pattern sciatica with a corresponding examination is indicative of a recurrent herniation at the same level, and a new pattern of pain with dissimilar findings on physical examination is consistent with a new herniation at a new level. The presence of a tension sign is critical for operative indications. Gd-enhanced MRI is the test of choice once 6 months have elapsed from the original surgery (5,36).

Stenosis

Back and leg pain can both be significant complaints caused by spinal stenosis in the previously operated patient. The causes of this condition include progression of preexisting degenerative disease, prior inadequate decompression, or overgrowth of a previous posterior fusion causing new stenosis. Depending on the etiology, the pain-free interval is variable. Aside from the history of the pain-free interval, the history and physical examination of the patient with stenosis after failed back surgery is not dissimilar from that seen in a patient with no history of surgery who has stenosis. Leg pain is usually but not always exacerbated by walking and standing and relieved by flexion maneuvers. Tension signs are generally negative, and the static neu-

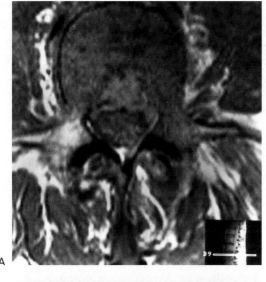

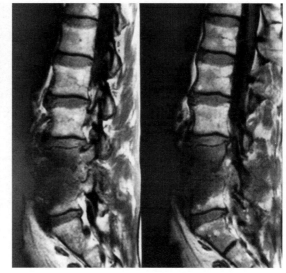

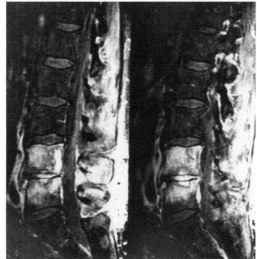

FIGURE 9. Magnetic resonance imaging (MRI) of a 38-year-old man with pain 6 weeks after diskectomy. Initial postoperative MRI was nondiagnostic. At 3 months, an MRI with gadolinium was obtained. **A:** The axial image shows enhancement of disk material centrally and peripherally. Sagittal T1- **(B)** and T2- **(C)** weighted images show enhancement of the disk space and the adjacent vertebral bodies consistent with a postoperative disk space infection.

rologic examination is normal in most patients. Neurogenic claudication can sometimes be seen, with a positive stress test reproducing the patient's symptoms.

Plain radiography reveals facet degeneration, spondylosis, decreased interpedicular distance, decreased sagittal canal diameter, and disk space degeneration. Spondylolisthesis is also a commonly associated finding at the postoperative level or may be seen at its most common level, L4-5. CT scan, especially with postmyelographic images, can be very helpful in evaluating the bony pathology of stenosis, including the lateral recesses and neural foramina. MRI with Gd enhancement shows dural compression at the involved levels; however, care must be taken in reading the postoperative MRI, because scar tissue can coexist and make interpretation difficult. Gd enhancement allows better differentiation of scar tissue and typical stenosis caused by hypertrophy of normal soft tissue structures such as the ligamentum flavum or the facet capsule.

Surgical results are favorable when strict criteria for stenosis are met and conservative therapy has been exhausted. If true bony compression exists, a laminectomy is indicated. In the case of epidural fibrosis and scar tissue, operative intervention usually yields poor results (28). Fusion with or without instrumentation is needed in the cases of concomitant instability, spondylolisthesis, or significant scoliosis.

Arachnoiditis

Nonmechanical causes of recurrent leg pain include arachnoiditis and epidural fibrosis. Inflammation of the pia-arachnoid membrane can vary from involvement of one single nerve root (type I), to multiple nerve roots (type II), to the whole subarachnoid space at a particular level, with loss of patency of the central spinal fluid–filled space (48). Patients usually present with leg and sometimes back pain after a pain-free interval of 1 to 6 months.

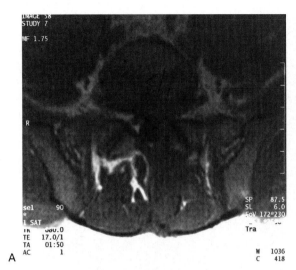 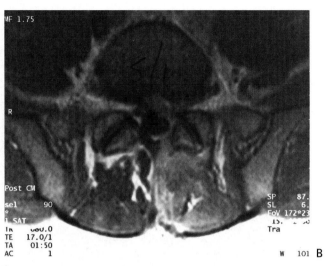

FIGURE 10. Magnetic resonance imaging performed with and without gadolinium–diethylenetriamine pentaacetic acid approximately 4 months after lumbar diskectomy in a 29-year-old man with recurrent leg pain. **A:** Without contrast a soft tissue mass is demonstrated, consistent with either recurrent disk herniation or epidural fibrosis. **B:** After contrast, enhancement of the soft tissue mass is demonstrated, confirming that it is epidural fibrosis and not disk.

Risk factors for postsurgical arachnoiditis include preoperative oil-based myelography, intraoperative dural tears, and postoperative infection. The test of choice is Gd-enhanced MRI, which is the most sensitive test after 6 months (7). Myelography and postmyelography CT scanning can also be used. Surgery is not an effective treatment modality. Nonoperative management varies from physical conditioning and narcotic detoxification to epidural steroids and electrical stimulation. Antidepressant medicines may also be helpful.

Epidural Fibrosis

Symptomatic epidural scar formation or fibrosis presents with leg pain and back pain after a variable pain-free interval ranging from 3 months to several years. The onset of pain is gradual and exacerbated by activity. Physical examination is nonspecific unless the fibrosis has caused nerve compression, at which point positive tension signs may be seen (23). Again, Gd-enhanced MRI is an excellent tool for differentiating epidural fibrosis from HNP (Fig. 10). Treatment similar to that of arachnoiditis is suggested, whereas surgical decompression is usually unsuccessful (36).

Extraspinal

Finally, the failed back patient may have symptoms and persistent back problems from extraspinal causes. Diabetes, the commonest cause of peripheral neurop-

athy, can be mistaken for radiculopathy and can be easily differentiated by EMG and NCV testing (38). Other common causes of back pain that can be medically addressed include abdominal aortic aneurysm, pancreatitis, kidney stones, and pelvic disorders. In patients with a history of cancer or in patients older than 50 years of age with recent weight loss or pain at rest, metastatic disease should be ruled out. Finally, psychosocial disorders such as drug abuse, alcoholism, depression, or secondary gain (litigation, worker's compensation) should always be evaluated before surgery to improve results.

ALGORITHM

In the workup of the complicated failed back patient, many physicians find an algorithmic approach to be a good way to evaluate efficiently, in stepwise fashion, the important aspects of these patients. The failed back algorithm provides a sensible approach that helps to deal reasonably well with the mass of information, potential tests, and possible diagnoses (Fig. 11). It uses a logical approach to help synthesize a large amount of information so that patients are treated in a reproducible pattern to help maximize favorable outcomes. The workup of all failed back patients should begin with a thorough medical evaluation that, if positive, leads to appropriate medical treatment.

Similarly, consideration of the presence of a significant psychosocial abnormality should be routinely

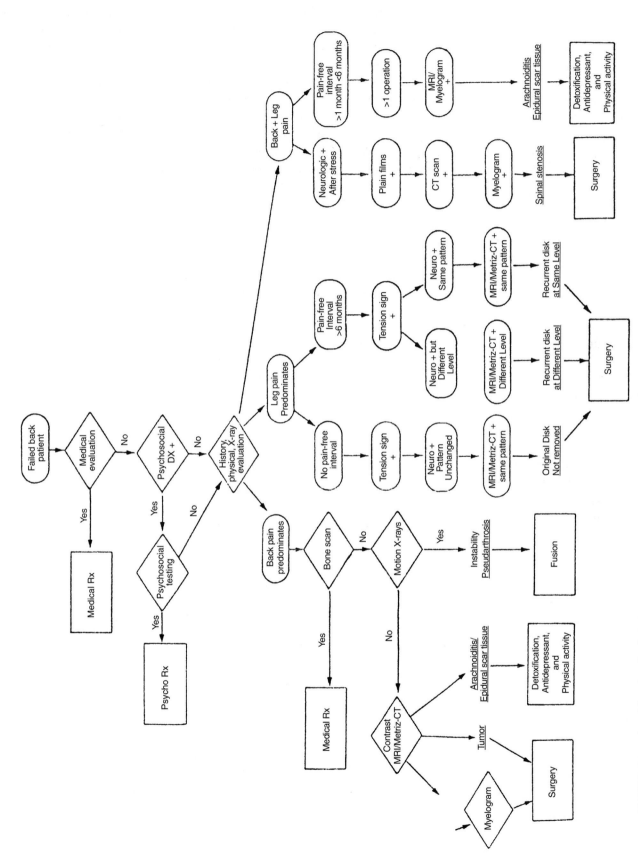

FIGURE 11. Algorithm for the failed back. CT, computed tomography; Dx, dianosis; MRI, magnetic resonance imaging; Rx, therapy.

made. In the case of questionable pathology, formal psychological testing should be pursued, leading to the appropriate treatment when positive. The remainder of information gleaned from the history and physical examination should place the patient into one of three categories: back pain, leg pain, or both back and leg pain.

In the patient with back pain, a bone scan can identify early vertebral osteomyelitis, metastatic disease, or sacral insufficiency fractures, which are treated with a nonsurgical approach. The patients who do not fall into these categories require dynamic radiographs to rule out instability or pseudarthrosis that is treated with a fusion. Patients who do not fall into the above categories are not candidates for further evaluation and are treated with detoxification, antidepressant medication, and physical therapy. MRI in these individuals may demonstrate arachnoiditis or epidural fibrosis or, rarely, an intraspinal neoplasm.

In the patient with leg pain, the pain-free interval is used to divide individuals into three groups: no pain-free interval, a pain-free interval of less than 6 months, and a pain-free interval of greater than 6 months. In the patient with no pain-free interval with a positive tension sign and an unchanged neurologic examination, MRI usually reveals a retained HNP that can benefit from surgical intervention. In the patient with a pain-free interval of greater than 6 months, a positive tension sign, and a new neurologic abnormality, an MRI should be obtained. A recurrent disk at the same level is likely if the neurologic pattern is the same as before the initial surgery, whereas a recurrent disk at a new level is indicated by a new neurologic pattern. After failed conservative treatment in either setting, operative intervention is indicated. Patients with a pain-free interval of 1 to 6 months typically have more back pain and usually have arachnoiditis or epidural fibrosis.

In the patient with back and leg pain, a good history is elicited. If the symptoms are exacerbated with walking and imaging studies reveal stenosis, the patient usually benefits from operative decompression if conservative therapy fails.

CONCLUSION

With the amount of spine surgery in the United States increasing yearly, the number of failed back patients has seen steady increases over the last two decades. Because the chance for a successful outcome for these patients declines with each operation, a sys-

tematic, thoughtful approach is required in evaluating the failed back patient. Preventing failure by adhering strictly to appropriate indications for the initial surgery is the most important step. Once these patients do present, a thorough history and physical examination should be obtained. Diagnoses that need to be entertained include mechanical and nonmechanical causes. After an adequate course of nonoperative treatment, imaging modalities such as MRI or CTM should be obtained. It should be stressed that the presence of a condition that is sometimes treated surgically, such as disk herniation, stenosis, or segmental instability, does not mean that surgery is automatically warranted; indeed, the majority of patients with prior failed operations, even with these diagnoses, are best treated initially with an aggressive nonoperative approach. Surgery is rarely indicated in the patient with nonmechanical reasons for pain. It is hoped that, by adhering to this approach, the physician will see improved results in the multiply operated back patient.

REFERENCES

1. Aminoff MJ. Clinical electromyography. In: Aminoff MJ, ed. *Electrodiagnosis in clinical neurology*, 2nd ed. New York: Churchill Livingstone, 1992:231–263.
2. Bircher MD, Tasker T, Crashaw C, et al. Discitis following lumbar surgery. *Spine* 1988;13:98–102.
3. Blumenthal SL, Gill K. Can lumbar spine radiographs accurately determine fusion in postoperative patients *Spine* 1993;18:1186–1189.
4. Boden SD, Davis DO, Dina TS, et al. Abnormal magnetic resonance scans of the lumbar spine in asymptomatic subjects. *J Bone Joint Surg Am* 1990;72A:403–408.
5. Boden SD, Davis DO, Dina TS, et al. Contrast-enhanced MRI performed after successful lumbar disk surgery; a prospective study. *Radiology* 1992;182:59–64.
6. Brodsky AE, Kovalsky ES, Khalil MA. Correlation of radiographic assessment of lumbar spine fusions with surgical exploration. *Spine* 1991;16:261–265.
7. Burton CV. Lumbosacral arachnoiditis. *Spine* 1978;3:24–30.
8. Byrd SE, Cohn ML, Biggers SL, et al. The radiographic evaluation of the symptomatic post-operative lumbar spine patient. *Spine* 1985;10:652–661.
9. Coin CG. Cervical disc degeneration and herniation: diagnosis by CT. *South Med J* 1984;77:979–982.
10. Craig FS. Vertebral-body biopsy. *J Bone Joint Surg* 1956; 38(A):93–102.
11. Dall BE, Rowe DE, Odette WG, et al. Postoperative discitis; diagnosis and management. *Clin Orthop* 1987; 224:138–148.

12. Dooley JF, McBroom RJ, Taguchi T, et al. Nerve root infiltration in the diagnosis of radicular pain. *Spine* 1988;13(1):79–83.

13. Finnegan WJ, Fenlin JM, Marvel JP, et al. Results of surgical intervention in the symptomatic multiply operated back patient. *J Bone Joint Surg Am* 1979;61(A):1077–1082.

14. Frymoyer JW. Magnitude of the problem. In: Weinstein JN, Wiesel SW, eds. *The lumbar spine.* Philadelphia: WB Saunders, 1990:32–38.

15. Gertzbein SD, Robbins SE. Accuracy of pedicular screw placement in vivo. *Spine* 1990;15:11–14.

16. Grubb SA, Lipscomb HJ, Gilford WB. The relative value of lumbar roentgenograms, metrizamide myelography, and discography in the assessment of patients with chronic low back syndrome. *Spine* 1987;12:282–286.

17. Hazlett JW, Kinnard P. Lumbar apophyseal process excision and instability. *Spine* 1982;7:171–174.

18. Hochhauser L, Kieffer SA, Cacayorin ED, et al. Recurrent postdiscectomy low back pain; MR-surgical correlations. *AJNR Am J Neuroradiol* 1988;9:769–774.

19. Holt E. The question of lumbar discography. *J Bone Joint Surg* 1968;50A:720–726.

20. Horton W, Daftari T. Which disc as visualized by MRI is actually a source of pain? A correlation between MRI and discography. *Spine* 1992;17:164–171.

21. Hueftle JG, Modic MJ, Ross JS, et al. Lumbar spine: postoperative MRI with Gd-DTPA. *Radiology* 1988;167:817–824.

22. Jackson RP, Cain JE, Jacobs RR, et al. The neuroradiographic diagnosis of lumbar herniated nucleus pulposus. *Spine* 1989;14:1356–1367.

23. Langensky A, Kiviluoto O. Prevention of epidural scar formation after operations on the lumbar spine by means of free fat transplants. *Clin Orthop* 1976;115:92–95.

24. Lauerman WC, Bradford DS, et al. Results of pseudarthrosis repair. *J Spinal Disord* 1992;5(2):149–157.

25. Lee CK. Accelerated degeneration of the segment adjacent to a lumbar fusion. *Spine* 1988;13:375–377.

26. McCulloch J, Transfeldt EE. *McNab's backache.* Baltimore: Williams & Wilkins, 1997.

27. Mooney V. Position statement on discography. *Spine* 1988;13:1343.

28. Nasca RJ. Surgical management of lumbar spinal stenosis. *Spine* 1987;12:809–816.

29. O'Brien JF, Evans G. Surgical removal of ruptured lumbar discs. A five-year follow-up. *Pain Topics* 1978;7:5.

30. Ottolenghi CE. Aspiration biopsy of the spine: technique for the thoracic spine and results. *J Bone Joint Surg Am* 1969;51(A):1531–1544.

31. Palestro CJ. Radionuclide imaging after skeletal interventional procedures. *Semin Nucl Med* 1995;25:3–14.

32. Paris SV. Physical signs of instability. *Spine* 1985;10:277–279.

33. Reilly JP, O'Leary PF. *Complications of lumbar spine surgery in the lumbar spine.* New York: Raven Press, 1987: 357–372.

34. Ross JS, Modic MT. Current assessment of spinal degenerative disease with MRI. *CORR* 1992;279:68–81.

35. Ross JS, Delamarter R, Hueftle MG, et al. Gadolinium-DTPA enhanced MRI of the postoperative lumbar spine: time course and mechanism of enhancement. *AJNR Am J Neuroradiol* 1989;10:1251–1254.

36. Ross JS, Masaryk TJ, Modic MT, et al. Lumbar spine: postoperative assessment with surface-coil MRI. *Radiology* 1989;164:851–860.

37. Rothman RH, Simeone FA. *The spine.* Philadelphia: Harcourt Brace Jovanovich, 1992.

38. Simpson JM, Silveri CP, Balderston RA, et al. The results of operations on the lumbar spine in patients who have diabetes mellitus. *J Bone Joint Surg Am* 1993;75(A):1823–1829.

39. Slizofski WJ, Collier BD, Flatley TJ, et al. Painful pseudarthrosis following lumbar spinal fusion: detection by SPECT. *Skeletal Radiol* 1987;16:136–141.

40. Stanley D, McLaren MI, Euinton HA, et al. A prospective study of nerve root infiltration in the diagnosis of sciatica. *Spine* 1990;15(6):540–543.

41. Teplick JG, Haskin ME. CT of the postoperative lumbar spine. *Radiol Clin North Am* 1983;21:395–420.

42. Waddell G. Failures of disc surgery and repeat surgery. *Acta Orthop Belg* 1987;53:300–302.

43. Waddell G, Kummel EG, Lotto WN, et al. Failed lumbar disc surgery and repeat surgery following industrial injuries. *J Bone Joint Surg Am* 1979;61(A):201–207.

44. Waddell G, McCullock JA, Kummel E. Non-organic physical signs in low back pain. *Spine* 1980;5:117–125.

45. Walsh T, Weinstein J, Spratt K, et al. Lumbar discography in normal subjects. A controlled prospective study. *J Bone Joint Surg Am* 1990;72A:1081–1088.

46. White AA, Panjibi MM. *Clinical biomedicines of the spine.* Philadelphia: JB Lippincott Co, 1990:349–362.

47. Wilbourn AJ. The value and limitations of electromyographic examination in the diagnosis of lumbosacral radiculopathy. In: Hardy RW, ed. *Lumbar disc disease.* New York: Raven Press, 1982:65–109.

48. Wilkinson HA. Adhesive arachnoiditis. In: Weinstein JN, Wiesel SW, eds. *The lumbar spine.* Philadelphia: WB Saunders, 1990:1872–1876.

49. Yoo JU, Ghanayem A, Petersilge C, et al. Accuracy of using CT to identify pedicle screw placement in cadaveric human lumbar spine. *Spine* 1997;22:2668–2671.

LUMBAR SPINE: NONOPERATIVE TREATMENT

HOWARD I. LEVY

Nonoperative management options for failed lumbar surgery pain are based on the presence of pain. Most treatments are not determined by the type of pain or even what structures are affected (save for the possibility of using injections for particular pain and antiseizure medications and antidepressant medications for radicular pain). For the purposes of this chapter, it is assumed that patients benefit from a trial of the most conservative options followed by more aggressive and invasive approaches. This chapter addresses nonoperative management options for patients who recently had surgery. It assumes that surgically correctable lesions [such as recurrent herniated nucleus pulposus (HNP) in the early postoperative period, pseudarthroses, and iatrogenic instabilities] are best managed surgically. Late symptoms, such as a recurrent HNP after more than 1 year, are managed as new HNPs without regard to prior surgery. Likewise, adjacent segment degeneration is managed as new symptoms with similar expectations as degeneration from natural history. The assumption is that patients with successful surgery will present with new symptoms after a period of relief. Thus, the surgery should not be considered a failure. No study has demonstrated the natural history for patients with failed lumbar surgery. One of the great benefits of the National Spine Network database, a collection of data from centers of excellence for spine care, is that in the future this issue can be studied. Failed lumbar surgery patients who have no surgically correctable lesion and do not benefit from nonoperative care are most likely going to end up with a chronic pain syndrome.

The most important use for pain medication and injections, or the soft tissue modalities of physical therapy, is their ability to control pain and allow patients to embark on an active exercise program, which serves to modulate pain, in part by inducing endogenous endorphin secretion (70). Psychological issues are mainly pursued by chronic pain programs. This chapter addresses most other routinely used options.

Patients with low back pain and sciatica that are persistent after lumbar surgery have the same conservative treatment options as patients who have never had surgery. Although occasionally influenced by the type of surgery, most treatment is prescribed on the basis of pain symptoms rather than prior surgery. The natural history for resolution of back pain may be less favorable for patients who have had back surgery. The counseling of such patients concerning conservative treatment options stresses that these help to contain and ease the pain but do not necessarily eliminate it. Conservative treatment, however, does provide the patient with the possibility of a better functional outcome. The clinician should explain to patients, during the course of conservative treatment, that appropriate graded activity increases pain tolerance and stamina.

When patients increase their activity, they also increase their ability to walk longer distances and to participate in activities that are typical of daily living, such as shopping or gardening. Some patients do not realize that they can still indulge in these activities even though they have low back pain. Counseling patients may settle some of the anxiety associated with failed back surgery patients (74). Clarifying the distinction between "hurt" that may be tolerable and "harm" that implies further tissue damage is very reassuring in this regard.

MEDICATION

Medications given for failed back surgery syndromes consist of those for pain relief, muscle relaxation, and sedation. Typically, the medications include nonsteroidal antiinflammatories, narcotics, muscle relaxants, tricyclic antidepressants, and antiseizure medication. A topically applied ointment that is a substance P analogue, capsaicin, can be used for pain syndromes in failed back pain surgery. Most medications lose their efficacy for pain control when used over extended periods of time. Consequently, a patient who has had multiple medications may find the more commonly used drugs ineffective and, thus, must seek other medications that can be used for chronic pain syndromes. Patients with failed back syndrome are almost always taking some medication. Some adopt drug-seeking behaviors that must be addressed when prescribing medications. Ensuring that there is only one prescribing physician is of paramount importance when prescribing medications for patients with persistent pain syndromes. When patients manage to get more and more medication from different prescribers, they have earlier loss of ability to get relief with a given medication and, thus, must change medication more frequently.

Aspirin, salsalate, or nonacetylated salicylates and nonsteroidal antiinflammatory drugs (NSAIDs) are the most commonly used medications for the treatment of failed back surgery pain syndromes. These medications have the attributes of being antiinflammatory and analgesic (55). Currently, many nonsteroidal antiinflammatories are available, and although there can be a great variation in individual responses, no study has demonstrated the efficacy of one over another (8). Typically, they are chosen because of their costs and side-effects profile and a history of prior success or failure to respond. Nonsteroidal antiinflammatories have a local and central effect for pain relief (17,55,79). They act by blocking cyclooxygenase in the arachidonic acid pathway. This prevents the synthesis of prostaglandins that are local mediators for the release of inflammatory agents and amplify the effects of inflammatory agents (8,79). NSAIDs also act on the central nervous system for pain control (17,53,55).

NSAIDs are known for their adverse effect on the gastrointestinal system, the urinary tract, and platelet aggregation (8,79). The antiinflammatory medication has a direct harmful effect on the gastric mucosa and also blocks the synthesis of prostaglandins that aid in secretion of acid-neutralizing products. The antiinflammatory medications also complicate the gastrointestinal side effects by inhibiting platelet aggregation and prolonging bleeding time (8,79). The deleterious combined effects on gastric mucosa and bleeding time can lead to the severe complication of gastric hemorrhage; thus, caution must be observed when prescribing, especially in elderly patients. Because of the primarily urinary excretion of NSAIDs, papillary necrosis, interstitial nephritis, and hematuria may also occur (8,79). The costs and side-effects profile become important in prescribing these medications, as no single antiinflammatory medication has distinguished itself as a clear, better medication for pain control and antiinflammatory effects, despite the fact that there are several chemical classes of NSAIDs (36). Nabumetone (Relafen) has

been identified for being somewhat better tolerated in the gastrointestinal tract (62,68). Sulindac (Clinoril) is repeatedly metabolized by the liver and has a large percentage excreted fecally (8,79). Thus, it may have some benefit in patients with renal disease. Ketorolac (Toradol) has the unique property for intramuscular usage (17). Acetaminophen (Tylenol) and possibly cyclooxygenase 2 (COX 2) inhibitors can be used for NSAID-intolerant patients (88,89).

One interesting new development regarding antiinflammatories is the use of the COX 2 inhibitors. It has been found that cyclooxygenase exists as two isomers termed *COX 1* and *COX 2*. NSAIDs exert their prostaglandin-blocking effects on cyclooxygenase. The two isomers have distinctly different properties, with COX 1 affecting the gastric mucosa, the kidneys, and hemostasis (76). COX 2 mediates inflammation (76). By selectively blocking COX 2, inflammation may be stopped without the side effects of gastric irritation. However, recent studies have demonstrated renal effects may persist.

Antiinflammatory medication should be prescribed initially on a scheduled basis for at least 2 weeks. Once pain has been controlled or is better tolerated, the medication can be withdrawn and used on an as-needed basis. The risk for adverse effects and complications arises with the extended use—generally more than 4 weeks—of antiinflammatory medications. Blood studies monitoring renal, hepatic, and platelet function should be taken at a minimum every 3 months in patients on chronic antiinflammatory medication. Medication dosage should be titrated from a minimum dosage up to an effective dosage, being careful not to exceed the maximum recommended dosage. If the maximum recommended dosage does not provide pain relief, the medication should be switched to a different chemical class.

Muscle Relaxants

Muscle spasm and irritation from failed back surgery may arise from direct trauma to the muscle tissue during surgery or from irritation of the nerve fibers that supply muscles. Direct trauma results from cutting directly through the muscular tissue or from traction applied to the muscle tissue during exposure for operative procedures. The traction may have the double effect of having local mechanical tissue destruction along with ischemic consequences. Nerve fibers that supply these muscles can be irritated through traction applied during surgery or from scarring that may occur in the surrounding tissues after surgery. Muscle relaxants can be used to treat the spasm as a result of this trauma. Most of the muscle relaxants commonly used, such as carisoprodol or cyclobenzaprine, have no direct effect on the muscle; rather, they act on the central nervous system either through the brain or spinal cord (62).

Side effects from muscle relaxants include dizziness, dry mouth, drowsiness, and tachycardia (62). The drowsiness can be used to help patients with sleep difficulty after failed back surgery. Initially, because of the drowsiness, patients should be cautioned on operation of motor vehicles when they are under the influence of the medications.

Muscle relaxants are prescribed for the times when the patient feels the muscle spasms the most. Very rarely are they used on a scheduled basis. Typically, the author suggests patients use them at night to facilitate sleep. The minimal effective dose is prescribed, and the medications are switched if the maximum recommended dosage is ineffective. Some studies have demonstrated greater efficacy when used in combination with an NSAID (3,6), and generally, this is the best bet when using muscle relaxants.

Narcotics

Narcotic medications have tremendous efficacy as analgesics. They are most commonly used for acute pain syndromes of relatively short duration, such as after surgery, and for such chronic painful conditions as arise from cancerous conditions. The use of narcotic agents in failed back surgery patients must be approached with a great deal of caution. Tolerance and dependence are seen in chronic usage of these medications.

Narcotic analgesics use the same opiate receptors in the central nervous system as endorphins (32). In addition to the side effects of constipation, nausea, and vomiting, tolerance to these drugs may develop, tempting patients to take more medication. This is very troublesome for failed lumbar surgery patients, as their expectations for pain relief are higher than those who have not had surgery.

Patients with failed back syndrome who need acute pain relief may benefit from the occasional use of narcotics; however, they are not strongly advocated for chronic pain associated with failed back surgery. Some circumstances may occur in which chronic narcotic analgesics should be used. Before embarking on long-term therapy, patients must sign an informed consent (83). They must have a contract that outlines the requirements for them to continue medication prescription and that must include a statement that the patient receives medication from only one physician (83). Narcotic therapies should be used in combination with other types of therapies that anticipate a probable reduction in the medication at some point. Should tolerance develop to the narcotic medication, a change in the class of narcotic medication is preferred to increasing dosages. Narcotic therapy for chronic pain is best managed by specialists, and typically, the patient would be referred to a chronic pain therapy center.

Tramadol (Ultram) is an opiate receptor agonist. Its benefit is pain control without addiction and other untoward narcotic effects. It is as effective as and a useful alternative to acetaminophen with codeine in elderly patients (64) and as effective as narcotic analgesia postoperatively (42,78). Some tendency toward habituation, drowsiness, and constipation may occur (62).

Oral Corticosteroids

Prednisone and methylprednisolone can be used for acute flare-ups from failed back surgery that appear to be mediated more by inflammation. Pain relief from corticosteroids is primarily from their antiinflammatory effects, although there are some direct neuroanalgesic effects (22). As with NSAIDs, corticosteroids act by inhibiting the synthesis of arachnoidic acid (32). They also act by stabilizing the cell membrane to inhibit the release of inflammatory mediators (32).

Chronic administration of corticosteroids should be avoided. The adverse side effects of corticosteroid administration include gastric ulceration, hyperglycemia, osteoporosis, water retention, adrenaline insufficiency, and thinning of the skin (32). A particularly worrisome side effect of steroid administration is avascular necrosis of the femoral heads. These side effects must be weighed against the relative benefits of the medication.

The steroid preparations are typically prescribed for acute severe exacerbations as a decreasing dosage that lasts for 6 days, such as methylprednisolone (Medrol Dosepak). Prednisone can also be prescribed in decreasing dosages or the same dosages over a relatively short period, such as 5 to 7 days.

Tricyclic antidepressant medications affect the neurogenic pain pathways in the central nervous system (9,18,31,73). Typically, these medications are used for chronic pain syndromes associated with failed back syndromes. Amitriptyline (Elavil) and nortriptyline (Pamelor) are two of several that can be used. The sedating effects of these medications can have the added benefit of enhancing sleep in addition to relieving the pain, but this can have the troublesome side effects of daytime drowsiness, confusion, and greater risk of falling (62).

Antiseizure medication such as carbamazepine (Tegretol) and gabapentin (Neurontin) is suitable for patients with sciatica as a result of neuritic pain syndrome and epidural scarring. These medications act by stabilizing the neural membrane, thereby modulating the pain. The doses are titrated to the best effect not exceeding the maximum antiseizure dose.

Capsaicin, a synthetically manufactured substance P analogue (12), can be used topically to control painful symptoms in patients with failed back surgery syndrome. Capsaicin acts by displacing substance P in nerve endings and relieving local irritation (12,14). The cream can be applied in areas of pain, including the graft harvest sites and along the external scars. The efficacy of this medication has been found in studies of osteoarthritis in which patients have had decreased pain symptoms when using capsaicin (19,58).

LUMBOSACRAL CORSETS

A lumbosacral corset with metal stays can be prescribed for patients with failed lumbar surgery. Although there is no study to document its efficacy in this situation, some studies have demonstrated effectiveness for other back pain syndromes (1,59). It is a low-cost alternative for treatment if it is helpful. Most patients are instructed to wear the corset when they are up and about. Little concern need be shown for dependence or deconditioning; it is more important that the corset is providing patients with relief. Typically, obese patients cannot be fitted from off-the-shelf sizes. The author does not believe that they would gain support from a custom corset, and, thus, it is never prescribed.

PHYSICAL THERAPY

The physical therapy used for failed back syndromes has two components: passive modalities and active exercise programs. The goal should be to place patients on active exercise programs that allow them to be mobilized and active. During the first few weeks of treatment, modalities such as hot packs, electrical stimulation, and ultrasound can be used to relieve soreness and to loosen the soft tissue spasm. However, there are no proven long-term effects; thus, passive modalities should only be used for analgesic effects early in the course of treatment or for acute exacerbation to facilitate the patient's ability to progress in an exercise rehabilitation program. As patients develop a series of home exercises that can be advanced as their condition improves, they are discharged to their home exercise program. A gym program coupled with those exercises is ideal.

Manipulation has been found to have some efficacy with uncomplicated acute low back syndromes (72). However, its use in chronic pain syndromes has never been successfully documented (72). Patients with failed back syndromes who have an acute episode or an exacerbation of pain may benefit from a trial of one or two sessions of manipulation. Probably it is best used to mobilize facet joints or sacroiliac (SI) joints in patients with symptoms from these areas with failed back pain.

Lumbar traction has been found to reduce intradiskal pressure, although studies of lumbar traction have not documented any significant decrease in pain and recovery (85). Traction for disk-generated pain in failed back surgery is only used as a passive modality for the initial treatment period. It may be helpful in the treatment of persistent foraminal stenosis, but this diagnosis is more than likely a surgically correctable lesion.

Active exercise has been reported in the literature to increase functional level in patients with chronic pain (45). One study concluded that patients with increased exercise tolerance had greater functional capacity, without any change in the pain level (63). However, exercise is understood to increase endorphins and may allow tolerance of pain (70). Mixed evidence has been found that strengthening the spine can prevent future episodes (39,45); however, it appears that, at the very least, it dispels possible disabling habituation (56).

A series of stretches for spinal musculature and for limb and pelvic musculature may begin the active exercise routine. This may be followed by a McKenzie exercise program for pain control. The McKenzie exercise program, a series of maneuvers aimed at controlling pain by repeated lumbar movements, has been advocated for disk-generated pain syndromes (24). Its efficacy for pain control has some support in the literature (24); however, it cannot be considered a universal exercise program for all patients with failed back surgery. It may be contraindicated for patients with spondylolisthesis and spinal stenosis.

Dynamic lumbar stabilization is an active exercise program that has been used to treat many types of low back pain syndromes (69). It relies on finding a neutral position for the lumbar spine that is pain free for the patient. This neutral position may be different for every patient who is treated, but the series of exercise programs accommodates for the differences in neutral postures. The patients then are taken through a series of progressively more difficult exercises, using the limbs while maintaining the axial skeleton in a neutral posture. As the exercises get more and more difficult, the lumbar spine gets more and more strengthening, corseted by the abdominal and the extensor musculature. These exercises also have a functional component in which patients are given specific tasks to simulate the daily activities of living and various job functions that they can perform well while maintaining a neutral position of the lumbar spine.

The success of aquatherapy arises from the water's buoyancy, which unloads the spine. The patients can exercise with less weight on the disks and the facet joints, and thus they are able to tolerate more exercise. The Arthritis Foundation in Georgia sponsors an aerobic aquatic program throughout the state that charges a minimal fee for participation. Patients find it to be not only a good exercise program but also a social outlet to aid in recovery from failed back syndromes.

Low-impact aerobic activities such as stationary cycling and swimming are recommended for patients who can tolerate a more aggressive exercise. These activities have the benefit of aerobic activity without pounding the spine while developing cardiovascular fitness and providing assistance with weight control.

WORK HARDENING AND FUNCTIONAL RESTORATION

Work hardening is a set of task-motivated exercises that are designed to return a patient to work. By strengthening patients in an ergonomically accurate program that simulates the work environment, they are thought to have a better chance to return to a functional lifestyle (66). Studies have demonstrated that exercises of strengthening can decrease pain (65,66). Several programs have been developed for functional recovery. Probably the most successful work-hardening programs have a normal work schedule of 8 hours a day, 5 days a week. Patients have functionally oriented tasks to perform and are assessed for functional capacity at various times during the program. Patients in these programs are encouraged to return to work, not necessarily to the previous job function but at a level proven by a functional capacity evaluation; this allows them to resume being contributing members of society (4,47,66). Most studies of work-hardening programs demonstrate functional gains; however, a key element in determining return-to-work rates is the amount of time spent out of work (27). Those with shorter times off return more frequently than those with longer out-of-work status.

The multidisciplinary approach of functional restoration to treating patients with chronic back pain is based on the premise that patients with chronic back pain require multiple areas of expertise to be successful in returning to the work force (40). It assumes that patients with spinal pain have psychological, functional, and vocational issues that need to be resolved. The key components of the functional restoration program include an interdisciplinary staff (to address psychological, functional, and vocational issues), a low staff-patient ratio that allows for individual attention, and the measurement of capabilities before, during, and after the program (16,40). Physical training with active exercise without modalities is performed that includes the whole body for flexibility, strengthening, and endurance (16,40,50,57,60); there are also components that simulate work. Psychological, cognitive, and vocational counseling are included. Some studies have shown psychological improvement in patients undergoing functional reconstruction (38,41). Although prospective studies still have not proven the efficacy of functional reconstruction (40,82), other studies have shown an 80% reemployment rate for patients who have had chronic back pain with a total commitment to this type of program. Evidence has also shown that all parameters addressed during the program improve (16,40,50,57,60).

Functional restoration and work hardening are the centerpiece for patients with failed back syndrome for return to work. The goal-oriented therapy appears to be ideal for placing injured workers into jobs in which their capabilities are functionally adequate.

INJECTION PROCEDURES

Spinal injection procedures can be attempted as a more aggressive and invasive nonoperative management. Facet injections are injections of the zygapophyseal joints under fluoroscopy. A spinal needle is placed within the facet joint, and radiographic contrast is injected to outline the joint. A small amount of local anesthetic and steroid is then injected to relieve the pain. The efficacy of these injections is not clearly supported in the literature (30,44,46,61); however, anecdotal reports of success indicate that they may have some utility (26,30). Once the patient has clearly been shown to have facet-mediated pain with a series of differential posterior primary rami blocks along with interarticular injections, ablation of the posterior primary rami (of the level that is being affected as well as of the level above) may allow for extended relief of facet joint–mediated pain (26,54,64). Studies have shown greater efficacy in the cervical spine than the lumbar spine, but further research is needed.

For failed low back pain surgery patients with radicular and sciatic pain, epidural steroid injections may have some usefulness in treating pain. Although only four of the nine (7,11,13,15,23,49,67,75,86) published controlled studies document any relief from radicular pain, a trial of injections for sciatica is usually performed. The steroid injections should be done under fluoroscopy and attempts made to place the injection in the area where the pain is generated. Our institution advocates the use of transforaminal injections, as they tend to place more medication anterior to the thecal sac as compared to interlaminar injections. This has some support from anatomic studies (10,87) and has demonstrated effective pain relief in approximately 84% of patients (90). Although patients with persistent sciatica do not have any clear indication for chronic use of epidural steroid injections, one or two can be attempted to try to mediate some of the pain while the patients enter an exercise program.

Lumbar root sleeve injections can be done from a similar approach as a transforaminal epidural steroid injection. The spinal needle is placed within the root sleeve just caudad to the pedicle. Radiographic contrast is injected to confirm needle placement, followed by injection of anesthetic and steroid. During needle placement or injection of the contrast or medication, the patient may experience reproduction of radicular symptoms. In addition to the therapeutic effects, depending on concordant or discordant radicular symptoms, diagnostic information may be gained from this injection (20,21,25,51,52,77,80).

Trigger point injections can be attempted for myofascial pain. The injections of local anesthetic with or without steroid are injected into the most tender point of the muscle. The needle can be withdrawn and reinserted in an attempt to "break up" the trigger point. Controlled studies have failed to demonstrate the effectiveness of medication over dry needling (37). The injections can be used to ease pain temporarily to allow patients to engage in an active exercise program.

Acupuncture has long been used throughout the Far East for treatment of pain syndromes (43). It has recently gained favor in the West, as more traditional

medical practices are accepting alternative approaches to pain. Additionally, acupuncture has more and more support in the lay press. Its acceptance into this culture has been based on the conclusion that its widespread use in Eastern communities argues for its success and effectiveness. However, few data are available demonstrating its clinically relevant importance in this matter. Acupuncture is based on an idea developed by traditional Chinese medicine that the body has energy that is known as *chi*. This chi is in balance throughout the body and flows along meridians, which are lines that divide the body in a vertical manner. Pain is the result of a deficiency of chi, and acupuncture facilitates the flow of chi (18).

Studies have shown that acupuncture raises beta-endorphin levels in the brain and bloodstream (5). In addition, sympathetic nervous system effects can be found (46). Acupuncture also stimulates nerve fibers, improving symptoms through the "gate control" theory for pain (84). Thus, there is a biochemical basis for its use in addition to the traditional Chinese medicine rationale.

Acupuncture needles are placed at acupuncture points spelled out in Chinese medical literature. Most acupuncture treatments last 20 to 30 minutes at intervals of one or two times a week for a course of 2 to 4 months. As an adjunct to acupuncture treatment, electrical stimulation or a process called *moxibustion*, which uses burning incense around the acupuncture needle under a glass cover, can be applied.

The usefulness of acupuncture has not been clearly supported, but in patients who have chronic pain syndromes, when the standard techniques cannot supply them with any significant relief, acupuncture may be an avenue for relief. Additionally, acupuncture may be of benefit in patients with chronic trigger points in place of giving any injection of medication. This is supported by studies that have shown that needling a trigger point with an empty hypodermic needle may have the same effect or better as injecting medication (37). Empirically, it can be considered as an alternative treatment that can be tried for chronic pain syndromes. The risks and complications are relatively few. It appears to be a relatively safe procedure that may be relatively cost-effective compared to other long-term chronic therapies.

PIRIFORMIS SYNDROME AND SACROILIAC JOINT PAIN

Two uncommon causes for low back pain and sciatica may manifest themselves as sources for pain from failed back surgery. These diagnoses, piriformis syndrome and SI joint pain, are made in the absence of any other sources for pain (48). Clearly, these syndromes need to be evaluated in patients with failed back surgery syndromes who have unremitting sciatica despite an appropriate nonoperative plan.

Piriformis Syndrome

Patients with piriformis syndrome have pain resulting from the compression of the sciatic nerve within the sciatic notch. The nerve can be pinched by passing over, above, or through the piriformis muscle. Fibrous bands may be attached to the muscle that encircle the nerve, causing the development of symptoms. The piriformis fossa can be palpated by placing the patient in an abducted, flexed, and internally rotated position for the hip. Piriformis pain can be considered when patients have leg pain with tenderness along the muscle from the greater trochanter into the sciatic notch when all imaging studies and diagnostic tests have ruled out any spinal sources for pathology. Patients with piriformis syndrome may also have a simulated straight-leg raise, diminished reflexes at the ankle simulating sciatica (2). Diagnosis of piriformis syndrome can be confirmed by nerve conduction studies (33). A slowing of the H-wave in the stressed, abducted, flexed, and internally rotated hip position may indicate evidence for piriformis syndrome (33). Although other authors have advocated rectal examinations for the diagnosis of piriformis syndrome, the absence of any spinal pathology with tenderness in the piriformis fossa and a confirmatory electromyographic study are sufficient tools to make a presumptive diagnosis in our practice. If one is suspicious of a pelvic tumor causing irritation of the piriformis muscle or sciatic nerve, the rectal or vaginal examination should be performed in addition to the appropriate diagnostic tests.

Treatment for piriformis syndrome consists of analgesic medications, including antiinflammatories and, occasionally, a tricyclic antidepressant or one of the antiseizure medications. Muscle relaxants are used on occasion. A series of exercises have been developed for treatment of piriformis syndrome [Fishman L. Personal communication, 1993]. The exercises consist of deep soft tissue massage and a stretching program, actively and passively, that stretch the piriformis muscle. Occasionally, surgery to divide the portion of the piriformis muscle impinging on the sciatic nerve is performed (33). However, most patients tend to respond to a conservative exercise program (33).

Sacroiliac Leg/Joint Pain

Pain that arises from the SI joint may be a source for persistent symptoms despite successful disk surgery (71). The hallmark for diagnosing SI joint pain is on the basis of nonconcordant imaging studies and a series of provocative maneuvers that may elicit presumed SI joint pain. The physical examination for patients with suspected SI joint pain is compounded by negative as well as positive findings (28,29). The straight-leg raise test can be positive or negative, and, when positive, it should not necessarily be attributed to a true radicular sign. The patient may have pain with Patrick's maneuver in the SI joint region. The SI joint shear test (performed by placing the palm of one hand on the wing of the ilium and the other hand on the base of the sacrum and thrusting them together) can reproduce pain in the SI joint by producing a shear force across the joint. An additional provocative maneuver is the Gaenslen's maneuver, which consists of having the patient drop the symptomatic leg off the table while the opposite-side leg, knee, and hip are flexed and held by the patient's hand. The examiner stabilizes the patient by placing one hand on the contralateral anterior superior iliac spine and applying a small amount of stress downward on the affected leg. The patient should experience pain in the area of the SI joint that reproduces his or her common complaints.

Confirmatory diagnosis is made by interarticular SI injections (34,35). Under fluoroscopy a spinal needle is placed into the SI joint, and a small amount of radiographic contrast is injected to confirm placement into the joint. It may reproduce the patient's symptoms, at which point 3 mL of the solution containing a local anesthetic, with or without a corticosteroid, is injected. After the injection procedure, the patient should experience at least a 50% reduction of pain in that region for diagnostic purposes in addition to therapeutic effects.

In addition to the injections, treatment of SI joint pain consists of mobilization or manipulation of the SI joint, or both, by a skilled physical therapist, followed by exercises that aim to stabilize the joint. NSAIDs and analgesics should be retried. Occasionally, SI belts are used. Another method of treatment may use a shoe lift under the symptomatic side at a height that feels comfortable to the patient.

ORGANIZED APPROACH TO FAILED LUMBAR SURGERY

With an understanding of the most commonly used nonoperative management options, an organized

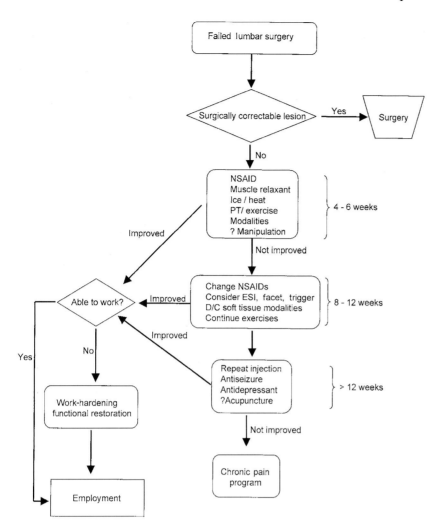

FIGURE 1. An organized nonoperative approach to failed lumbar surgery. D/C, discontinue; ESI, epidural steroid injection; NSAIDs, nonsteroidal antiinflammatory drugs; PT, physical therapy.

approach can be developed. Figure 1 is an algorithm that can be followed to treat failed back pain. At the outset it is crucial to rule out potentially surgically correctable causes for failed lumbar surgery. The need for surgery may be emergent, such as with postoperative infections or iatrogenic instability, or it may be elective for inadequate decompression. Either scenario for surgery must be presented to the patient. My assumption is that patients may have already made the decision for surgery and are to elect surgery over a trial of nonoperative care. For those who do not want surgery and those with no surgical options, the first step in an organized nonoperative approach for conservative care begins with counseling the patient. Additionally, an antiinflammatory medication is begun on a scheduled basis, coupled with a muscle relaxant for any spasm. Patients also can be given a lumbosacral corset and are encouraged to use it any time that it provides relief. McKenzie and lumbar stabilization exercises are begun. Up to 2 weeks of passive modalities, such as heat, ice, ultrasound, electrical stimulation, and/or manipulation,

can be used. At 4 to 6 weeks, those patients who improve can return to their usual activities or can be placed in a job-specific exercise program with reemployment as the end point. For those who do not improve or are worse, an injection procedure (trigger, facet, or epidural steroid) can be performed. The understanding should be that the injection may not provide permanent relief; however, it may facilitate the exercise program. The antiinflammatory can be changed. The patient is continued on the exercise program.

At 8 to 12 weeks, the injections can be attempted again. At this point patients who are improved are placed in a job-specific exercise program or are reemployed, or both. Those who are no better or are worse can be started on tricyclic antidepressant or antiseizure medication. Chronic pain programs are considered at any point after this. Most patients with no improvement at this time benefit from a comprehensive pain program. This type of program addresses psychosocial issues that are sure to have arisen, in addition to the pain problem.

EMPLOYMENT

For patients with failed lumbar surgery, the goals for employment become narrowed. Sedentary to light work may be the norm. Even patients who have had lumbar surgery that was successful may not be able to return to heavy work (81). For example, patients who were previously involved in construction or heavy manual work may be relegated to sedentary activities such as being a night watchman. By quizzing the patients as to their daily activities around the house, the clinician is able to evaluate the type of future employment. In some cases, the barriers to specific work may not only be from a functional level. Psychosocial issues may intervene. However, prolonged out-of-work status may prevent return to work. Employment opportunities can be explored using vocational counselors to assess the patient's abilities and needs. Vocational counselors can also assist in finding employers who are willing to accommodate the special needs of patients with failed back surgery, such as rest periods and frequent position changes throughout the day.

CONCLUSION

Nonoperative care for failed lumbar surgery builds on a pattern for recovery. The medications, modalities in physical therapy, and injection procedures all serve to reduce pain enough to allow the patient to embark on an exercise program. These exercise programs have as a goal the return to a functional lifestyle that allows patients to return to work at some appropriate level. Counseling patients that this is the end point can aid in their recovery and dissuade the notion of disability.

REFERENCES

1. Ahlgren SA, Hansen T. The use of lumbosacral corsets prescribed for low back pain. *Prosthet Orthot Int* 1978;2:101–104.
2. Barton PM. Piriformis syndrome: a rational approach to management. *Pain* 1991;47:345–352.
3. Basmajian JV. Acute back pain and spasm: a controlled multicenter trial of combined analgesic and antispasm agents. *Spine* 1989;14:438–439.
4. Beissner KL, Saunders RL, McManis BG. Research report: factors related to successful work hardening outcomes. *Phys Ther* 1996;76:1188–1201.
5. Bianchi M, Jotti E, Sacerdote P, et al. Traditional acupuncture increases the content of beta-endorphin in immune cells and influences mitogen induced proliferation. *Am J Chin Med* 1991;19:101–104.
6. Borenstein DG, Lacks S, Wiesel SW. Cyclobenzaprine and naproxen versus naproxen alone in the treatment of acute low back pain and muscle spasm. *Clin Ther* 1990;12:125–131.
7. Breivik H, Hesla PE, Molnar I, et al. Treatment of chronic low back pain and sciatica. Comparison of caudal epidural injections of bupivacaine and methylprednisolone with bupivacaine followed by saline. In: Bonica JJ, Albe Fessard D, eds. *Advances in pain research and therapy.* New York: Raven Press, 1976:917–932.
8. Brooks PM, Day RO. Nonsteroidal antiinflammatory drugs—differences and similarities. *N Engl J Med* 1991;324:1716–1725.
9. Bryson HM, Wilde MI. Amitriptyline. A review of its pharmacological properties and therapeutic use in chronic pain states [review]. *Drugs Aging* 1996;8:459–476.
10. Burn J, Guyer P, Langdon V. The spread of solutions injected into the epidural space: a study using epidurograms in patients with lumbosciatic syndrome. *Br J Anaesth* 1973;45:338–345.
11. Bush K, Hillier S. A controlled study of caudal epidural injections of triamcinolone plus procaine for the management of intractable sciatica. *Spine* 1991;16:572–575.
12. Capsaicin: a topical analgesic. *Med Lett Drugs Ther* 1992;34:62–63.
13. Carette S, Leclaire R, Marcoux S, et al. Epidural corticosteroid injections for sciatica due to herniated nucleus pulposus. *N Engl J Med* 1997;336:1634–1640.
14. Cordell GA, Arajuo OE. Capsaicin: identification, nomenclature, and pharmacotherapy [review]. *Ann Pharmacother* 1993;27:330–336.
15. Cuckler J, Bernini P, Wiesel SW, et al. The use of epidural steroids in the treatment of lumbar radicular pain. *J Bone Joint Surg Am* 1985;67-A:63–66.
16. Curtis L, Mayer TG, Gatchel RJ. Physical progress and residual impairment quantification after functional restoration. Pt III: Isokinetic and isoinertial lifting capacity. *Spine* 1994;19:401–405.
17. Dahl J. Care of the terminally ill patient: effective pain management in terminal care. *Clin Geriatr Med* 1996;12:279–300.
18. Davis AE. Primary care management of chronic musculoskeletal pain. *Nurse Practitioner* 1996;21:72,75,79–82, passim.
19. Deal CL, Schnitzer TJ, Lipstein E, et al. Treatment of arthritis with topical capsaicin: a double-blind trial. *Clin Ther* 1991;13:383–395.
20. Derby R. Diagnostic block procedures: use in pain localization. *Spine: State of the Art Reviews* 1986;1:47–64.
21. Derby R, Kine G, Saal J, et al. Response to steroid and duration of radicular pain as predictors of surgical outcome. *Spine* 1992;17[Suppl]:S176–S183.
22. Devor M, Govrin-Lippmann R, Raber P. Corticosteroids suppress ectopic neural discharge originating in experimental neuromas. *Pain* 1985;22:127–137.

23. Dilke TFW, Burry HC, Grahame R. Extradural corticosteroid injection in the management of lumbar nerve root compression. *Br Med J* 1973;2:635–637.

24. Donelson R. The McKenzie approach to evaluating and treating low back pain. *Orthop Rev* 1990;19:681–686.

25. Dooley J, McBroom R, Taguchi T, et al. Nerve root infiltration in the diagnosis of radicular pain. *Spine* 1988;13:79–83.

26. Dreyer SJ, Dreyfuss P, Cole AJ. Zygapophyseal (facet) joint injections: intra-articular and medial branch block techniques. *Phys Med Rehabil Clin North Am* 1995;6:715–741.

27. Reference deleted.

28. Dreyfuss P, Dryer S, Griffin J, et al. Positive sacroiliac screening tests in asymptomatic adults. *Spine* 1994;19:1138–1143.

29. Dreyfuss P, Michaelsen M, Pauza K, et al. The value of medical history and physical examination in diagnosing sacroiliac joint pain. *Spine* 1996;21:2594–2602.

30. Dreyfuss PH, Dreyer SJ, Herring SA. Contemporary concepts in spine care: lumbar zygapophyseal (facet) joint injections. *Spine* 1995;20:2040–2047.

31. Dubner R, Hargreaves KM. The neurobiology of pain and its modulation [review]. *Clin J Pain* 1989;5[Suppl 2]:S1–S4 + discussion S4–S.

32. Fisher N, Westfall T. Neuromuscular blocking agents and anti-spasticity drugs. In: Craig CR, Stitzel RE, eds. *Modern pharmacology*. Boston: Little, Brown and Company, 1982:203–213.

33. Fishman LM, Zybert PA. Electrophysiologic evidence of piriformis syndrome. *Arch Phys Med Rehabil* 1992;73:359–364.

34. Fortin JD, Aprill CN, Ponthieux B, et al. Sacroiliac joint: pain referral maps upon applying anew injection/arthrography technique. Pt II: Clinical evaluation. *Spine* 1994;19:1483–1489.

35. Fortin JD, Dwyer AP, West S, et al. Sacroiliac joint: pain referral maps upon applying a new injection/arthrography technique. Pt I: Asymptomatic volunteers. *Spine* 1994;19:1475–1482.

36. Furst DE. Are there differences among nonsteroidal antiinflammatory drugs? Comparing acetylated salicylates, nonacetylated salicylates, and nonacetylated nonsteroidal antiinflammatory drugs [review]. *Arthritis Rheum* 1994;37:1–9.

37. Garvey TA, Marks MR, Wiesel SW. A prospective, randomized, double-blind evaluation of trigger-point injection therapy for low-back pain. *Spine* 1989;14:962–964.

38. Gatchel RJ, Mayer TG, Capra P, et al. Quantification of lumbar function. Pt 6: The use of psychological measures in guiding physical functional restoration. *Spine* 1911;11:36–42.

39. Hansen FR, Bendix T, Skov P, et al. Intensive, dynamic back-muscle exercises, conventional physiotherapy, or placebo-control treatment of low-back pain: a randomized, observer-blind trial. *Spine* 1993;18:98–108.

40. Hazard RG. Spine update: functional restoration. *Spine* 1995;20:2345–2348.

41. Hazard RG, Fenwick JW, Kalisch SM, et al. Functional restoration with behavioral support. A one-year prospective study of patients with chronic low-back pain. *Spine* 1989;14:157–161.

42. Houmes RM, Voets MA, Verkaaik A, et al. Efficacy and safety of tramadol versus morphine for moderate and severe postoperative pain with special regard to respiratory depression. *Anesth Analg* 1992;74:510–514.

43. Hsu DT. Acupuncture: a review. *Reg Anesth* 1996;21:361–370.

44. Jackson RP, Jacobs RR, Montesano PX. 1988 Volvo Award in Clinical Sciences. Facet joint injection in low-back pain: a prospective statistical study. *Spine* 1988;13:966–971.

45. Jackson CP. Physical therapy for lumbar disc disease. *Semin Spine Surg* 1989;1:28–34.

46. Ketorolac tromethamine. *Med Lett Drugs Ther* 1990;32:79–81.

47. King PM. Outcome analysis of work-hardening programs. *Am J Occup Ther* 1993;47:595–603.

48. Kirkaldy-Willis WH, Hill RJ. A more precise diagnosis for low-back pain. *Spine* 1979;4:102–109.

49. Klenerman L, Gareenwood R, Davenport HT, et al. Lumbar epidural injections in the treatment of sciatica. *Br J Rheumatol* 1984;23:35–38.

50. Kohles S, Barnes D, Gatchel RJ, et al. Improved physical performance outcomes after functional restoration treatment in patients with chronic low-back pain. Early versus recent training results. *Spine* 1990;15:1321–1324.

51. Krempen J, Smith B. Nerve-root injection. *J Bone Joint Surg Am* 1974;23:35–38.

52. Larsson U, Choler U, Lidstrom A, et al. Auto-traction for treatment of lumbago-sciatica: a multicentre controlled investigation. *Acta Orthop Scand* 1980;51:791–798.

53. Long DM, Filtzer DL, BenDebba M, et al. Clinical features of the failed-back syndrome. *J Neurosurg* 1988;69:61–71.

54. Lord SM, Barnsley L, Wallis BJ, et al. Percutaneous radio-frequency neurotomy for chronic cervical zygapophyseal-joint pain. *N Engl J Med* 1996;335:1721–1726.

55. Malmberg AB, Yaksh TL. Hyperalgesia mediated by spinal glutamate or substance P receptor blocked by spinal cyclooxygenase inhibition. *Science* 1992;257:1276–1278.

56. Manniche C, Skall HF, Braendholt L, et al. Clinical trial of postoperative dynamic back exercises after first lumbar discectomy. *Spine* 1993;18:92–97.

57. Mayer T, Tabor J, Bovasso E, et al. Physical progress and residual impairment quantification after functional restoration. Part I: Lumbar mobility. *Spine* 1994;19:389–394.

58. McCarthy GM, McCarty DJ. Effect of topical capsaicin in the therapy of painful osteoarthritis of the hands. *J Rheumatol* 1992;19:604.

59. Million R, Nilsen KH, Jayson MI, et al. Evaluation of low back pain and assessment of lumbar corsets with and without back supports. *Ann Rheum Dis* 1981;40:449–454.

60. Mitchell RI, Carmen GM. The functional restoration approach to the treatment of chronic pain in patients with soft tissue and back injuries. *Spine* 1994;19:633–642.

61. Moran R, O'Connell D, Walsh MG. The diagnostic value of facet joint injections. *Spine* 1988;13:1407–1410.

62. *Physicians' Desk Reference*, 51st ed. Montvale, NJ: Medical Economics Co, 1997.

63. Rainville J, Ahern DK, Phalen L, et al. The association of pain with physical activities in chronic low back pain. *Spine* 1992;17:1060–1064.

64. Rauck RL, Ruoff GE, McMillen JI. Comparison of tramadol and acetaminophen with codeine for long-term pain management in elderly patients. *Curr Ther Res* 1994;55:1417–1431.

65. Risch SV, Norvell NK, Pollock ML, et al. Lumbar strengthening in chronic low back pain patients: physiologic and psychological benefits. *Spine* 1993;18:232–238.

66. Robert JJ, Blide RW, McWhorter K, et al. The effects of a work hardening program on cardiovascular fitness and muscular strength. *Spine* 1995;20:1187–1193.

67. Rogers P, Nash T, Schiller D, et al. Epidural steroids for sciatica. *Pain Clinic* 1992;5:67–72.

68. Roth SH. Nabumetone: a new NSAID for rheumatoid arthritis and osteoarthritis [rev]. *Orthop Rev* 1992;21:223–227.

69. Saal JA. Dynamic muscular stabilization in the nonoperative treatment of lumbar pain syndromes. *Orthop Rev* 1990;19:691–700.

70. Schwarz L, Kindermann W. Changes in beta-endorphin levels in response to aerobic and anaerobic exercise [review]. *Sports Med* 1992;13:25–36.

71. Schwarzer AC, Aprill CN, Bogduk N. The sacroiliac joint in chronic low back pain. *Spine* 1995;20:31–37.

72. Shekelle PG, Adams AH, Chassin MR, et al. Spinal manipulation for low-back pain [review]. *Ann Intern Med* 1992;17:590–598.

73. Shimm DS, Logue GL, Maltbie AA, et al. Medical management of chronic cancer pain. *JAMA* 1979;241:2408–2412.

74. Sikorski JM. A rationalized approach to physiotherapy for low-back pain. *Spine* 1985;10:571–579.

75. Snoek W, Weber H, Jorgensen B. Double blind evaluation of extradural methyl prednisolone for herniated lumbar discs. *Acta Orthop Scand* 1948;48:635–641.

76. Spangler RS. Cyclooxygenase 1 and 2 in rheumatic disease: implications for nonsteroidal anti-inflammatory drug therapy. *Semin Arthritis Rheum* 1996;26:436–448.

77. Stanley D, McLaren M, Euinton H, et al. A prospective study of nerve root infiltration in the diagnosis of sciatica. A comparison with radiculography, computed tomography and operative findings. *Spine* 1990;15:540–543.

78. Sunshine A, Olson NZ, Zighelbolm I, et al. Analgesic oral efficacy of tramadol hydrochloride in postoperative pain. *Clin Pharmacol Ther* 1992;51:740–746.

79. Swingle K, Kvam DC. Anti-inflammatory and anti-rheumatic agents. In: Craig CR, Stitzel RE, eds. *Modern pharmacology.* Boston: Little, Brown and Company, 1982:951–967.

80. Tajima T, Furukawa K, Kuramochi E. Selective lumbosacral radiculography and block. *Spine* 1980;5:68–77.

81. Taylor ME. Return to work following back surgery. A review. *Am J Ind Med* 1989;16:79–88.

82. Teasell RW, Harth M. Functional restoration. Returning patients with chronic low back pain to work—revolution or fad? [review]. *Spine* 1996;21:844–847.

83. Tennant FSJ, Uelman GF. Narcotic maintenance for chronic pain: medical and legal guidelines. *Postgrad Med* 1983;73:81–83, 86–88, 91–94.

84. Urba SG. Care of the terminally ill patient: nonpharmacologic pain management in terminal care. *Clin Geriatr Med* 1996;12:301–311.

85. van der Heijden GJ, Beurskens AJ, Koes BW, et al. The efficacy of traction for back and neck pain: a systematic, blinded review of randomized clinical trial methods. *Phys Ther* 1995;75:93–104.

86. White AH, Derby R, Wynne G. Epidural injections for diagnosis and treatment of low-back pain. *Spine* 1980;5:78–86.

87. Williams NE, Hardy PAJ, Evans AF. Spread of local anaesthetic solutions following sacral extradural (caudal) block: influence of posture. *J Spinal Disord* 1989;2:249–253.

88. McMurray RW, Hardy KJ. Cox-2 inhibitors: today and tomorrow. *Am J Med Sci* 2002;323(4):181–189.

89. Anonymous. Valdecoxib (Bextra)—a new cox-2 inhibitor. *Med Lett Drugs Ther* 2002;44(1129):34–40.

90. Vad VB, Bhat AL, Lutz GE, et al. Transforaminal steroid injections in lumbosacral radiculopathy: a prospective randomized study. *Spine* 2002;27(1):11–16.

LUMBAR SPINE: DEGENERATIVE DISEASE

ASHISH D. DIWAN, HARVINDER S. SANDHU, SAFDAR N. KHAN,
HARI K. PARVATANENI, AND FRANK P. CAMMISA, JR.

Degenerative conditions of the lumbar spine include degenerative disk disease, herniated nucleus pulposus (HNP), lumbar canal stenosis, and degenerative instability. Nearly 15% of patients with operations on the lumbar spine for degenerative causes may end up requiring another operation of the lumbar spine (40). Failed degenerative lumbar spine surgery does not imply a failure of surgery but includes development of new back and leg symptom(s) due to causes related to the surgery or as the natural progression of degenerative disease or due to an adverse alteration in the natural progression of lumbar degeneration, or both.

Operations for degenerative conditions of the lumbar spine are decompression alone, decompression and fusion procedures, or fusion of vertebrae alone. Different operations may lead to separate causes that are responsible for new symptoms in patients who have undergone low back surgery. The size of the pool of patients requiring reoperation is likely to increase with time due to the increasing rates of primary lumbar surgery. Further, as the lumbar region or lower back is the most commonly operated region of the spine and the most common cause for lower back surgery is a degenerative disorder, failure after lumbar spine surgery leads to a separate subgroup of patients.

These patients require a different approach to the understanding and management of their new set of problems when compared to their problems before the index surgery. Typically, surgeons are required to see these patients, as it is believed that surgeons know best how to evaluate the region that was visualized and dealt with by them. This chapter discusses causes that may lead to symptoms after degenerative lumbar spine surgery operations—that is, after either decompression or fusion of the lumbar spine. We attempt to summarize some recent epidemiologic information available from *International Classification of Diseases, Ninth Revision* (*ICD-9*) coding–based studies at the outset and overall results of reoperation for lumbar spine degeneration toward the later part. Sections are devoted to special situations involving osteoporotic spinal column and smokers and newer technologies that may improve quality of revision surgery, making these revision operations safer and more efficacious.

EPIDEMIOLOGY

Spinal decompression alone is performed most frequently, followed by a combination of decompression and fusion operation. Fusion of vertebral bodies as an isolated procedure is the least frequently performed operation for degenerative conditions. Patients undergoing fusion surgery have a marginally higher rate of reoperation when compared to patients undergoing decompression of the lumbar spine alone (Table 1).

PATIENT PROFILE: AGE

The spectrum of reasons for reoperation on the back depends on the type of index operation. Data from a large population-based cohort studied by Hu et al. (28) revealed that young individuals (younger than 45 years of age) are more likely to undergo diskectomy; fusion is commonly carried out as the first operation for patients in the 45- to 65-year age group, whereas people older than 65 years of age are likely to have a laminectomy performed. Their data indicated that diskectomy was associated with fewer complications than laminectomy but the elderly are 25% less likely to undergo a reoperation; hence, over a 3-year period the reoperation rate for all three groups was approximately 10%. The overall aims of reoperation are either further decompression, addition of fusion, or augmentation of fusion. The relative proportion of decompression or fusion as the second operation in the three categories is shown in Table 2.

FAILED SPINE AFTER DECOMPRESSIVE SURGERY

Revision Diskectomy

The long-term results of simple disk excision are comparable with nonoperative management for HNP when residual pain and disabilities are compared over a 15- to 20-year period. However, a simple surgical excision of a frankly prolapsed or sequestered disk

TABLE 1. FIVE-YEAR REOPERATION RATES FOR DEGENERATIVE LUMBAR SURGERY[a]

Study	Rate	Decompression	Decompression with Fusion	Fusion Alone
Washington study (40) (n = 6,376)	Annual surgical rate	83.7	10.9	5.4
	Reoperation rate	14.6	18.2[b]	
Ontario study (28) (n = 4,722)	Annual surgical rate	78.3	13.5	8.1
	Reoperation rate	9.5[c]	10.2	9.2

[a]Rates of spinal operation and reoperation in population-based cohorts studied longitudinally for 5 years. Annual surgical rate is the percent of n, and the reoperation rate is the percent in that group undergoing revision surgery. The Washington study (40) (1998) excluded federal hospitals in the state. The Ontario study (28) (1990–1991) covered all residents of Ontario (population, 10 million).
[b]Combined reoperation rate for fusion alone and decompression with fusion groups.
[c]Majority of reoperations in the Ontario decompression alone group consisted of diskectomy. In the decompression alone group, laminectomy had a 60% higher chance of leading to a complication than a diskectomy. More than two-thirds of the patients undergoing laminectomy were older than 60 years of age, whereas 60% of the patients undergoing diskectomy were between 30 years and 49 years of age.

that is causing significant leg pain or neurologic deficit, or both, provides extremely gratifying results for management of pain for the patient and for the surgeon in the short to medium term. After disk excision, a recurrence of HNP at the same site, from the same disk on the contralateral side, or from an adjacent disk can occur in up to 10% of patients (11).

In the prospective study of 365 consecutive patients, Cinotti et al. (11) report 30 patients who presented with recurrence of same-side leg pain after at least a 6-month pain-free interval following the index operation. Of these patients, 26 (7.1%) required surgery. In their case control study, Cinotti et al. (11) found that recurrence was precipitated by injury, patients with recurrence had more severe preindex-surgery-degeneration as determined by magnetic resonance imaging (MRI), early results following revision decompression for recurrence were similar to those of controls who did not have recurrence, and recurrence of nucleus pulposus did not affect the psychological status of the patients.

Peridural fibrosis following decompression surgery is referred to in the literature as a *cause* of persistent sciatica, although a direct cause-effect relationship between clinically significant pain and the peridural scar tissue has not been established. Jönsson and Strömqvist (31) found significantly poor results for reoperation of the lumbar spine after decompression surgery for degeneration in patients in whom they found fibrosis at revision surgery. Further, they report deterioration in the clinical results with time in these patients with peridural fibrosis. On the other hand, in a study in which the amount of peridural fibrosis in MRI was quantified and then correlated to clinical outcomes, Nygaard et al. (44) found no correlation between the amount of fibrous tissue and patient outcome after revision surgery. It hence appears that the poorer outcomes in the Jönsson and Strömqvist series may be due to the difficulty encountered while operating around scar tissue and not due to the scar itself.

We believe that it is important to evaluate the amount and extent of fibrosis and dural ectasia before reoperation in the lumbar spine region, in anticipation of the degree of difficulty that may be encountered during revision surgery and not as an indicator of patient symptoms. A sufficient amount of experience and ability is required to operate around the dura and nerve roots in the presence of fibrosis. A helpful technique is to define the proximal and distal end of the fibrosis before embarking on separating it from the dural layer. If the scar tissue is not likely to cause compression after adequate deroofing, it may be left adherent to the dura.

Patients with recurrent HNP need meticulous clinical evaluation. The choice of investigation for these patients is an MRI (18). MRI evaluation can be augmented by the use of gadolinium to differentiate between infective granulation tissue and imma-

TABLE 2. OVERALL PROFILE OF REOPERATION FOR LUMBAR SPINE DEGENERATION[a]

Age (Yr)	Likely Primary Operation	Chance of Reoperation at 3 Yr (%)	Likely Reoperation (Decompression: Fusion)
<45	Diskectomy	9	3:1
45–65	Fusion	11	1:3
>65	Laminectomy	10	2:1

[a]Age distribution and most likely reoperation that are needed at 3 years after lumbar spine operation as assimilated from information in Tables 1, 3, and 5 in the study by Hu et al. (28).

ture scarring. Although myelograms can provide valuable central or lateral stenosis, their value in a recurrence is limited. A root cutoff that may not correlate to clinical findings is probably due to dural scarring. The usefulness of computed tomography (CT) scans in early recurrence is similarly restricted due to the inability of many CT scanners and their software to differentiate between scar tissue and a new HNP. In a situation in which there is a recurrence at the same level and the new MRI shows changes of degeneration in the adjacent level, a diskogram may be of help in determining the "new" symptomatic level.

Revision Microdiskectomy

The recurrence rate for sciatica or persistence of symptoms following microdiskectomy is in the range of 3% to 15% (14). A recurrent HNP at the same site is the most common cause of recurrence (up to 80% of all recurrences). Other causes include disk herniation at a new site and lateral recess stenosis.

The steep learning curve in patient selection and operative skills for microdiskectomy has been overcome due to the procedure now being incorporated as an essential technique to be acquired during training. It is, however, not uncommon to see an inadequate decompression either due to incomplete disk excision or missed fragments or incomplete attention to lateral recess stenosis. On the other hand, overzealous attempts at decompression through a small portal can result in instability following facet joint transgression or stress fracture occurring later on around the joint.

The majority of recurrences following microdiskectomy is seen during the first year. However, the results of reoperation in these patients are not as good as those for patients who present first after a year following the index operation (48). This may be due to different reasons for the recurrence of symptoms in the two groups.

Patients who present with recurrence after microdiskectomy should undergo a detailed neurologic examination and imaging studies. Revision exploration for persistent or recurrent sciatica is only indicated when the distribution of symptoms correlates with an identifiable disk herniation or stenosis on an imaging study. The majority of these reexplorations can be carried out using a microscope. Backache alone as a symptom following microdiskectomy is not an indication for reexploration. Rather, it should be managed by nonoperative means followed by further reevaluation for instability if symptoms persist. Only in the event that an extensive lateral decompression leads to instability should one consider a stabilization procedure.

Laminectomy

Decompressive laminectomy is a very rewarding procedure for moderate to severe lumbar canal stenosis and has been performed for a long period with overall gratifying results. Results of revision laminectomy are discussed in the section Functional Outcomes. However, the problems seen after simple laminectomy where fusion is not carried out include stress fracture of the pars, progressive instability indicated by spondylolisthesis, postlaminectomy kyphosis, and scar tissue formation as postlaminectomy membrane. These problems can be addressed by performing a fusion of the symptomatic levels as a revision procedure. One needs to consider the option of interbody fusion either anterior or posterior, as there is an absence of posterior elements following a laminectomy.

FAILED SPINE AFTER FUSION SURGERY

The index fusion operation for degenerative disease can be performed through the anterior approach, either by one of the laparoscopic techniques or via an open approach. From the posterior approach these interfacet with intertransverse fusions, referred to as *posterolateral fusions*, can either be instrumented or noninstrumented. All of these surgeries are usually done with a decompression of the canal at lesser, similar, or more levels than the fused segment. A third type of fusion, which can be performed from the posterior approach, is a posterior lumbar interbody fusion. A combination of the interbody fusions (either anterior or posterior) along with posterolateral fusion is a fourth type of fusion known as *360-degree fusion*.

Failures of any four of these fusion techniques vary in their details; however, the common causes of failure are discussed below. Examples of failed lumbar spine following fusion are shown in Figures 1 to 5.

Pseudarthrosis

The term *pseudarthrosis* in spinal fusion is applied when there is a failure of osseous bridging within the fusion mass as evaluated by plain x-rays, tomograms, stress films, CT scans, or CT scans with sagittal reconstruction. One year after surgery is the accepted time when a lack of fusion can be labeled as pseudarthrosis. A failure of bridging bone across vertebral bodies in anterior lumbar interbody fusion or posterior lumbar interbody fusion and across facet joints in posterolateral lumbar fusion is also referred to as *pseudarthrosis*. The most common cause of pseudarthrosis is continued smoking by the patient following surgery. The

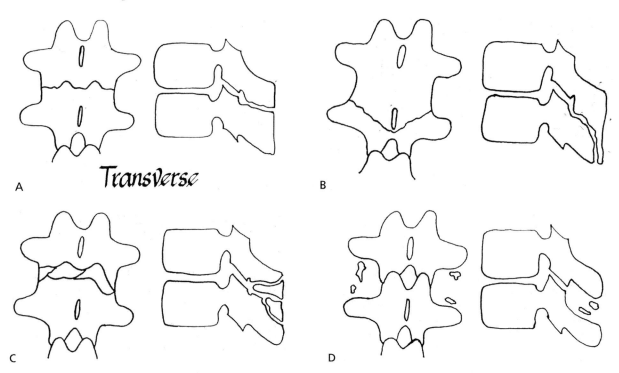

Transverse

FIGURE 1. Various types of pseudarthrosis, as described by Heggeness et al. (25).

reported rate of pseudarthrosis following lumbar surgery varies considerably in the literature (Table 3).

Heggeness et al. (25) histologically evaluated specimens from 35 patients undergoing revision surgery for failed posterior spinal fusion. No bursal structures as described for long bone pseudarthrosis were found. Dense fibrous tissue stroma between bone ends and the presence of necrotic bone pieces were

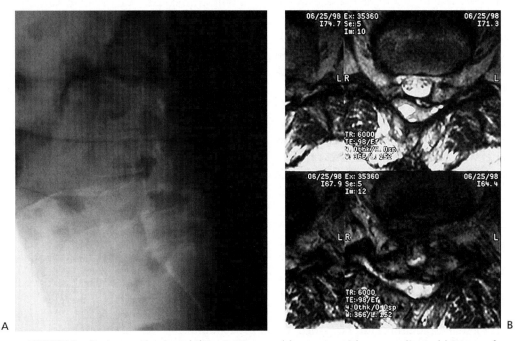

FIGURE 2. Postoperative instability. A 53-year-old woman with a complicated history of several back operations over a 2-year period presented with disabling back pain and left leg pain. Index operation was an L4-5 decompressive laminectomy followed by revision decompression and instrumented fusion. This was complicated by a dural tear and infection, which were addressed by multiple procedures. On presentation to us, she had a gross L4-5 instability with spondylolisthesis **(A)** and plain films with canal stenosis **(B)** myelogram. *(continued)*

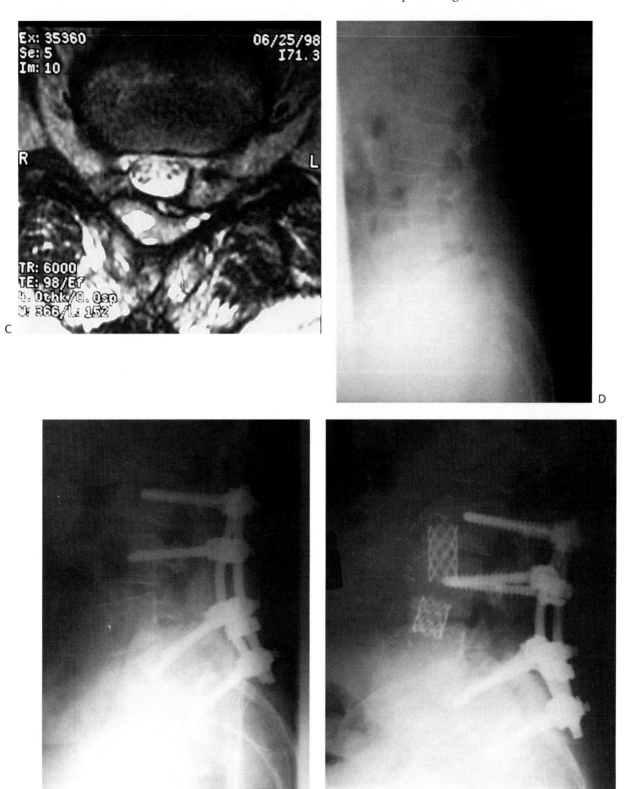

FIGURE 2. (*continued*) On presentation, she also had a persistent durocoele with granulation tissue magnetic resonance imaging **(C)**. The listhesis reduced partially on the operating table **(D)**. She underwent a three-stage procedure. The first was a biopsy and débridement, the second was a posterior decompression and fusion using pedicle screw instrumentation and iliac crest bone grafting **(E)**, and the third was a procedure to achieve anterior interbody fusion for L-2 to S-1 **(F)**. She was asymptomatic at 2.5 years after revision surgery.

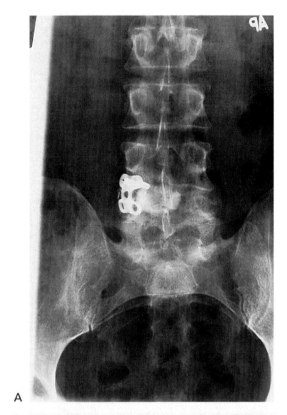

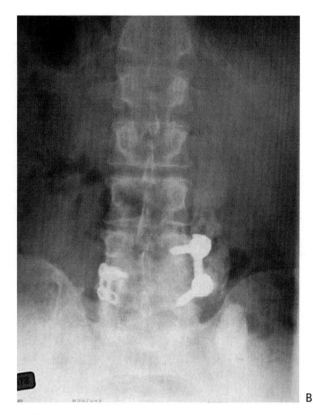

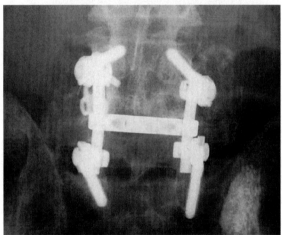

FIGURE 3. Painful implant, adjacent degeneration. A 55-year-old man presented with disabling low back pain. His index operation was an L4-5 laminectomy in March 1994, followed by an anterior fusion from the left **(A)** 2 years later and then a posterior spinal fusion **(B)** after an interval of 2 years. Initial evaluation by us revealed no abnormal movement in flexion/extension and lateral radiographs. No stenosis was seen on magnetic resonance imaging, and a nonpainful disk was present at L2-3, L3-4, and L-5 to S-1 diskography. However, the patient was greatly relieved by local anesthetic injection around the implant. Removal of implant was an option, but in due course, his pain became severe and unresponsive to local anesthetic injection. He was managed nonoperatively for 12 months. When a repeat diskogram of L-5 to S-1 demonstrated concordant pain, revision fusion from L-4 to S-1 was performed 6 months after operation, and radiographs revealed excellent bone formation.

the hallmarks of fusion mass pseudarthrosis. Further, none of the specimens stained positive for S100 protein, which is a neural tissue marker. It hence may be possible that structures other than the pseudarthrosis may be painful due to continuing movement or instability. Heggeness and Esses (26) further analyzed 85 pseudarthroses and proposed four morphologic types: transverse (Fig. 1A), shingle (Fig. 1B), complex (Fig. 1C), and atrophic (Fig. 1D).

It is difficult to diagnose pseudarthrosis. One looks for a possible pseudarthrosis in patients who present with persistent pain. However, one should remember that a large number of pseudarthroses remain pain free, and, further, when a pseudarthrosis is present with pain, the pain can also arise from other structures

in the back (e.g., adjacent level disk). A complete evaluation of such a patient for the source of pain before planning a repair of the pseudarthrosis is, therefore, mandatory. One should also look for potentially correctable host factors. These include anemia, phosphate depletion secondary to antacid (ab)use, vitamin D abnormalities, malabsorption syndrome, and excessive tobacco and alcohol use.

Flat Back

The term *flat back* refers to a decrease in the lumbar lordosis or a frank kyphosis of the lumbar spine. It can be caused by distraction instrumentation placed posteriorly (such as Harrington rods), multiple or

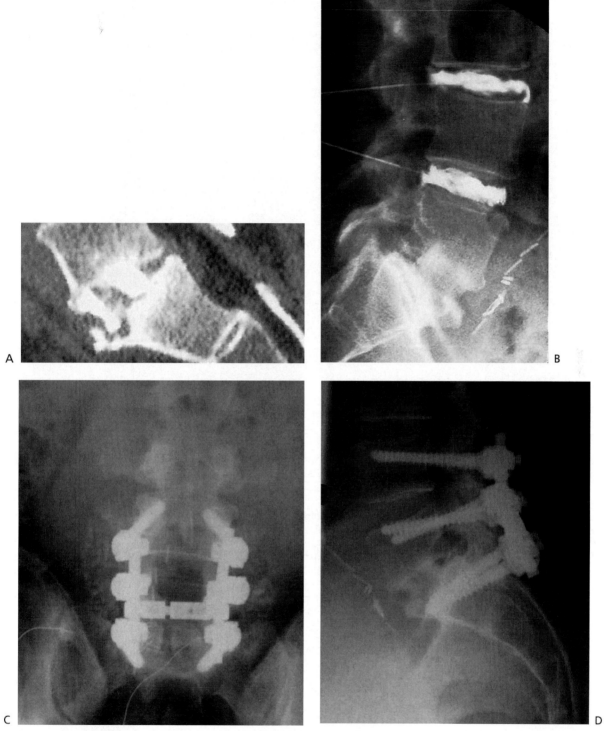

FIGURE 4. Pseudarthrosis following anterior lumbar interbody fusion. A 50-year-old man underwent a laparoscopic transperitoneal anterior lumbar interbody fusion at L-5 to S-1 using two threaded allograft cortical dowels with autograft packed within in February 1998 for long-standing degenerative disk disease. One year later, he continued to have pain. Computed tomography scan **(A)** shows a failure of anterior lumbar interbody fusion pseudarthrosis. One month later, right-sided radiculopathy developed, with magnetic resonance image showing evidence of a degenerative disk bulge at L3-4 and L4-5 with L4-5 lateral foraminal stenosis. A diskogram **(B)** revealed concordant pain for L4-5 disk injection. A posterolateral instrumented fusion **(C, D)** from L-4 to S-1 with an L4-5 decompression was performed using frameless image-guided stereotactic guidance and demineralized bone matrix augmented autograft.

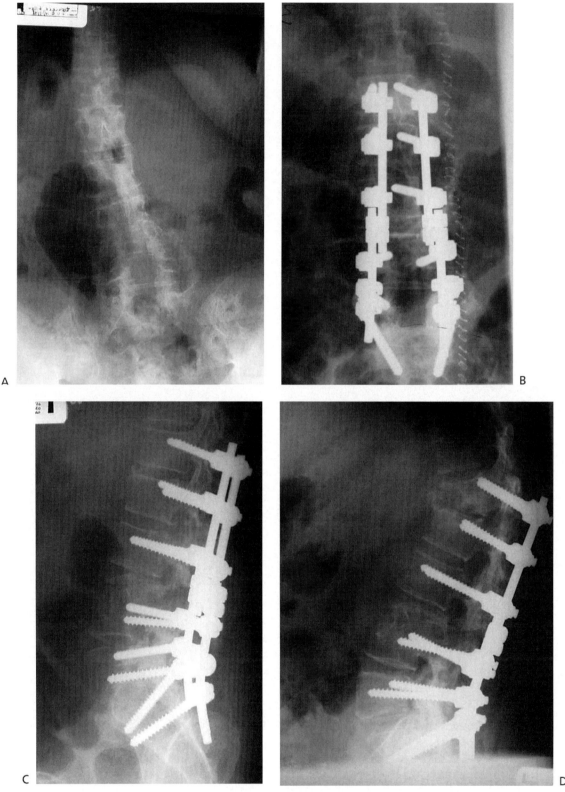

FIGURE 5. Flat back juxtafusion kyphosis. A 49-year-old woman presented with severe back pain and flat back **(A)** after instrumented decompression fusion of the lumbar spine that was complicated by infection. Instrumentation was removed, leading to L3-4 disk space collapse. Preoperatively, she was diagnosed as having osteoporosis, and antiosteoporotic medication was initiated. Anterior surgery was ruled out because of morbid obesity and scarring. A one-stage posterior decancellation osteotomy at L-3 with fusion from T-12 to S-1 was performed **(B)**. The patient did well in the postoperative period; however, 9 months after surgery a junctional kyphosis developed with wedge compression of the T-12 vertebra due to osteoporosis **(C)**. This was corrected by proximal extension of fusion.

TABLE 3. INCIDENCES OF PSEUDARTHROSIS AFTER LUMBAR SURGERY

Fusion Type	Incidence Range
Intertransverse	3.0–25.5%
Anterior interbody	4–68%
Posterior interbody	6–27%

Modified from Steinmann JC, Herkowitz HN. Pseudarthrosis of the spine. *Clin Orthop* 1992;284:80–90.

single level disk space collapse (due to degeneration or infection following surgery) leading to kyphosis, and postlaminectomy kyphosis. Flat back is a disabling condition, as the patient may flex the hips during stance to prevent the upper trunk from pitching forward. Hip flexion in these patients is then compensated for by knee flexion, associated with fatigability, decreased walking distance, and knee pain.

Most patients with flat back need a surgical solution for their problem. If the deformity is correctable passively as revealed by hyperextension films, posterior instrumentation in the correct position followed by anterior intervertebral body fusion can be carried out. If the deformity is fixed, anterior multiple-level diskectomies with structural grafts in the corrected position combined with a posterior instrumentation-fusion procedure should be carried out. If the deformity is associated with bony fusion across most of the lumbar spine, osteotomies in the front or back or pedicle subtraction osteotomies from the posterior aspect alone can be performed.

Adjacent Level Failures

The problems in the adjacent regions of the fusion mass, cephalad as well as caudad, can be kyphosis, scoliosis, degenerative, or a combination of these problems. Juxtafusion issues arise from an abrupt transition from a mobile to a fused segment. One should be aware of these problems when evaluating a patient who has undergone fusion of the lumbar spine.

Juxtafusion Kyphosis

Juxtafusion kyphosis occurs at the cephalic end of the fusion mass, probably because of abnormally high loading associated with an increased mobility in this region. The kyphosis can occur as a result of a compression fracture of the last unfused vertebra, collapse of the terminal unfused disk anteriorly, wedge compression of the proximalmost fused vertebral body, or a combination of these. Juxtafusion kyphosis may appear in a dramatic fashion when it is associated with bony wedge compression, or it may be insidious when

associated with degeneration of the disk. While evaluating patients with juxtafusion kyphosis, one needs to (a) remember that the apex of the thoracic kyphosis is normally in the region of the T-7 vertebra and (b) evaluate the quality of bone, specifically looking for osteoporosis. As osteoporosis is a major challenge and closely related to juxtafusion kyphosis, we discuss this again later in this chapter.

Bracing to prevent juxtafusion kyphosis has no role in clinical practice. Juxtafusion kyphosis, which is small, pain free, and nondisabling, can be managed nonoperatively by activity modification and use of a hyperextension brace. Dramatic juxtafusion kyphosis or one that is painful and disabling has to be addressed surgically by proximal extension of the fusion either through the approach previously used (most commonly posterior), an anterior approach, or a combined anterior-posterior procedure. One should, however, not stop the proximal extension either at or just below the kyphosis at T-7 vertebra.

Juxtafusion Scoliosis

As in the case of juxtafusion kyphosis, juxtafusion scoliosis can occur if the collapse of the body or disk structures occurs laterally. In correcting the deformity, care must be taken to address compensatory curves and to include at least the end vertebra in the extension of fusion. When a surgical option is exercised, more often than not an anterior spinal fusion is recommended with posterior realignment and extension of fusion.

Juxtafusion Degeneration

Degenerative changes in the facets and disk adjacent to the fusion mass usually occur in the caudal region. Injury to these structures can occur during surgery, especially the posterior facet joints, or later on due to increased mobility around the first intervertebral disk caudad to the fusion. These degenerative conditions can present as degenerative disk, HNP, retrolisthesis, canal stenosis, facet arthritis, or a combination of these. Although there is a paucity of data to definitely state whether this juxtafusion degeneration is a natural, age-related phenomenon of the lumbar disks or is an accelerated degeneration due to adjacent fused segments, it is a robust clinical observation that this degeneration adjacent to the fusion mass occurs as a result of the altered mechanics in the region of the fused-unfused segment.

The plan for managing this intricate problem is related to the patients' symptoms. Initially, nonoperative treatment must be stressed for these individuals. A failure of nonoperative measures calls for surgical intervention, which on rare occasions may be decompression alone. More frequently, an extension of fusion is carried out.

Failures under Fusion

A painful disk under a posterolateral fusion may lead to a "failed back surgery." This can be evaluated by diskography. An anterior disk excision and fusion using an anterior interbody device (metallic or cortical bone graft) can be used.

Symptoms of radiculopathy may persist or arise afresh under a fusion mass. If imaging studies discover significant canal stenosis, it may necessitate a decompression of the canal.

Insufficiency fractures of vertebral bodies within a fused segment are known to occur. These may remain painful for a long time, as collapse of the body is prevented by the fusion mass, thereby delaying union. External bone stimulators and chronic pain management strategies with antiosteoporotic medication can be initiated.

Broken, Loose, or Painful Implants

The safety of using pedicle screws, hooks, rods, plates, sublaminar wires, and interbody devices is well established in various clinical settings. Modern day implants are strong enough to withstand repetitive cyclical loading. However, if fusion is delayed, the stress may overcome the forces at the fixation point of screws and hooks or the strength of rods and plates, leading to loosening or breakage. Indications for revision are pain or instability, or both, due to pseudarthrosis. Loose and broken sublaminar wires have the potential to cause neurologic damage, especially if a pseudarthrosis is present, and thus need to be removed in such situations.

Implants can become painful when they are prominent and can be palpated, specifically in the lumbosacral junction. This can be avoided by using low-profile implants. Implant protuberance may form a bursa that may get inflamed and cause pain. These bursas also have the potential to become infected. Hardware in deeper tissue may give rise to pain, possibly because of aseptic inflammation in response to fretting corrosion. Diagnosis can be confirmed by infiltrating local anesthetic around the implant and assessing for relief of pain. Trimming or removal of the implant is indicated for very painful implants, impending infection of a bursa associated with an implant, or a frankly infected implant with solid fusion.

SPECIAL CONSIDERATIONS

Revision Lumbar Spine Surgery and Osteoporosis

Osteoporosis can be classified as either primary or secondary (35). Primary osteoporosis is due to the inevitable physiologic changes associated with aging along with environmental factors. Secondary osteoporosis is due to a disease process or agent that accounts for a change in bone mineral density—for example, primary hypothyroidism, family history, males with hypogonadism, oral glucocorticoid use for greater than 3 months, and so forth. Smoking, alcohol, sedentary lifestyle with low dietary intake of calcium and vitamin D, low body weight (<127 lb), anticonvulsants, antineoplastic agents, and heparin are also implicated in the development of osteoporosis (32,35). The World Health Organization has defined osteoporosis as a bone mineral density value of more than 2.5 standard deviations below peak bone mass (32,35).

As the life expectancy and quality of life in elderly patients have increased, so has their desire to remain pain free and active in everyday life. As a result, surgeons have seen an increase in older patients who are willing to undergo surgery for a variety of painful spine conditions—for example, spinal stenosis, spondylolisthesis, degenerative disk disease, and so forth—with a high expectation of pain relief and functional recovery.

Preoperatively, most of these patients are osteoporotic as well as poorly nourished, are functionally impaired, or have a debilitating chronic disease. It is important to see these patients as part of an interdisciplinary team for their medical management. Intraoperative difficulties with instrument fixation or postoperative instrument failure can be a significant problem in these patients. Postoperatively, osteoporosis also contributes to junctional failure as well as juxtafusion fractures. In these difficult scenarios, it is evident that spine surgeons must be cognizant of revision strategies and outcomes for spine surgery in osteoporotic individuals.

A combined approach that accommodates the anterior and the posterior columns must be taken when dealing with osteoporotic patients. Appropriate instrumentation is critical, and segmental instrumentation allowing multiple points of fixation-like pedicle screws, laminar hooks, or sublaminar wires is usually indicated in these patients.

Intraoperative Failure of Fixation

Inadequate bone quality that is evident during drilling or probing the pedicle, leading to poor purchase of pedicle screws, is the most common example of mechanical failure due to osteoporosis. Failure of pedicle screw fixation in relation to bone mineral density has been demonstrated in numerous studies. Axial pullout of pedicle screws has been directly implicated with decreased bone mineral density (12,23,46,64). However, pedicle screws inserted with laminar hooks appear to provide the greatest resistance to pullout. This is attributed to the fact that the laminae, being more cortical than cancellous, are more slowly affected by osteoporosis. However, this is not always possible due to a concomitant decompressive laminectomy performed in these patients. Progressive osteoporosis leads to thinning of the cortex and widening of the medullary canal, resulting in a wider inner diameter of the pedicle (28). As a result, failure of pedicle screw fixation in osteoporotic patients has also been attributed to poor fit of the screw within the pedicle. In terms of technique, lateral shifting of the instrumented motion segment can be prevented by nonparallel placement of the screws in an upward and inward direction (34,65). Insertion of sublaminar wires or cables can also strengthen the construct.

Augmentation vertebroplasty has been described to improve the fixation of the unanchored screw. In this procedure, 2 to 3 mL of pressurized methylmethacrylate is injected into the vertebral body through the drilled or probed pedicle. This procedure has been contraindicated when the outer pedicle cortex has been breached due to the danger of extrusion of the methylmethacrylate out of the vertebral body and into the foramen or spinal canal (54).

When fixation at a particular segment is impossible, the surgeon has two options. The first is to perform an uninstrumented *in situ* fusion with the patient using external bracing. The second, more radical approach is to extend the fusion above or below the preexisting fusion mass so that adequate fixation can be achieved.

Postoperative Failure of Fixation

The signs of immediate postoperative hardware failure include sudden pain, deformity, and subcutaneous prominence of the instrumentation. A change in position or radiolucency around the hardware signifies hardware pullout. Hardware prominence and immediate pain are indications for revision surgery; change in position can usually be treated with conservative measures. Late hardware loosening may be a sign of pseudarthrosis and could necessitate revision fusion with instrumentation or augmentation with an anterior procedure, commonly an anterior release with strut graft-

ing. This may reduce the flexion/extension moments applied to the posterior instrumentation, hence sparing the pedicle screws from cyclical loading and loosening.

Correction of Deformity

Junctional kyphosis is a significant problem in osteoporotic patients. They usually have solid fusions but present with severe pain and a new deformity. Kyphotic deformities develop as a result of failure of the anterior column. Treatment usually involves an initial conservative course with bracing, analgesics, and medical management; however, surgical extension of the fusion is usually necessary. Kyphotic deformity due to anterior column deficiency can be surgically treated by either restoring the anterior column height or shortening the posterior and middle column to achieve the same effect. Restoring anterior column height with strut grafts may cause graft penetration into the thin vertebral bodies, thus achieving sagittal plane balance by shortening the posterior and middle column with an eggshell osteotomy; a posterior closing wedge osteotomy is more rewarding. In either case, it is essential for the surgeon to be gentle with the remaining bone stock at the fusion levels. Soft, osteoporotic bone may predispose to vertebral damage with mechanical distractive devices. The endplate may be violated in situations in which iliac crest strut grafts are used as they cut into the endplate. Considering that much of the anterior graft's mechanical support comes from the endplate, this could be devastating. As a result, allografts with larger surface areas such as tibial or femoral diaphyseal ring allografts tend to provide a greater surface area.

Autogenous bone grafting in revision osteoporotic patients certainly does not make life easier for the spine surgeon. Preoperative assessment of the location to harvest autogenous bone graft must be undertaken, as most patients at the revision stage already have had one previous autologous bone graft procedure performed. Preoperative CT scan to assess the possibility of harvesting the same iliac crest again is important. Insufficiency fractures through the pelvis may occur in patients with extensive fusion with more than one autogenous iliac crest bone harvest. Mixing demineralized bone matrix preparations or bone marrow aspirate with the available autograft is another option. The potential role of growth factors for osteoaugmentation is discussed below.

Revision Lumbar Spine Surgery in Smokers

The healing of spine fusions depends on many local and systemic factors (Table 4). These factors can

TABLE 4. FACTORS THAT AFFECT OUTCOME OF REVISION SPINAL SURGERY

Positive impact
  Identifiable cause of symptoms (e.g., compression by disk or osteophyte)
  Clinical and radiologic correlation
  Radicular or compressive symptoms predominant
  Definite period of improvement in symptoms after index surgery (particularly if >6 mo)
  Fewer surgical levels
  Successful repair of pseudarthrosis present at the time of revision surgery
  Stable spine
  High level of functioning preoperatively and a high level of motivation
  High level of understanding by the patient of his or her condition; a high level of education
Negative impact
  Scarring, fibrosis, arachnoiditis
  Pending litigation, worker's compensation, or other secondary gain issues
  Smoking (pack-years)
  Increasing age, significant comorbidities, obesity
  Abnormal psychological profile
  High number of prior surgical procedures

negatively and positively affect healing of the fusion mass. A positive or successful outcome of surgery is a good, solid fusion at the desired level, resulting in pain relief or abatement of preoperative symptoms. However, a spine surgeon is faced with a poor outcome, most commonly in the form of a pseudarthrosis. The most common cause leading to the failure of fusion is cigarette smoking. Nonunion rates increase to as much as fourfold in patients who smoke before surgery (3,24). Nicotine in cigarette smoke interferes with bone metabolism and prevents revascularization and osteogenesis. Brown et al. (6) compared 50 nonsmokers with 50 smokers who had undergone a two-level laminectomy and fusion. Follow-up after 1 to 2 years revealed that a pseudarthrosis had developed in 40% of smokers, whereas only 4% of nonsmokers failed to fuse.

Detailed history taking at the time of index and then revision surgery can alert the spine surgeon to patients who are smokers. They must be counseled before their revision surgery again to cease smoking completely, as it adversely affects their chances of a complete bony union. They must be made aware of the risks of continued cigarette smoking on bone healing. Time and patience must be invested in these patients, as modifying this aspect of their lifestyle can drastically affect the outcome of the surgery.

In the event of revision surgery due to continued smoking after index surgery, patients must again be counseled and directed to the fact that failure of fusion can be directly attributed to their persistent smoking. Surgical options are similar to those for pseudarthrosis due to any other reason. Additional measures include the use of internal and external electromagnetic stimulators.

Interest has been shown in the use of osteoinductive growth factors to reverse the inhibitory effect of nicotine. Silcox et al. (53) examined the effect of an osteoinductive bone protein extract on spinal fusion in the presence of nicotine in a rabbit model. A 100% fusion rate was achieved in the experimental group (with the bone protein plus autograft), whereas there was no fusion in the control group (autograft alone). The authors concluded that the inhibitory effect in an established nicotine-induced nonunion model could be overcome with the use of bone growth factors in an animal model. This study validated the use of growth factors in cases in which fusion was difficult to achieve. It remains to be seen how soon these growth factors can be used routinely in surgical practice as an adjunct to surgery.

NEW TECHNOLOGIES IN REVISION SURGERY

Computerized Frameless Stereotactic Image-Guidance

Computerized frameless stereotactic image-guidance technology has been available to spine surgeons for approximately 4 years. Modifications and updates to the various navigation systems as well as improvements in their usability have increased their applicability and usefulness. Presently, the most widely used modalities for data acquisition are CT scanning preoperatively or fluoroscopy intraoperatively. Consequently, for spine surgery, this technology is used predominantly for bony navigation. Numerous reports in the literature have documented high levels of accuracy of instrumentation in the lumbosacral spine (8,51), mainly relating to transpedicular instrumentation. Several of these reports compare instrumentation using traditional techniques to instrumentation using computerized image-guidance and demonstrate higher accuracy rates in the latter group.

Traditionally, localization of bony components of the spine and associated structures that are not visualized through standard surgical approaches has been achieved via estimation of their anatomic relationships to more prominent structures and landmarks. If instrumentation is necessary for an intervertebral level that has been previously operated on, the normal bony anatomic landmarks may not be present or are altered (e.g., by decompression or a prior attempt at fusion); fibrous scar tissue may further hamper the identification of these landmarks. Accuracy of transpedicular instrumentation is important in avoiding complications related to hardware placement (e.g., nerve root injury) as well as in providing a biomechanically advantageous construct to facilitate bony fusion.

In principle, computerized image-guided navigation systems provide interactive anatomic data in multiple planes that are not normally available to the surgeon intraoperatively. When they are combined with clinical judgment, the surgeon can effectively determine and use appropriate entry points, trajectories, and depths for insertion of hardware. Computerized image-guidance may thus have a significant role in the clinical scenario of instrumentation of a spine that has been operated on previously. We have reported the preliminary findings of an ongoing study looking at the accuracy of transpedicular instrumentation in patients undergoing revision lumbar spinal fusion (45). Approximately 95% of pedicle screws assessed using CT scans were found to be well placed, whereas approximately 5% were found to expand the lateral cortices of their respective pedicles. No screws were misplaced.

New Transfusion Technology

Prolonged surgical times as well as wider surgical exposures predispose patients undergoing revision surgery to increased intraoperative blood loss. The extent of additional blood loss in revision lumbar surgery is unclear but is expected to be more significant with increasing surgical levels, bony decompression, and instrumentation (28). Morbidity can be decreased if these factors are identified and accounted for perioperatively. Effective strategies for minimizing the effects of elevated blood loss include adequate autologous predonation, erythropoietin therapy preoperatively, intraoperative acute normovolemic hemodilution, hypotensive anesthesia, and autologous reinfusion via cell salvage.

Growth Factors

Bone healing is mediated by numerous growth factors, all of which play an essential role in osseous repair. These polypeptides are provided by the bone matrix itself and have become an important area of research in an effort to enhance all aspects of bone regeneration, be it fracture repair or osseous integration in spine fusions. They include transforming growth factor betas, bone morphogenetic proteins (BMPs), fibroblast growth factors, insulin-like growth factors, and platelet-derived growth factors.

Of these substances, BMP has been the most extensively investigated. Recombinant BMP has been produced through genetically modified cell lines as a singular molecular species in virtually unlimited quantities.

Many preclinical studies have been performed to establish the efficacy of BMP in orthotopic environments. The most significant of these studies have been those performed on nonhuman primates. Boden et al. (4) demonstrated anterior lumbar intervertebral fusions without autogenous bone graft in rhesus monkeys after implantation of a threaded, hollow fusion cage filled with a collagenous sponge containing rhBMP-2. Each of the primates implanted with the growth factor had histologically confirmed solid fusion 6 months after surgery. No fusions occurred under sham conditions in which the collagen carrier was implanted without rhBMP-2.

Based on the exciting results of preclinical investigations, several pilot human trials have been initiated within the past few years. Boden et al. (5) have reported on the efficacious osteoinductive capacity of rhBMP-2 for primary one-level human spinal fusion application when compared to autograft controls in a limited multicenter study involving 14 patients.

The development and success of these recombinant growth factors have ushered in a new era in the treatment of failed spine fusions. The study by Silcox et al. (53) clearly demonstrated the efficacy of growth factors in the face of a difficult healing environment (i.e., the presence of systemic nicotine). Currently, rhBMP-2 is being studied in a variety of spinal clinical trials. As promising data continue to come in, spine surgeons wait eagerly for approval for the use of growth factors not just in primary spine fusions but in difficult revision spine cases.

SAFETY AND EFFICACY OF REVISION LUMBAR SPINAL SURGERY

Complications (Safety)

Reoperation on the lumbar spine is typically associated with a higher level of complexity than with primary surgery. This is mostly due to the presence of fibrous scar tissue, dural adhesions, altered anatomy, and poor tissue quality. Revision surgery can hence be expected to predispose patients to higher rates of complications.

The rates of misplaced pedicle screws for revision lumbar surgery vary in the reported literature but continue to be high (10,59), and rates of associated neurologic injury have been reported at 2% (61) and 3.2% (52). Complications of improper hardware placement (e.g., neurologic injury), especially with transpedicular instrumentation, are more likely in revision spine cases because of the greater challenge posed by alteration of surgical anatomy by previous surgical decompression or attempts at fusion. This must be carefully considered when the surgeon makes decisions regarding the surgical procedure and hardware to be used for treatment. Increased intraoperative vigilance, including the use of neurologic monitoring, helps to avoid or detect complications. Applicability of computerized image-guidance technology in this setting is described in Computerized Frameless Stereotactic Image-Guidance.

Deep wound infections complicating spine surgery have been reported to occur in approximately 2.1% of cases (59). The incidence varies with the procedure being performed (39,41,49) but has been shown to be lowest with diskectomy (approximately 1%) and highest with posterior instrumented fusion (3.2–7.2%). Increased length of surgery, more extensive exposures, greater amounts of fibrous scar tissue, and poorer tissue quality (decreased vascularity) are all associated with revision surgery, and all predispose to wound infection. Wound infections complicating revision surgery that are treated using standard protocols of parenteral antibiotics and surgical débridement are expected to have similar outcomes as for primary surgery.

Dural tears are undesired complications in spine surgery and are a significant source of anxiety for spine surgeons. Goodkin and Laska (22) found that dural tears were the second most frequent reason for litigation relating to spine surgery. Reports have, however, demonstrated that long-term results of spine surgery are unchanged by the occurrence of dural tears when treated appropriately (7,30,57). Cammisa et al. (7) have demonstrated higher rates of dural tears in revision spine surgery when compared to primary surgery, with rates being highest in decompression surgery. Fibrous scar tissue, dural adhesions, and greater difficulty in visualization during exposure all contribute to a higher rate of dural injury. An indefinite relationship was observed between dural tears and wound infection. A higher rate of deep wound infection was noted in surgery complicated with dural tears when compared to the overall infection rate for all surgeries (8.1% vs. 2.1%). No conclusions could be drawn regarding this, but this finding may be attributable to the higher rates of dural tears in revision surgical cases, which in turn predispose patients to wound infections. All of these findings underscore the importance of preoperative consideration of the numerous factors that make revision operation a surgical challenge.

Functional Outcomes

Several challenges are faced by the spine surgeon during the identification of specific surgical problems of the lumbar spine, correlation of clinical and laboratory findings with symptomatology, selection of suitable surgical candidates, and determination of ideal surgical interventions on an individual basis. These challenges increase significantly in patients who have had prior surgery, especially with failed back surgery. The symptomatology becomes less specific and less distinguishable (particularly with nonradicular problems), imaging of the spine is impaired by scar tissue and instrumentation, secondary gain issues cloud true clinical symptoms, and postfusion problems such as instability and pseudarthrosis may lead to more extensive revision or salvage procedures.

In reviewing the literature related to repeat lumbar spine surgery, several important parameters that have an impact on outcomes are highlighted. These are summarized in Table 4. These factors have varying impact from case to case but, in patients in whom they are applicable, seem to have significant correlation with outcomes.

Several reports of outcomes after revision surgery are summarized in Table 5. Good results after revision surgery have been reported to occur in approximately 25% to 80% of cases (2,16,36–38,50,60,62). The reported success rates for spine surgery vary significantly from series to series, but, overall, revision surgery is reported to have poorer outcomes than primary surgery. Additionally, the outcomes vary according to the procedure being performed, with better results reported with revision decompressive procedures including diskectomy than with revision fusion cases. Nasca (42) has reported better results after lumbar spinal stenosis surgery when performed primarily than when done as part of revision surgery (79.2% vs. 59.4% good results).

Cammisa et al. (68) have compared clinical outcomes of patients who underwent primary diskectomy (n = 30) to those who underwent revision diskectomy (n = 27). Except for frequency and severity of residual lower limb numbness (greater in the revision group), symptomatic outcomes and patient functioning were similar between groups. Additionally, patient satisfaction with surgery was similar between the two groups, with 80% or more of patients deriving significant improvement in their condition.

In one of the earliest reports on recurrent disk herniation treated with laminectomy and diskectomy without fusion, Epstein et al. (15) reported an

TABLE 5. OUTCOMES FOLLOWING REVISION SPINAL SURGERY BY PROCEDURE TYPE

Study (Yr)	No. of Patients	Mean Follow-Up (Mo)	Good or Excellent Outcome (%)
Revision lumbar decompression (including diskectomy)			
Jönsson and Strömqvist (31) (1993)[a]	91	24	45.1 (excellent)
Herron (27) (1994)[b]	46	54	69 (good)
Ozgen et al. (47) (1999)[c]	114	41.2	69.2 (good)
Revision lumbar surgery involving fusion and decompression			
Lehmann and LaRocca (38) (1981)[d]	36	36	56 (satisfactory)
Biondi and Greenberg (2) (1990)[e]	45	29	47 (good)
Carpenter et al. (9) (1996)[f]	72	51	26 (good or excellent)
Revision lumbar surgery—all types			
Finnegan et al. (17) (1979)[g]	67	48	11.9 (good)
Kim and Michelsen (33) (1992)[h]	50	59	66 (significant improvement)
Bernard (1) (1993)[i]	45	28.2	82 (successful)
Stewart and Sachs (56) (1996)[j]	39	48	72 (successful)
Curylo et al. (13) (2000)[k]	63	88	89 (good or excellent)

[a]Patients with disk herniation (n = 19) or stenosis (n = 37) had significantly better results than those with fibrosis (n = 35): 62.5% vs. 17.1%.

[b]All patients had recurrent disk herniations. Patients with pending litigation or work-related injuries had poorer outcomes (38.5% good).

[c]Patients with disk herniation (n = 89) had better results than those with fibrosis or arachnoiditis (n = 18).

[d]Better outcomes were noted in patients with >18 mo between primary and revision surgery vs. those with <18 mo (76% satisfactory outcome vs. 36%). Pseudarthrosis, as the sole indication for revision surgery, was reported to be associated with poorer outcomes. Objective preoperative findings of a surgically correctable lesion were associated with best results.

[e]Factors significantly associated with poor results were worker's compensation, <6 mo pain-free interval between surgeries, high degree of fibrosis, and male gender.

[f]All patients underwent revision surgery for pseudarthrosis, and 94% went on to fuse. Smoking had a significant negative effect on results, whereas cessation preoperatively had a significantly positive effect.

[g]Mechanical compression, instability, and pain-free intervals of >1 yr between surgeries correlated with better outcomes. Fibrosis and pending litigation/worker's compensation cases correlated with poorer results.

[h]Disk herniation (86.7% successful vs. 57.1% successful for other diagnoses), successful fusion of pseudarthroses (81.3% successful vs. 23.1% successful for nonfusion), and intervals of >24 mo between surgeries had a positive impact on outcomes.

[i]Factors with positive impact on outcomes were return to occupation, fusion, and noncompensable/nonlitigious injury.

[j]Factors with positive impact on outcomes included return to occupation, younger age, initial period of symptomatic improvement, and fewer numbers of spinal levels at the index procedure.

[k]All cases involved same-level revisions. The trend was toward better outcomes with surgery for recurrent herniated nucleus pulposus or degenerative deformity than for recurrent stenosis. Also, better outcomes were attained with fusion surgery (with or without decompression) than with decompression surgery alone.

81% rate of good outcomes. It is clear from reports that revision surgery is associated with better results when done for true disk herniations than for symptoms that are thought to be arising from fibrotic scar tissue. Additionally, fusion is not indicated as a routine adjunct to revision diskectomy unless intervertebral instability or other confounding factors are present.

For cases that involve decompression and fusion, the long-term outcomes have been reported to be worse than the outcomes for revision surgery involving decompression only. A short symptom-free interval, pseudarthrosis as the surgical indication, and smoking all have a negative impact on outcome. Stronger indications for fusion (e.g., instability) were associated with better outcomes. Glassman et al. (20) demonstrated that patients undergoing primary lumbar fusion with high preoperative scores on the SF-36 questionnaire in terms of social functioning and pain were less likely to undergo revision surgery than patients with lower scores in these two categories.

Glassman et al. (21) also demonstrated that, in patients who were undergoing lumbar fusion after a prior lumbar diskectomy, significant improvements occurred in physical function, social function, and bodily pain as obtained with the use of the SF-36 questionnaire at 1 year after surgery. Negative effects in several parameters were associated with pending worker's compensation or litigation cases, lower educational levels, and patients younger than 50 years of age.

Frymoyer et al. (19) reviewed 45 patients who required revision surgery at 10 or more years after the index surgery. They found that patients who underwent revision decompression only or those who underwent fusion after having undergone decompression only during the index surgery did significantly better than those who underwent revision of any sort after having undergone fusion during the index surgery. They concluded that revision after failure of fusion has a significantly worse prognosis than revision after failure of simple disk excision.

CONCLUSION

Significant back and leg symptoms develop in approximately 10% to 15% of patients who have undergone a spinal decompression procedure and approximately 15% to 20% of patients who have had a spinal fusion procedure for degenerative disease of the lumbar spine during the next 3 to 5 years so that they require revision lumbar surgery. The cause for their symptoms has to be diligently sought, as this is a main predictor of good outcome following revision surgery. Good history taking, including a detailed old-chart review; repeat physical evaluation; and input from therapists—physical and psychological, neurologists, and other caregivers—should be sought. These, together with an intelligent use of investigations, go a long way in helping to establish a cause for failure. Further, developing a revision surgical strategy is an intellectual exercise when a simple algorithmic approach may not always work. The process of evaluation and surgical management for failed lumbar degeneration is a science and an art requiring a great deal of understanding and commitment on the part of the surgeon. The temporal trend of improving outcomes is aided in part by emerging technologies; however, we have to be constantly aware of simple facts such as factors that influence outcome. The use of published literature and the experiences of our peers help us to offer appropriate surgical intervention while improving the long-term results of revision surgery of the lumbar spine.

REFERENCES

1. Bernard TN. Repeat lumbar spine surgery. Factors influencing outcome. *Spine* 1993;18:2196–2200.
2. Biondi J, Greenberg BJ. Redecompression and fusion in failed back syndrome patients. *J Spinal Disord* 1990; 3:362–369.
3. Blumenthal SL, Baker J, Dossett A, et al. The role of anterior lumbar fusion for internal disc disruption. *Spine* 1988;13:566–569.
4. Boden SD, Martin GJ, Horton WC, et al. Laparoscopic anterior spinal arthrodesis with rhBMP-2 in titanium interbody threaded cage. *J Spinal Disord* 1998;11:95–101.
5. Boden SD, Zdeblick TA, Sandhu HS, et al. The use of rhBMP-2 in interbody fusion cages: definitive evidence of osteoinduction in humans. *Spine* 2000;25:376–381.
6. Brown CW, Orme TJ, Richardson HD. The rate of pseudoarthrosis (surgical nonunion) in patients who are smokers and patients who are nonsmokers: a comparison study. *Spine* 1986;11:942–943.
7. Cammisa FP, Girardi FP, Sangani PK, et al. Incidental durotomy in spine surgery. *Spine* 2000;25:2663–2667.
8. Cammisa FP, Girardi FP, Voos K, et al. Direct repair of pars defect utilizing image guidance. *Syllabus of the Third Annual North American Program on Computer Assisted Orthopaedic Surgery.* Pittsburgh, 1999:214–219.
9. Carpenter CT, Dietz JW, Leung KYK, et al. Repair of pseudoarthrosis of the lumbar spine. *J Bone Joint Surg Am* 1996;78-A:712–720.
10. Castro WHM, Halm H, Jerosch J, et al. Accuracy of pedicle screw placement in lumbar vertebrae. *Spine* 1996;21:1320–1324.
11. Cinotti G, Roysam GS, Eisenstein SM, et al. Ipsilateral recurrent lumbar disc herniation—a prospective controlled study. *J Bone Joint Surg Br* 1998;80-B:825–832.
12. Coe JD, Warden KE, Herzig MA, et al. Influence of bone mineral density on the fixation of thoracolumbar implants: a comparative study of transpedicular screws, laminar hooks and spinous process wires. *Spine* 1990; 15:902–907.
13. Curylo LJ, Ragab AA, Bohlman HH. Same level revision lumbar surgery: an analysis of outcomes in 63 patients with a 2 to 21 year follow-up. In: Main C, ed. Annual Meeting of the International Society for Study of the Lumbar Spine. Adelaide, Australia: ISSLS, 2000.
14. Ebeling U, Kalbarcyk H, Reulen HJ. Microsurgical reoperation following lumbar disc surgery. Timing, surgical findings, and outcome in 92 patients. *J Neurosurg* 1989;70:397–404.
15. Epstein JA, Lavine LS, Epstein BS. Recurrent herniation of the lumbar intervertebral disc. *Clin Orthop* 1967;52:169–178.
16. Fager CA, Freidberg SR. Analysis of failure rates and poor results of lumbar spine surgery. *Spine* 1980;5:87–94.
17. Finnegan WJ, Fenlin JM, Marvel JP, et al. Results of surgical intervention in the symptomatic multiply-operated back patient. Analysis of sixty-seven cases followed for three to seven years. *J Bone Joint Surg Am* 1979; 61A:1077–1082.
18. Forristall RM, Marsh HO, Pay NT. Magnetic resonance imaging and contrast CT of the lumbar spine. Comparison of diagnostic methods and correlation with surgical findings. *Spine* 1988;13:1049–1054.
19. Frymoyer JW, Matteri RE, Hanley EN, et al. Failed lumbar disc surgery requiring second operation. A long-term follow-up study. *Spine* 1978;3:7–11.
20. Glassman SD, Dimar JR, Johnson JR, et al. Preoperative SF-36 responses as predictor of reoperation following lumbar fusion. *Orthopedics* 1998;21:1201–1203.
21. Glassman SD, Minkow RE, Dimar JF, et al. Effect of prior lumbar discectomy on outcome of lumbar fusion: a prospective analysis using the SF-36 measure. *J Spinal Disord* 1998;11:383–388.
22. Goodkin R, Laska LL. Unintended "incidental" durotomy during surgery of the lumbar spine: medicolegal implications. *Surg Neurol* 1995;43(1):4–12.
23. Halverson TL, Kelly LA, Thomas KA, et al. Effects of bone mineral density on pedicle screw fixation. *Spine* 1994;19:415–420.
24. Hanely EN, Levy JA. Surgical treatment of isthmic lumbosacral spondylolisthesis: analysis of variables affecting results. *Spine* 1989;14:48–50.
25. Heggeness MH, Esses SI, Mody DR. A histologic study of lumbar pseudoarthrosis. *Spine* 1993;18:1016–1020.
26. Heggeness MH, Esses SI. Classification of pseudoar-

throsis of the lumbar spine. *Spine* 1991;16:S449–S454.

27. Herron L. Recurrent lumbar disc herniation: results of repeat laminectomy and discectomy. *J Spinal Disord* 1994;7:161–166.

28. Hu RW, Jaglal S, Axcell T, et al. A population-based study of reoperation after back surgery. *Spine* 1997;22:2265–2271.

29. Reference deleted.

30. Jones AAM, Stambough JL, Balderston RA, et al. Long-term results of lumbar spine surgery complicated by unintended incidental durotomy. *Spine* 1989;14:443–446.

31. Jönsson B, Strömqvist B. Repeat decompression of lumbar nerve roots. A prospective two-year evaluation. *J Bone Joint Surg Br* 1993;75B:894–897.

32. Kendler DL. Risk factors in osteoporosis. *Br Col Med J* 1996;38:263–264.

33. Kim SS, Michelsen CB. Revision surgery for failed back surgery syndrome. *Spine* 1992;17:957–960.

34. Krag MH, Van Hal ME, Beynnon BD. Placement of transpedicular vertebral screws close to anterior vertebral cortex: description of methods. *Spine* 1989;14:879–883.

35. Lane JM. Osteoporosis: diagnosis and treatment. *J Bone Joint Surg* 1996;78A:618–632.

36. Law JD, Lehman RAW, Kirsch WM. Reoperation after lumbar intervertebral disc surgery. *J Neurosurg* 1978;48:259–263.

37. Lehmann TR, LaRocca HS. Repeat lumbar surgery. A review of patients with failure from previous lumbar surgery treated by spinal canal exploration and lumbar spinal fusion. *Spine* 1981;6:615–619.

38. Lehmann TR, LaRocca HS. Repeat lumbar surgery. A review of patients with failure from previous lumbar surgery treated by spinal canal exploration and lumbar spinal fusion. *Spine* 1981;6:615–619.

39. Levi AD, Dickman CA, Sonntag VK. Management of postoperative infections after spinal instrumentation. *J Neurosurg* 1997;86:975–980.

40. Malter AD, McNeney B, Loeser JD, et al. 5-year reoperation rates after different types of lumbar spine surgery. *Spine* 1998;23:814–820.

41. Massie JB, Heller JG, Abitbol JJ, et al. Postoperative posterior spinal wound infections. *Clin Orthop* 1992;284:99–108.

42. Nasca RJ. Surgical management of lumbar spinal stenosis. *Spine* 1987;12:809–816.

43. Reference deleted.

44. Nygaard OP, Kloster R, Dullerud R, et al. No association between peridural scar and outcome after lumbar microdiscectomy. *Acta Neurochir (Wien)* 1997;139:1095–1100.

45. Obedian RS, Cammisa FP, Parvataneni HK, et al. Stereotactic image guidance for placement of pedicle screws in revision fusion of the lumbar spine. In: Main C, ed. Annual Meeting of the International Society for the Study of the Lumbar Spine. Adelaide, Australia: ISSLS, 2000: 115.

46. Okuyama K, Sato K, Abe E, et al. Stability of transpedicle screwing for the osteoporotic spine: an in vitro study of mechanical stability. *Spine* 1993;19:240–245.

47. Ozgen S, Naderi S, Ozek MM, et al. Findings and outcome of revision lumbar disc surgery. *J Spinal Disord* 1999;12:287–292.

48. Patel N, Pople IK, Cummins BH. Revisional microdiscectomy: an analysis of operative findings and clinical outcome. *Br J Neurosurg* 1995;9:733–737.

49. Picada R, Winter RB, Lonstein JE, et al. Postoperative deep wound infection in adults after posterior lumbosacral spine fusion: incidence and management. *J Spinal Disord* 2000;13:42–45.

50. Quimjian JD, Matrka PJ. Decompression laminectomy and lateral spinal fusion in patients with previously failed lumbar spine surgery. *Orthopedics* 1988;11:563–569.

51. Sandhu HS, Kanim LEA, Kabo JM, et al. Effective doses of recombinant bone morphogenetic protein-2 in experimental spinal fusion. *Spine* 1996;21:2115–2121.

52. Scoliosis Research Society. *Mortality and morbidity committee report.* Park Ridge, IL: SRS, 1987.

53. Silcox DHR, Boden SD, Schimandle JH, et al. Reversing the inhibitory effect of nicotine on spinal fusion using an osteoinductive protein extract. *Spine* 1998;23:291–297.

54. Soshi S. An experimental study on transpedicular screw fixation in relation to osteoporosis of the lumbar spine. *Spine* 1991;16:1135–1141.

55. Reference deleted.

56. Stewart G, Sachs BL. Patient outcomes after reoperation on the lumbar spine. *J Bone Joint Surg Am* 1996;78-A:706–711.

57. Wang JC, Bohlman HH, Riew DK. Dural tears secondary to operations on the lumbar spine: management and results after a two-year-minimum follow-up of eighty-eight patients. *J Bone Joint Surg Am* 1998;80A:1728–1732.

58. Reference deleted.

59. Weinstein MA, McCabe JP, Cammisa FPJ. Post operative spinal wound infection. 11th Annual Meeting of the North American Spine Society. Vancouver: NASS, 1996: 254.

60. Weir KA, Jacobs GA. Reoperation rate following lumbar discectomy: an analysis of 662 lumbar discectomies. *Spine* 1980;5:366–370.

61. West JLI, Ogilvie JW, Bradford DS. Complications of variable screw plate pedicle screw fixation. *Spine* 1991;16:576–579.

62. Wiesel SW. The multiply operated lumbar spine. *Instr Course Lect* 1985;34:68–77.

63. Reference deleted.

64. Zdeblick TA, Kunz DN, Cooke ME. Pedicle screw pullout strength: correlation with insertional torque. 1993;18:673–676.

65. Zindrick MR. A biomechanical study of interpedicular screw fixation in the lumbosacral spine. *Clin Orthop* 1986;203:99–112.

LUMBAR SPINE: DEFORMITY

KEITH H. BRIDWELL AND OHENEBA BOACHIE-ADJEI

Adult patients with lumbar deformity who have undergone previous unsuccessful surgery usually present with one of the following complaints: pain, deformity, or neurologic problems. Patients may have had surgery to decompress a stenotic region of the spinal canal in the lumbar spine, in which case the deformity was not addressed, and the patient presents with progressive instability, decompensation, and dynamic stenosis related to activities such as standing, walking, bending, and twisting. For these patients, diagnostic evaluation using radiographs, magnetic resonance imaging (MRI) studies, computed tomography myelogram (CTM) scans, and diskography to assess painful levels is essential.

DECISION MAKING

Who Should Have Surgery?

Dickson et al. (18) have found that, for patients with substantial deformities, surgical treatment improves the natural history compared to a group of patients who were offered surgery and declined. He found that the group that had surgery functioned at a higher level and with less pain. Undoubtedly, many of these curves were lumbar deformities, and the surgeries were generally performed in an era with Harrington instrumentation. This is our best evidence that surgical treatment improves the natural history. If these kinds of results can be accomplished with Harrington instrumentation, our results should be much better with the modern-day systems that segmentally fix the spine and also do a better job of restoring sagittal lordosis in the lumbar spine.

A "typical" normal spine has 50 to 60 degrees of lumbar lordosis. The segmental contribution to lordosis increases with each caudal level in the normal spine. In the spine with substantial scoliosis, we usually see that degenerative disk disease occurs more quickly than in the spine without deformity. Therefore, the adult lumbar spine with significant deformity is usually very hypolordotic or frankly kyphotic (8,11). Correction of the coronal and sagittal com-

ponents of the deformity is usually necessary to achieve patient satisfaction.

When deciding to perform a surgical procedure on a patient with spinal deformity, it is necessary initially to define the goals and expectations. What is the patient's principal complaint? Is it the cosmesis of the deformity? Is it axial back pain? Is it referred radicular pain?

In assessing whether or not the surgery is going to be a "success," it is important to establish those goals and to discuss them extensively with the patient and the patient's family. Several factors contribute to whether those goals are achieved. One of those factors is the successful technical completion of the surgery. Other factors include the patient's comorbidities, the patient's understanding of the problem, and the patient's compliance and motivation. Minor and major complications need to be discussed with the patient and the patient's family. If it is the surgeon's perception that the patient or patient's family is going to become highly emotional when any minor complications occur, surgery should be deferred.

Determination of Fusion Levels

Determination of the fusion levels for surgical treatment and instrumentation does not follow the same criteria that are usually used for adolescent idiopathic scoliosis. However, it is critical to be able to take into consideration factors such as the stable vertebrae and transition zones that demonstrate instability and significant disk degeneration. Anteroposterior and lateral upright radiographs, followed by supine bending x-rays, provide information as to the overall coronal and sagittal balance and flexible levels of the lumbar curve and, more importantly, the lumbosacral fractional curve, if one decides to spare the lumbosacral region. On plain radiographs, the Cobb angles should be obtained using the traditional methods of assessment. The T-1 to S-1 plumb line assesses coronal plane decompensation. Areas of instability, characterized by spondylo-, retro-, or rotational listhesis, also should be evaluated. If the patient has had previous surgery such as a laminectomy, the area of decompression should be evaluated and considered for inclusion in the reconstruction procedure.

On the standing lateral radiographs, the standard kyphosis-lordosis measurements and the overall sagittal balance should be assessed. The T-1 to S-1 plumb line should fall slightly anterior to or behind the midsacral body. It is critical that the lateral radiographs in the upright position be obtained with the patient standing with the knees fully locked to assess the extent of flat back deformity resulting from loss of lumbar lordosis. In determining the fusion levels, one should consider factors such as painful areas from degenerative facets and disks, pseudarthrosis, postlaminectomy instability, and junctional degeneration of stenotic regions that need to be decompressed. All these levels should be included in the anticipated fusion. This is most critical in the distal end of the fusion, especially the lower lumbar and lumbosacral regions. Another factor to be considered in the extent of the fusion distally is the integrity of the bone density at the selected fusion levels. Proximal fusion levels should extend beyond the end of the curve into a normal zone to provide an overall balanced spine over a level pelvis. Patients with major lumbar curves who have had previous surgery may have had an operation into the thoracic region, in which case the surgery should be extended to the thoracic levels. If no previous surgery has been performed in the thoracic region, the proximal extent should take into account the normalcy of the levels in this area. The upper instrumented level is best stopped at the upper lumbar or lower thoracic region, avoiding extensions to the kyphotic apex of the thoracic spine, to reduce the chances of functional kyphotic deformity. If the fusion has to be extended proximally to the apex of the thoracic spine at T7-8, one should consider extending beyond the apex, to T3-4, to avoid the problem of junctional kyphosis, which commonly develops when the fusion is stopped at the midthoracic spine. This is more important if a patient presents with a hyperkyphotic thoracic spine, especially for postmenopausal or osteoporotic patients.

MRI scans help to determine the integrity of the intervertebral disks at the levels to be considered at the caudal end of the fusion. Degenerative levels should be included in the fusion to prevent progressive degeneration, instability, pain, and stenosis below the fusion. If the MRI is equivocal and the patient presents with distal lumbar pain that extends beyond the anticipated end of the fusion, pain-provocative diskography is helpful to determine the integrity of the disks below the fusion and the extent

of degeneration (23,29). Positive diskograms indicate a possible source of pain, and these levels usually should be included in the fusion levels.

In patients with severe scoliosis, rotation and instability are difficult to evaluate on an MRI study. In such instances, the myelogram with a CT scan evaluation is quite helpful. However, if a patient presents with symptoms of neurogenic claudication and spinal stenosis, or possible postsurgical epidural fibrosis and arachnoiditis, the MRI scan with gadolinium or the CTM of the lumbar spine clarifies the integrity of the spinal canal, nerve root canal, and evidence of arachnoiditis. Patients with dynamic instability may not demonstrate stenosis on the MRI scan in the supine position, but it is quite evident on the CTM scan performed with the patient in a semiupright position and also with flexion and extension views. For these patients, all stenotic regions should be decompressed during the posterior approach.

Having considered all the above factors, the bending films show whether there is a flexible or fixed lumbosacral fractional curve, in which case substantial correction of the lumbar curve may produce significant coronal plane imbalance. Therefore, fixation may have to be extended to the sacropelvic region to provide overall balance in the coronal plane. A mild lumbosacral fractional curvature of less than 20 degrees may not need to be instrumented, provided that the L4-5 and L-5 to S-1 disks are relatively normal on MRI studies and the patient has minimal distal lumbar back pain and has had no previous surgical procedures performed in this area. In some cases, coronal balance can be well achieved by adequate realignment and horizontalization of L-4 over the sacrum with distal pedicle screw fixation.

Determination of Fixation

The types of instrumentation and implants that are considered in the patient with failed lumbar deformity surgery depend on factors such as (a) extent of laminectomy; (b) previous surgery levels, with or without laminectomy; and (c) type of existing instrumentation and mode of its failure. A variety of implants, including hooks, wires, and pedicle screws, can be used in combination to provide the optimal balance correction (2,5,7). In patients who have had extensive laminectomies in the lumbar spine, wires or hooks are out of the question, because there are no posterior elements for fixation and, therefore, pedicle screws provide the best fixation method. The number of fixation points needed depends on the extent of the reconstruction. For a major lumbar curve with a large thoracic scoliosis or hyperkyphosis, the thoracic spine certainly can be instrumented with proximal hook fixation or a combination of intermediary wires and hooks. The lumbar spine is reconstructed with distal pedicle screws to better horizontalize the distal end fusion levels, with intermediary hooks or wires, or both, for coronal plane balance (7).

In the authors' experience, distal bilateral pedicle screw fixation provides a distal foundation for support and is ideal to horizontalize and optimally balance the lower-end instrumented vertebra in the coronal plane. Distal convex pedicle screws in the lumbar spine at the apical and periapical vertebrae for a major lumbar deformity provide the lordosing effect during the convex rod rotation maneuver. Concave sublaminar wires provide the necessary translational forces needed to correct major lumbar deformity. Proximally, in the thoracolumbar spine, pedicle screw placement in patients with adequate pedicle sizes provides the best three-dimensional stabilization effect. Hook-claw constructs placed in supralaminar-infralaminar positions provide an excellent alternative for the upper end instrumented vertebrae. However, the potential for junctional kyphosis should always be considered when one stops at the thoracolumbar junction with supralaminar-infralaminar claw constructs. If the fusion has to be extended to the sacropelvic region, several studies have shown the reliability and the biomechanical integrity of the Galveston construct (13,19,28). The traditional Galveston rods, prebent, or a modified, intrailiac screw using the CD or CD Horizon (Medtronic Sofamor Danek, Memphis, TN) or Isola system (DePuy AcroMed, Raynham, MA), supplemented with sacral pedicle and distal lumbar screws for a distal foundation, provide the best lumbosacral pelvic fixation (2–7,24). One also can consider the intrasacral, Jackson-type technique for distal sacral fixation whereby the sacroiliac joint is spared. A biomechanical study by Bradford et al. has shown the superiority of the Jackson fixation combined with an anterior column support in a structural graft to the traditional Galveston method (7,19). The study is yet to be supported with clinical data.

It is critical to note that the operation being considered here is the arthrodesis, and meticulous arthrodesis techniques should be performed to achieve a solid fusion, without which any instrumentation system will eventually fail (6). Therefore, thorough decortication of all existing facet joints (unless they have been removed), the lamina, and the transverse processes should be undertaken either with a gouge

or a high-speed burr. Previously fused levels should be extensively decorticated to bleeding, cancellous bone to generate enough bone graft material for the subsequent fusion.

Bone Graft

The best bone graft is the patient's own bone. The source can be from the iliac crest, or, if the patient has a significant thoracic deformity, a thoracoplasty can be performed to provide additional bone for the fusion.

Patients who are undergoing reconstruction for failed lumbar deformity surgery usually are considered for concomitant anterior fusion, in which case allograft can be considered anteriorly. Allograft anteriorly with autograft posteriorly is useful. Fusions that extend to the midlumbar region or to the lower lumbosacral spine should be considered for an anterior fusion and, in long constructs, the addition of anterior column support (23,24). Available structural supports for grafting anteriorly at L4-5 and L-5 to S-1 include femoral ring allograft, tricortical autograft, or allograft and titanium cages, which provide good structural support with the addition of morselized autograft. Long fusions to the sacrum should always be supplemented with anterior column structural support, as has been shown in many studies as the optimal fixation (6,9,15,23,24).

SINGLE OR COMBINED/CONTINUOUS OR STAGED SURGERY

In the idiopathic adolescent patient, it is common that the deformity can be corrected and a definitive fusion can be accomplished with a single-stage anterior or single-stage posterior surgery. However, in the adult patient, often the lumbar deformities in particular require circumferential surgery (27).

In adults, many curves between 45 and 70 degrees with normal segmental sagittal measurements can be treated with a posterior-only operation. In particular, most thoracic curves and most double major curves in young adults that do not require fusion below L-4 can be treated with a single stage.

It is more likely that combined anterior and posterior surgery is going to be required for stiff thoracic curves over 75 degrees; thoracic kyphosis over 75 degrees; thoracolumbar and lumbar curves with subluxation or significant segmental hypolordosis, or both; all long fusions to the sacrum; most lumbar pseudarthroses, especially if there is a component of hyperkyphosis; all cases with a "significant" anterior column gap if the weight-bearing line does not fall behind the posterior fusion; and most postlaminectomy deformities in the lumbar spine. Other factors that play a role are the size of the curves, the sagittal alignment of the curves, the biology of the patient, the extent of degenerative changes, osteoporosis, and whether it is a revision or a primary surgery.

The advantages of a simultaneous same-day combined approach are early postoperative mobilization, short hospitalization, and presumed decreased likelihood of complications such as deep venous thrombosis, pneumonia, muscle weakness, and osteoporosis. Disadvantages of the simultaneous same-day combined approach are surgeon and staff fatigue, excessive blood loss, increased fluid shifts/imbalances, pressure sores, and perhaps neurologic risk (27).

Indications for combined surgery in the same day are surgery that can be accomplished in less than 12 hours, a patient who can tolerate only one anesthetic, when doing one side of the spine can destabilize it to the point that loss of fixation occurs, and when the anticipated blood loss is not too great. Indications for staging the anterior and posterior surgery are procedures that last longer than 12 hours, a significant anticipated blood loss somewhat related to the number of segments being done, and when intercurrent halo traction is being considered.

We consider hyperalimentation or preoperative multiple lumen catheter placement, or both, if an extensive ileus is anticipated along with extensive blood loss, staged surgeries, and marginal patient nutrition. If surgeries are being staged, we generally prefer doing them 5 days rather than 2 weeks apart, as 2 weeks is closer to the nutritional nadir.

For the middle-aged or older adult who requires a long fusion and instrumentation to the sacrum, there are at least four minimal requirements for having any hope of getting a solid fusion. First, the patient must be in neutral or slightly negative sagittal balance, with a plumb dropped from C-7 falling through or behind the posterior aspect of the lumbosacral disk. Segmental fixation must be present at L-3, L-4, L-5, and the sacrum without any jumps or gaps. Four-point fixation of the sacrum and pelvis is advisable with bilateral S-1 screws and either two additional sacral screws, two additional iliac screws, or Jackson

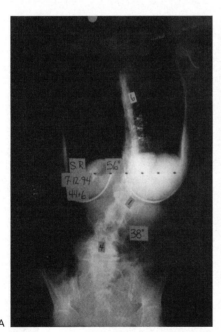
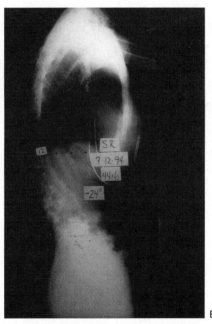

FIGURE 1. Series of photos of a woman in her 40s who had surgery many years ago consisting of a fusion without instrumentation from T-6 to L-1. With time, her deformity added on, and increasing degenerative changes developed in her lumbar spine. She had a very marked thoracolumbar kyphosis and was in slightly positive sagittal balance. She was treated with a posterior instrumentation extended down to the sacrum. This was an inadequate operation. She had only two-point fixation in the sacrum. She did not have adequate segmental fixation in the lumbar spine, there was no change in her sagittal balance, and no anterior procedure was performed. She therefore experienced failure of the implant and increasing deformity. She required revision that included anterior and posterior surgery, three-column osteotomy posteriorly, restoration of sagittal balance, four-point fixation in the sacrum and pelvis, and additional fixation points in the lumbar spine. Note her sagittal appearance before and after her last round of surgery. (Case performed by Dr. Bridwell.) **A:** Standing coronal radiograph in 1994. **B:** Standing sagittal radiograph in 1994. (*continued*)

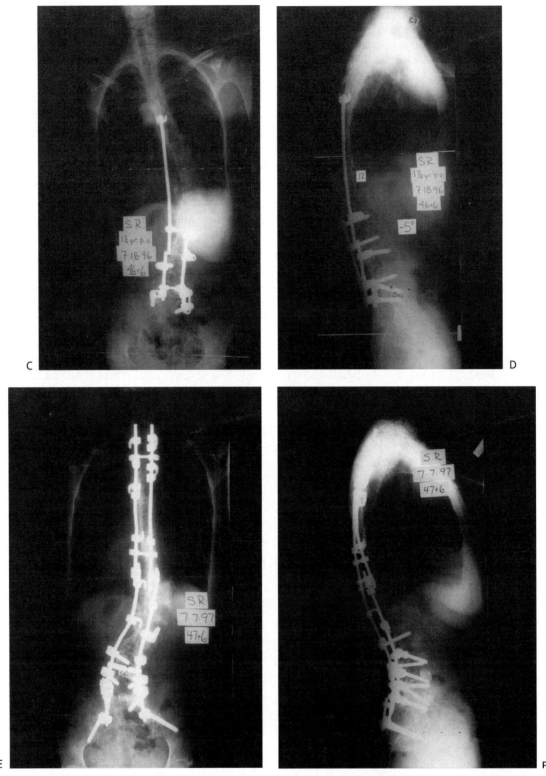

FIGURE 1. (*continued*) **C:** Standing coronal radiograph in 1996. **D:** Standing sagittal radiograph in 1996. **E:** Standing coronal radiograph in 1997 following surgical reconstruction. **F:** Standing sagittal radiograph in 1997 following revision reconstruction. Not enough time has passed since the revision surgery to determine whether the fusion is totally solid. At this time, the patient's pain and appearance are markedly improved over what they were preoperatively. (*continued*)

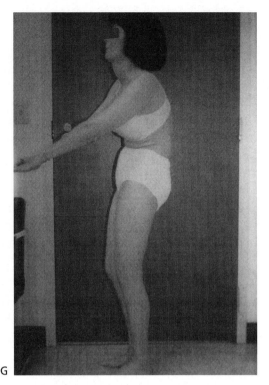
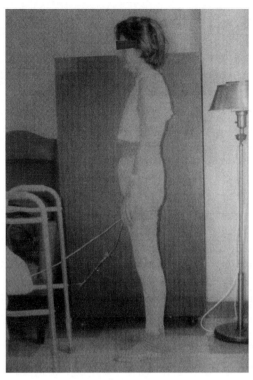

FIGURE 1. (*continued*) **G:** The clinical appearance of the patient demonstrating a marked flat back syndrome in early 1996. **H:** Sagittal clinical appearance of the patient following revision later in 1996. In 2002, the patient is 5 ½ years postoperative with solid fusion and no loss of correction.

intrasacral fixation. Also, an anterior fusion of each segment in the lumbar spine should be accomplished, preferably with structural grafting at least at L4-5 and L-5 to S-1. Dekutoski et al. (16) have documented the importance of sagittal balance. Saer et al. (28) have impressed on us the importance of adequate pelvic fixation to control the sacropelvic moment arm and to achieve a solid fusion to the sacrum. They have also emphasized that the results are much better and pseudarthrosis rates are much lower if anterior fusion is included on long fusions to the sacrum (Fig. 1).

COMPLICATIONS

The complications of lumbar deformity surgery include (a) inadequate correction, (b) continued pain, (c) junctional kyphosis above, (d) junctional kyphosis below, (e) pseudarthrosis and implant failure, (f) coronal decompensation, (g) sagittal decompensation, (h) neurologic deficit, (i) deep wound infection, and (j) systemic complications.

Adults undergoing complex reconstructions for failed lumbar deformities are expected to have higher complication rates than patients who undergo primary procedures. A review of adults undergoing reconstructive surgery reveals a total complication rate of approximately 71% in a study by Cummine et al. (15). The most frequent complications were pseudarthrosis (17%), infection (17%), and hematoma (12%).

Pseudarthrosis/Implant Failure

Patients who have spinal fusion and instrumentation for lumbar deformity may experience pseudarthrosis and implant failure. In most cases, the pseudarthrosis means increased pain and increasing deformity (especially increasing kyphosis) and, therefore, requires revision, bone grafting, and revision instrumentation. Occasionally, pseudarthrosis occurs at junctional levels on the top or the bottom and does not cause much in the way of symptomatology. If the pseudarthrosis is asymptomatic, that is, does not cause pain and does not lead to loss of correction, a "stable" pseudarthrosis can be left alone.

A relative indication for combined surgery is that of needing to repair a pseudarthrosis in the lumbar spine, especially if that segment has fallen into kyphosis. It is more effective to apply compression across the pseudarthrosis than neutralization or distraction forces. It is particularly important to realign the lumbar spine in a position of physiologic sagittal lordosis to repair the pseudarthrosis and get a solid fusion. (See Fig. 1 for an illustration of these points.)

Neurologic Deficit

Perioperative neurologic deficits with spinal deformity surgery can occur as a result of spinal cord compression from extradural pressure. Potential etiologies include retropulsed bone, disk, wires, and hooks. Any source of extradural compression should be identifiable on a myelogram. A second potential etiology for neurologic deficit is that of distraction of the spinal canal to the point that the nerve roots or spinal cord are stretched. A stretch of the neural elements secondarily reduces their blood supply. At Barnes-Jewish Hospital, we determine whether the spinal canal has been lengthened by performing a "string test." We place a string in the sagittal plane along the posterior vertebral body line the length of the fusion and instrumentation, adjust for magnification, and compare it preoperatively to postoperatively. In the coronal plane we place the string in the midportion of the vertebral bodies the length of the fusion and instrumentation, adjust for magnification, and compare preoperatively to postoperatively. The corrective force on the lumbar spine should never be distraction from the posterior side of the spine. All forces on the posterior spine should be either translational or cantilever or compression on the convexity. The only acceptable distraction force in the lumbar spine should be that applied to the anterior column at the time of the anterior procedure. After taking out the disks anteriorly, it is often helpful to open up the disk space with spreaders and place structural graft or cages anteriorly to increase anterior column height. This may at times increase middle column height somewhat also.

The third potential etiology for neurologic deficit is that of a purely vascular injury. This is unlikely to occur with simply a posterior approach. It is most likely to occur with an anterior and a posterior approach if all the anterior vessels are being harvested. The risk of neurologic deficit from a purely vascular etiology might be increased if hypotensive anesthesia is used intraoperatively as well.

A myelogram and a string test can rule out the first two etiologies. If a perioperative neurologic deficit does occur, the surgeon must determine immediately which of the three etiologies has caused the neurologic deficit and act quickly. Clearly, if a neurologic deficit occurs half an hour after instrumentation has been placed, this implicates the instrumentation. If the surgeon is unsure of etiologies, it is best to remove all the instrumentation and plan to return later for the definitive instrumentation.

Somatosensory potentials, motor evoked potentials, clonus tests, and Stagnara wake-up tests are all potential ways of monitoring the neural elements during surgery.

Quite a bit of dispute is still going on regarding which motor evoked potential method is most accurate in monitoring the motor tracks. Many case reports have suggested that somatosensory potentials do not globally monitor the spinal cord and can miss motor deficits. Thus, clinical correlates such as a clonus test or a Stagnara wake-up test do have a role along with the electronic monitoring. At Washington University in St. Louis, we have had four major neurologic deficits over the last 10 years. All four of those cases were combined surgeries, all four were principally thoracic operations, and all four were associated with a component of hyperkyphosis (12). To date, we have not had any neurologic deficits in adult lumbar deformity surgeries.

Coronal Plane Imbalance

Spinal surgery for adult lumbar deformity can result in imbalance in either the coronal or sagittal plane, or a combination. Coronal plane imbalance with translation of the trunk laterally is usually associated with rotational deformity. The patient also may have a slight shift forward or be twisted more to one side. The most common presentation is the patient's inability to maintain an upright posture, and, in some patients, the rib cage margin may extend down to the pelvic region and impinge on the iliac crest. Significant translation also can lead to traction or compression, or both, on lumbar nerve roots, resulting in radiculopathy, which can interfere with functional activities, including standing and walking (22). Patients may have neurologic deficit on physical examination but also usually present with an entirely normal neurologic examination (20).

Coronal plane imbalance can result from (a) juxtafusion disk degeneration with loss of disk height and progressive instability, (b) severe facet degeneration, and, at times, (c) facet joint or pars interarticularis fracture. Dislodgment of instrumentation, either a hook or a broken pedicle screw at a distal fusion level, can also produce coronal plane imbalance. This may or may not be associated with pseudarthrosis (21,22).

The best treatment for coronal plane imbalance is its prevention, and in the initial treatment, it is critical that proper levels are chosen and a strong, stable instrumentation be performed to produce balanced correction. Juxtafusion disk degeneration can be reduced if these levels are included in the index operation. Strong, stable, segmental instrumentation reduces the chances of failed or broken instrumentation that can result from inadequate fixation or pseudarthrosis. For long constructs, such as to the sacrum, an anterior load-sharing fusion with a structural graft reduces the chance of failed implants or pseudarthrosis (9). Distal pedicle

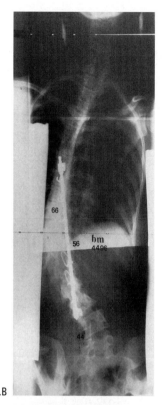 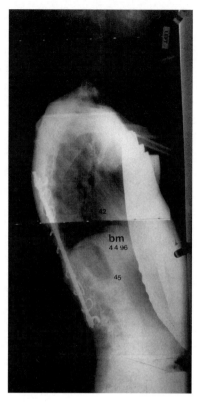 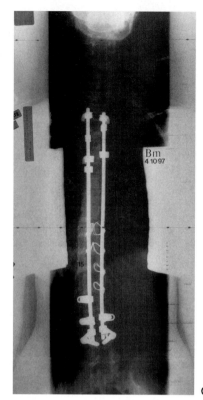

A.B

C

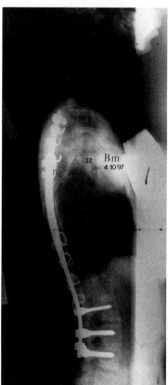

D

FIGURE 2. A 35-year-old woman with progressive coronal plane imbalance following a previous fusion with instrumentation. (Case performed by Dr. Boachie-Adjei.) **A:** Preoperative coronal radiograph showing the residual coronal plane imbalance. **B:** Preoperative sagittal radiograph showing thoracolumbar kyphosis. **C:** Postoperative coronal radiograph showing the restoration of coronal plane balance. **D:** Postoperative sagittal radiograph showing the restoration of sagittal plane balance.

screws in the lumbosacral spine provide better fixation than hook or wire fixation (7). For juxtafusion disk degeneration, extension of the fusion to include the diseased levels after appropriate diagnostic studies may be required. A herniated disk or stenosis at the juxtafusion level usually is a localized disorder with a radicular pain pattern. Treatment includes extension of the fusion with definitive decompression of the affected levels. If the primary fusion was to L4 or L5, an extension of the fusion to the sacropelvic region may be required.

Patients who present with failed instrumentations—either rods, pedicle screws, or dislodged hooks—require further surgery to revise the entire instrumentation or part thereof. In the presence of pseudarthrosis, anterior diskectomies and fusion, if previous anterior surgery has not been performed, increase the chances to obtain a successful arthrodesis. For severe lumbar deformities with significant coronal plane imbalance, a circumferential release with multilevel diskectomies and fusion, or osteotomies through an existing fusion mass at multiple levels, provides the desired balanced correction in the coronal plane without stressing the correction at a single level with one osteotomy (Fig. 2). In the presence of pseudarthrosis, the reconstruction should consider the use of autogenous bone graft via iliac crest or a rib thoracoplasty, supplemented with anterior structural grafts for distal lumbar or lumbosacral levels. An extension to the sacropelvic region is the best option for patients with significant coronal plane imbalance, especially in the presence of a significant oblique takeoff of L4-5 or junctional disk degeneration at L4-5, L-5 to S-1, for whom a long fusion past the thoracolumbar junction proximally is to be considered (6,7,13). This provides the best foundation in the distal segment to prevent loss of fixation at an L-4 or L-5 level.

Sagittal Imbalance

Etiologies of sagittal imbalance or flat back syndrome include posttraumatic kyphosis following fusion of the thoracolumbar spine in kyphosis; postfusion in the scoliosis patient, shortening the anterior column with Dwyer or Zielke instrumentation or lengthening the posterior column with Harrington instrumentation; degenerative, mainly fusing in segmental kyphosis without correction and then having the patient subsequently break down proximally; and associated systemic conditions such as juvenile rheumatoid arthritis and ankylosing spondylolysis and related disorders (25,26). Indications for osteotomy with flat back syndrome are either a fixed kyphosis or a patient who is out of balance, with C-7 plumb falling well anterior to the lumbosacral disk on the standing lateral radiograph.

The spectrum of the deformity is as follows: With a type I deformity, a patient is segmentally flat but globally in balance and able to compensate by hyperextending segments above and below. A type II patient is segmentally and globally flat and out of balance, with C-7 falling in front of the lumbosacral disk. The patient is unable to compensate by hyperextending segments below either because they are severely degenerated or fusion to the

sacrum has already been accomplished. The problems with fixed kyphosis are the terrible cosmesis, poor function, fatigue pain in the neck and hip extensors, and effect on levels above and below, predisposing to early degeneration.

The goal of surgical treatment is to restore coronal and sagittal balance so that the head is over the feet, with C-7 over the middle of the sacrum in the coronal plane and in the sagittal plane with C-7 over or just behind the posterior aspect of the lumbosacral disk. Strategies for the osteotomies include either a posterior-only approach for the type I deformity; anterior release, then posterior osteotomies; posterior osteotomies followed by structural grafting anteriorly; one or multiple osteotomies; and Smith-Petersen or transpedicular osteotomies. With a transpedicular osteotomy, one can usually achieve approximately 30 degrees of correction. With Smith-Petersen osteotomies, one can generally achieve approximately 1 degree of correction for every millimeter of bone resected through the posterior column.

A Smith-Petersen osteotomy is purely a posterior column osteotomy done between the pedicles. A transpedicular/pedicle subtraction/three-column osteotomy is performed from a posterior approach. A V is created through all three columns of the spine. The posterior and middle columns are shortened, and the anterior column is the hinge (Fig. 3). For Smith-Petersen osteotomies, the posterior column is shortened and the anterior column is opened up. Thus, with the Smith-Petersen osteotomies, in most cases it is going to be necessary to bone graft the anterior column.

At Washington University, we consider multiple Smith-Petersen osteotomies without anterior surgery if we are fusing short of the sacrum (usually a type I deformity) on a young patient with excellent bone stock. In this case, we are achieving mild to moderate correction at several levels if the disks anteriorly are relatively fat. We are trying to accomplish a physiologic segmental sagittal restoration.

Indications for anterior releases and morselized graft preceding multiple Smith-Petersen osteotomies are cases of narrow or partially calcified disks, pseudarthrosis, and considerable correction needed, usually a type II patient. If the weight-bearing line falls behind the osteotomies postoperatively with excellent fixation at all levels, it may not be necessary to structurally graft (Fig. 4). On the other hand, if there are big gaps anteriorly, if the weight-bearing line does not fall well behind the posterior fusion, or if we are extending the fusion caudally, structural grafting is also needed.

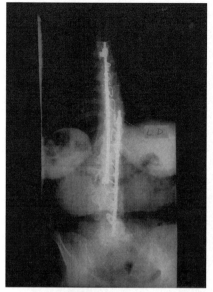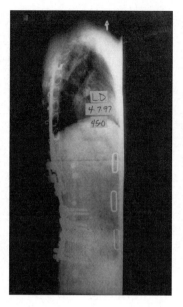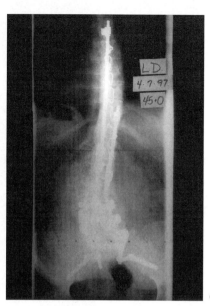

A,B

C

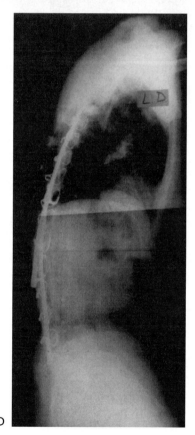

D

FIGURE 3. A female patient in her early 40s had previous Harrington instrumentation and fusion with sublaminar wires down to L-5. With time and aging, she has degenerated her L-5 to S-1 disk below and presents very pitched forward. Rather than performing the surgery used on patient CH (see Figure 4), we took a different approach. Because no pseudarthrosis was present anteriorly, rather than doing a thoracoabdominal approach we did a paramedian retroperitoneal approach and performed an anterior fusion at just L-5 to S-1 with cages and autogenous bone graft. In the posterior spine, we then did a three-column pedicle subtraction osteotomy in the midlumbar spine and revised the instrumentation by adding dominos to the Harrington rods, finding multiple fixation points in the lumbar spine, and then achieving four-point fixation in the sacrum and pelvis with two sacral screws and two iliac screws. In this case, the three-column pedicle subtraction osteotomy allowed us to achieve the same goals but with somewhat less invasive surgery for the patient. (Case performed by Dr. Bridwell.) **A:** Coronal standing radiograph preoperatively. **B:** Sagittal standing radiograph preoperatively. **C:** Standing coronal radiograph postoperatively. **D:** Standing sagittal radiograph postoperatively.

Decisions as to whether to perform one or several osteotomies are based on the degree of correction needed, whether there is concomitant coronal decompensation, and the patient's biology. It is best to perform most osteotomies in cauda equina territory below the conus. If the patient has an anterior and a posterior fusion, the options are either separate anterior and posterior osteotomies or a pedicle subtraction three-column osteotomy. Separate anterior and posterior procedures in that situation are more likely indicated if pseudos are present, anterior segmental spinal instrumentation is in place, extensive canal scarring exists, or more than 30 degrees of correction is needed.

The osteotomies should always be closing, never opening, wedges. It is best to plan them so that the osteotomy is closed tightly at the completion of correction with bone on bone.

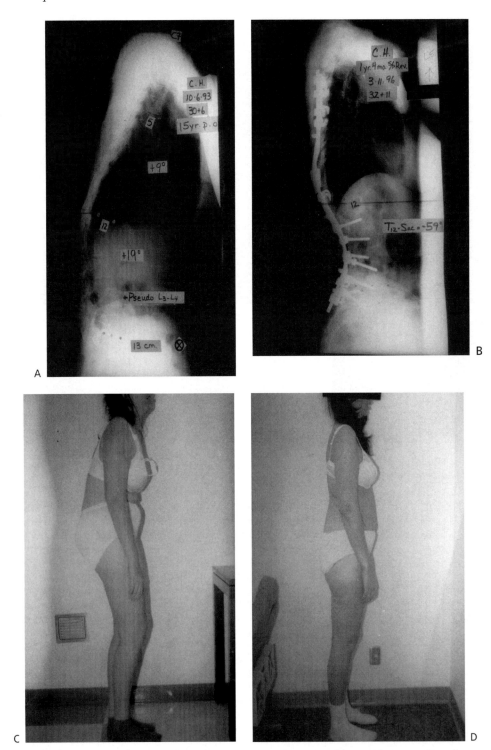

FIGURE 4. A young adult woman 15 years after her initial fusion for lumbar scoliosis. She was initially treated with Harrington instrumentation. See the retained alar hook on the sacrum. She was in marked positive sagittal balance, with her C-7 plumb line falling 13 cm in front of the lumbosacral disk, and she had a pseudarthrosis at L3-4. The patient was treated with an anterior approach, multiple diskectomies and fusion anteriorly with morselized grafting, then posterior Smith-Petersen osteotomies at multiple levels in the lumbar spine, and reconstruction in the fashion that is seen here. Because no significant gaps were created anteriorly, since multiple Smith-Petersen osteotomies were performed, and because the weight-bearing line fell well behind the posterior fusion, it was not necessary to structurally graft the segments anteriorly. (Case performed by Dr. Bridwell.) **A:** Sagittal radiograph of the patient preoperatively. **B:** Sagittal radiograph of the patient postoperatively. **C:** Clinical appearance of the patient preoperatively with a flat back syndrome. **D:** Clinical appearance of the patient postoperatively.

Principles of reconstruction are to instrument equal moment arms above and below the osteotomies. Dr. Bridwell and colleagues at Washington University usually use hooks above and screws below and find pedicles in the fusion mass with fluoroscopic assist; Dr. Bridwell's preference is to fix the whole fusion mass (10).

Between 1988 and 1996, one of us (Dr. Bridwell) was the surgeon or cosurgeon on 46 such procedures. Complications have included wound infection (patients with multiple previous surgeries) and spinal fluid leaks that are always a risk but have not been a problem. In particular, because the osteotomies are closed tightly, there is nowhere for the spinal fluid to leak. Blood loss is quite variable. Patients do recover slowly from the surgery because of the magnitude of the procedure. Fortunately, the author (Dr. Bridwell) has not had complications of loss of fixation or neurologic deficit in this group of patients. Patient satisfaction has been high if we have been able to restore physiologic sagittal balance and maintain coronal balance in a patient who is well motivated and has an excellent social situation. Satisfaction has not been as high if we have not fully restored sagittal balance, as was the case in one patient; if we do not maintain coronal balance, as was the case in two patients; or if complications such as wound infection occur or the patient's social situation is not ideal.

Miscalculation of Levels Chosen

One of the commonest causes of imbalance in the coronal plane occurs when inappropriate levels (in retrospect) are chosen during the index operation. This can result from too few or too many levels being fused, which may lead to progressive decompensation. Fusions can also be left short when the proximal extension does not include a major thoracic or thoracolumbar deformity. In this instance, correction of the lumbar curve may result in coronal plane imbalance. It is best to extend the fusion to involve major thoracolumbar or thoracic deformity for overall balance.

Care should be taken to factor the amount of correction that is needed to provide overall balance in the coronal plane. Magnitude of correction in these cases is not the relevant issue; balanced correction is critical. The use of distraction instrumentation in the lumbar spine commonly results in loss of lumbar lordosis. An associated coronal decompensation can result from use of such instrumentation because of the inability of the compensatory curves in the thoracic/thoracolumbar spine to correct spontaneously. If the patient presents later with a fused lumbar spine, overall imbalance, and an unfused thoracic/thoracolumbar curve, treatment involves spinal reconstruction using the anterior and posterior approaches (17,27). The anterior surgery consists of diskectomy and fusion of the lumbar or thoracolumbar deformity followed by posterior removal of the instrumentation, in its entirety in most cases, with multiple-level osteotomies and three-column realignment with segmental fixation. Care must be taken not to correct the lumbar deformity beyond the ability of the thoracic curve to compensate.

Patients with significant oblique takeoff of the lumbosacral spine whose fusions have not been extended to the sacrum can present with coronal plane decompensation from overcorrection of the lumbar spine and inability of a rigid lumbosacral fractional curve to correct spontaneously. Such instances are best treated by extending the fusion to the sacropelvic region, combined with an anterior column load sharing, via use of structural allograft or cages at L4-5 and L-5 to S-1. These grafts should be placed to maintain lumbar lordosis from L-4 to the sacral region. The inner canal of these cages or femoral rings should be packed carefully with autogenous cancellous bone before insertion to facilitate an arthrodesis. Fusion to the sacropelvic region is best for a patient with (a) a lumbar curve that extends to the sacrum; (b) a stiff, unbalanced lumbosacral fractional curve; and (c) lumbosacral pain secondary to degenerative disk disease below the lumbar curvature. In these cases, posterior arthrodesis alone, with instrumentation to the sacrum as a single procedure, does not produce the desired results. The incidence of pseudarthrosis, loss of lumbar lordosis, implant failure, and coronal plane decompensation is high in these patients, and, therefore, combined anterior and posterior spine fusion to the sacropelvic region should be considered (21).

In both authors' experience, anterior lumbar instrumentation usually has no added benefit in an older adult. However, the grafts can be transfixed with screw fixation to prevent their dislodgment during the posterior surgical reconstruction.

In a second stage or under the same anesthesia, posterior spine reconstruction using the transiliac fixation with a Galveston technique, or an iliac screw, extending the fixation to the upper thoracolumbar and lumbar spines is the preferred approach (17,27). Overcorrection of the lumbar deformity should be avoided, because a fixed pelvic obliquity and persistent coronal plane imbalance can result (Fig. 5).

Before the patient leaves the operating room, it is helpful to obtain a 3-foot coronal radiograph of the spine to be sure that the shoulders are balanced rela-

tive to the pelvis as they were on the standing preoperative radiograph. It is also helpful to sit the patient postoperatively in the operating room before going to the recovery room. Further, the surgeon should observe the patient standing on the first postopera-

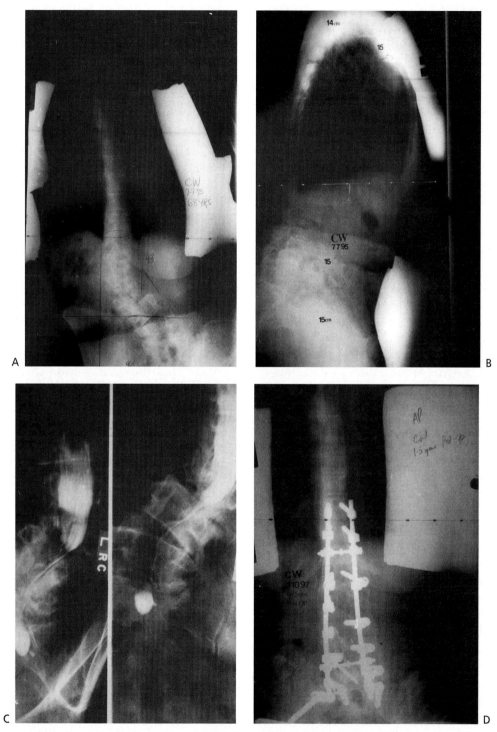

FIGURE 5. A 68-year-old woman with progressive decompensation following a previous laminectomy. Collapsing deformity developed with neurogenic claudication. Coronal and sagittal imbalance resulted. (Case performed by Dr. Boachie-Adjei.) **A:** Preoperative coronal radiograph shows the significant coronal plane imbalance. **B:** Sagittal deformity associated with this patient's symptoms. **C:** Preoperative myelogram; note segmental lumbar spinal stenosis. **D:** Postoperative coronal view showing restoration of coronal plane balance. *(continued)*

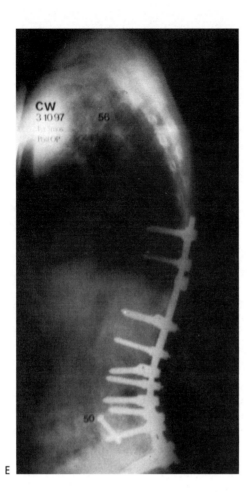

E

FIGURE 5. (*continued*) **E:** Postoperative sagittal view showing restoration of sagittal balance in the lumbar spine, although a proximal junctional kyphosis has developed. An apparent junctional kyphosis has remained unchanged 2 years after operation.

tive day. That way, if imbalance is detected, an early return to the operating room can be accomplished for correction.

In patients with fused thoracic and lumbar deformities, coronal plane balance can be achieved by osteotomies of the major curve to produce a balanced correction. Surgery for lumbar deformities is best performed in conjunction with anterior procedures. This reduces the potential for pseudarthrosis when multiple osteotomies are performed. Instrumentation anchors should be placed into the thoracic fusion mass.

Continued Pain

Pain is the most common presenting symptom in the patient with failed lumbar deformity surgery. It may be caused by prominent instrumentation, pseudarthrosis, degenerative disk disease, spinal stenosis, instability, or nerve root entrapment (1,14,15,20–22).

Painful disorders often can be localized by the patient and physician. Prominent or painful instrumentation is an example in which patients can localize pain directly over the offending instrumentation. Large, bulky instrumentations can be acutely prominent and painful and may require removal,

with replacement of the instrumentation and augmentation of the bone graft if fusion is not solid. Pseudarthrosis may be painful and may progress to instrumentation failure or progressive deformity, or both. The initial diagnosis may be difficult because of the overlying instrumentation. Plain radiographs with oblique views and tomograms can be helpful, but exploration of the fusion may be required to confirm diagnosis and treat the problem. During dissection, poor periosteal stripping of the fusion mass is a good indication of pseudarthrosis. Extensive decortication should be performed at the time of exploration, with débridement of the pseudarthrosis and revision of the fusion with rigid, compression-type instrumentation. Consideration of an anterior procedure, particularly at the level of the pseudarthrosis, increases the fusion rate, especially in the thoracolumbar and lumbosacral regions and in the presence of multiple pseudarthroses.

Juxtafusion disk degeneration with diskogenic pain also can be a source of local pain. This identification can be undertaken by radiographic studies such as MRI or diskography (20,29). Pain-provocative diskograms may indicate the source of pain. An extension of the fusion to include the juxtafusion level may be required. In a patient fused for lumbar spine deformity with a previously asymptomatic instability or spondylolisthesis in the lower lumbar or lumbosacral region, painful spondylolisthesis can subsequently develop. Treatment of the symptomatic spondylolisthesis with a posterior spine fusion without interfering with the intervening motion segments may be indicated. Instability can be demonstrated on flexion/extension radiographs. CTM can demonstrate nerve root entrapment. During treatment of painful disorders or postsurgical lumbar deformity, any attempt to merely decompress, fuse, and instrument without realignment usually leads to failure and may complicate eventual realignment and instrumentation.

In patients who have undergone extension to the sacropelvic region with an L rod or intrailiac screw fixation across the pelvis, sacroiliac pain may develop along with loosening of the iliac rod or screw. These complications may be lessened by use of a transverse connector across the two iliac rods over the sacral (S-1) level. If pain persists, the short end of the L rod or the iliac screw can be removed.

Infection

At Barnes-Jewish Hospital we reviewed wound infections in adult patients who had spinal fusion with segmental spinal instrumentation. We reviewed 519 consecutive adult patients. We had a total of 11 deep wound infections in ten patients. Seven were acute (occurring within the first 2 months after surgery), and four were delayed (occurring 1 to 3 years after the operative procedure). The seven acute infections were treated initially with irrigation, débridement, and closure over tubes. Five of the seven have subsequently gone at least 1 year since treatment without recurrence. One required posterior segmental spinal instrumentation removal with subsequent infection resolution, and one is still draining with the segmental instrumentation in place. For the four delayed infections, three presented with late sinuses and one with malaise and an increased sedimentation rate. The acute infections were treated with 6 weeks of intravenous antibiotics followed by oral agents. The delayed infections were treated with 2 weeks of intravenous antibiotics after removal of the instrumentation, and each has resolved. Of the ten patients, four were revisions, six were combined (anterior and posterior surgeries), and eight had medical risk factors. All of the wound infections were posterior. The infection rate for revisions was 4 of 147, for 2.7%. The rate for combined surgeries was 6 of 148, or 4.1%. Only one infection, which was a delayed infection, occurred in a patient without medical risk factors who had a primary single approach/stage surgery.

Risk factors for deep infection include revision surgery, combined anterior and posterior surgery, and medical risk factors. Without "risk factors," the likelihood of a deep, acute, or late wound infection is rather low (in our series, 1 of 519 patients and one of ten infections).

Those results should be discussed with the patient and patient's family preoperatively. It should be stressed that wound infection does not necessarily mean a failure of the surgery. With débridement and closure over tubes, the instrumentation usually can be salvaged. It is always a mistake to remove the instrumentation before the fusion is absolutely solid. In an adult patient, this inevitably leads to a pseudarthrosis if instrumentation is removed before 1 year after operation. Delayed infections are solved by simply removing the instrumentation. These all seem to be very low-grade infections with very low virulence organisms. To reduce the incidence of wound infection, it is important to débride all devitalized muscle and to close each fascial compartment tightly. Our preference is to drain each cavity with a Hemovac so that hematoma does not put undue tension on the fascial closure.

SUMMARY

The majority of adults who undergo revision surgery for failed lumbar deformity requires combined procedures, such as anterior multilevel diskectomy and fusion and posterior spine fusion with instrumentation or circumferential osteotomies at multiple levels, or single wedge resections. These procedures are technically challenging and very lengthy, with increased blood loss and a greater potential for complications.

Surgical treatment of failed adult lumbar deformity presents a challenge to the spine surgeon. Proper understanding of the etiology and pathophysiology of the underlying disorders and pain-generating factors is the first step toward treatment.

Meticulous surgical technique to achieve an arthrodesis combined with the use of rigid, low-profile, segmental instrumentation and intraoperative radiographs obtains a balanced correction postoperatively. For patients who are undergoing long fusions to the sacropelvic region, the best results have been reported with the use of sacral and iliac fixation combined with anterior column support at the lumbosacral junction.

CONCLUSION

Causes of "failure" in adult lumbar deformity surgery include

1. Inadequate correction
2. Continued pain
3. Junctional kyphosis above
4. Junctional kyphosis below
5. Pseudarthrosis and implant failure
6. Coronal decompensation
7. Sagittal decompensation
8. Neurologic deficit
9. Deep wound infection
10. Systemic complications
11. Counterproductive or inadequate social support

The prevention and management of postsurgical deformity and imbalance in the adult patient should include

1. Proper patient selection
2. Selection of appropriate fusion levels
3. Extensive preoperative planning, including appropriate diagnostic studies
4. Choice of procedure: posterior, anterior/posterior, osteotomies as necessary
5. Strong, stable, durable, low-profile segmental instrumentation
6. Posterior autograft supplemented with anterior allograft (structural) or cages packed with autograft for lumbosacral levels
7. Intraoperative radiographs
8. Postoperative external immobilization as deemed necessary

REFERENCES

1. Albert TJ, Purtill J, Mesa J, et al. Health outcome assessment before and after adult deformity surgery. A prospective study. *Spine* 1995;20:2002–2004.
2. Allen BL, Ferguson RL. The Galveston technique for L-rod instrumentation of the scoliotic spine. *Spine* 1982;7:276–284.
3. Asher MA. Isola spinal instrumentation: an update focusing on realignment and versatility. *Spine* 1994;8:355–401.
4. Asher MA, Strippgen WE, Heining CF, et al. Isola spinal implant system: principles, design and applications. In: An HS, Cotler JM, eds. *Spinal instrumentation.* Baltimore: Williams & Wilkins, 1992.
5. Balderston RA, Winter RB, Moe JH, et al. Fusion to the sacrum for nonparalytic scoliosis in the adult. *Spine* 1986;11:824–829.
6. Boachie-Adjei O, Dendrinos GK, Ogilvie JW, et al. Management of adult spinal deformity with combined anterior-posterior arthrodesis and Luque-Galveston instrumentation. *J Spinal Disord* 1991;4:131–141.
7. Bradford DS. The latest and best in sacral fixation. *Instr Course Lect* 1995;62:115–118.
8. Bridwell KH. Adult idiopathic and degenerative scoliosis. In: Garfin SR, ed. *Orthopaedic knowledge update: spine.* Rosemont, IL: American Academy of Orthopaedic Surgeons, 1997:161–171.
9. Bridwell KH. Load sharing principles: the role and use of anterior structural support in adult deformity. *Instr Course Lect* 1996;45:109–115.
10. Bridwell KH. Osteotomies for fixed deformities in the thoracic and lumbar spine. In: Bridwell KH, DeWald RL, eds. *The textbook of spinal surgery,* 2nd ed. Philadelphia: Lippincott–Raven Publishers, 1997:821–835.
11. Bridwell KH. Where to stop the fusion distally in adult scoliosis—L4, L5, or the sacrum? 1996;45:101–107.
12. Bridwell KH, Lenke LG, Baldus C, et al. Major intraoperative neurologic deficits in pediatric and adult spinal deformity patients: incidence and etiology at one institution. *Spine* 1998;23:324–331.
13. Camp JF, Caudle R, Ashmun RD, et al. Immediate complications of Cotrel-Dubousset instrumentation to the sacro-pelvis. A clinical and biomechanical study. *Spine* 1990;15(9):932–941.
14. Cochran T, Irstam L, Nachemson A. Long-term anatomic and functional changes in patients with adolescent idiopathic scoliosis treated by Harrington rod fusion. *Spine* 1983;8:576–584.
15. Cummine JL, Lonstein JE, Moe JH, et al. Reconstructive surgery in the adult for failed scoliosis fusion. *J Bone Joint Surg Am* 1979;61A:1151–1161.
16. Dekutoski MB, Cohen M, Schendel MJ, et al. Fusion to the sacrum in adult idiopathic scoliosis: the role of sagittal balance. *Orthop Trans* 1993;17:125–126.
17. Dick J, Boachie-Adjei O, Wilson M. One-stage versus two-staged anterior and posterior spinal reconstruction in adults. Comparison of outcomes including nutritional status, complication rates, hospital costs and other factors. *Spine* 1992;17:S310–S316.
18. Dickson JH, Mirkovic S, Noble PC, et al. Results of operative treatment of idiopathic scoliosis in adults. *J Bone Joint Surg Am* 1995;77A:513–523.
19. Glazer PA, Colliou O, Lotz JC, et al. Biomechanical analysis of lumbar fixation. *Spine* 1996;21:1211–1222.
20. Grubb SA, Lipscomb HJ, Conrad RW. Diagnostic findings in painful adult idiopathic scoliosis. Presented at the Meeting of the Scoliosis Research Society, Amsterdam, The Netherlands, September 1989.
21. Grubb SA, Lipscomb HJ, Suh PB. Results in surgical treatment of painful adult scoliosis. *Spine* 1994;19:1619–1627.
22. Jackson RP, Simmons EH, Stripinis D. Incidence and severity of back pain in adult idiopathic scoliosis. *Spine* 1983;8:749–756.
23. Kostuik JP. Treatment of the scoliosis in the adult thoracolumbar spine with special reference of fusion to the sacrum. *Orthop Clin North Am* 1988;19:371–381.

24. Kostuik JP, Hall BB. Spinal fusions to the sacrum in adults with scoliosis. *Spine* 1983;8:489–500.

25. Kostuik JP, Maurais JR, Richardson WJ, et al. Combined single staged anterior and posterior osteotomy for correction of iatrogenic lumbar kyphosis. *Spine* 1988;13:257–266.

26. LaGrone MO, Bradford DS, Moe JH, et al. Treatment of symptomatic flatback after spinal fusion. *J Bone Joint Surg Am* 1988;70A:569–580.

27. Ogilvie JW. Anterior and posterior spinal surgery: same-day, staged, anterior first, posterior first, or simultaneous? In: Pritchard DJ, ed. *Instr Course Lect* 1996;45:99–100.

28. Saer EH III, Winter RB, Lonstein JE. Long scoliosis fusion to the sacrum in adults with nonparalytic scoliosis: an improved method. *Spine* 1990;15:650–653.

29. Schellhas KP, Pollei SR. The role of discography in evaluation of patients with spinal deformity. *Orthop Clin North Am* 1994;25:265–273.

LUMBAR SPINE: TRAUMA

LOUIS G. JENIS AND HOWARD S. AN

A sound understanding of the anatomy of the thoracic and lumbar spine, the concept of stability, the pathomechanics of injury, and the pathoanatomy of neural compression are vitally important in the successful management of fractures and fracture/dislocations in this area. Proper preoperative planning and attention to surgical details can limit complications of treating such injuries. This chapter focuses on the prevention and management of complications related to the surgical treatment of thoracolumbar spinal fractures, including the problems of inadequate decompression; the development of late pain or paralysis, or both; posttraumatic kyphotic deformity; pseudarthrosis; and degeneration in adjacent vertebral levels.

INADEQUATE DECOMPRESSION

The treatment of the unstable fracture or fracture dislocation of the thoracolumbar and lumbar spine with neurologic compromise remains a controversial topic despite numerous publications advocating various treatment modalities (2,3,13,17,20,26,42,50,58,60,64). In addition, the specific treatment of the unstable fracture requires careful consideration of the neurologic status of the patient. A complete spinal cord injury is often managed by spinal stabilization to allow early patient mobilization and limit the consequences of prolonged bed rest. A complete injury is more common in the thoracic region. Neurologic outcome after decompression has not been shown to be significantly improved as compared to stabilization alone (5,10,50). In the thoracolumbar junction, most neurologic deficits are incomplete, involving the conus, cauda equina, or a combination of spinal cord and nerve roots.

In the presence of incomplete neurologic deficits, decompression and spinal stabilization can be beneficial in terms of neurologic recovery. The exact methods of management are numerous, and controversy prevails on the issue of an anterior versus posterior approach for patients with an incomplete spinal cord injury (4–6,17,21,29,38,42,53). A thorough history and examination are mandatory, along with radiographic evaluation, including plain films, com-

puted tomography (CT), and magnetic resonance imaging studies to define the fracture pattern. The contribution of canal compromise from bony fragment retropulsion and that from disk herniation should be determined and differentiated.

The spinal canal dimensions can be restored indirectly from a posterior approach via distraction instrumentation and ligamentotaxis (21,25) or directly via posterior transpedicular (31), posterolateral (24), or anterior decompression (42). Ligamentotaxis depends on the intact posterior longitudinal ligament or annular disk fibers and their bony attachments for reduction of the retropulsed fragments (14). An indirect posterior decompression requires that the reduction be performed within the first several days following the injury, as fracture hematoma can rapidly organize, allowing the fragments to slowly gain stability (66). Edwards and Levine (21) reported 32% canal clearance using Harrington rod instrumentation and sleeves when applied within 48 hours from the time of injury. Less clearance was achieved when they were applied after this time frame. Esses et al. (25) showed that canal clearance can be improved from the preoperative 44% compromise to 16% with the use of the Arbeitsgemeinschaft für Osteosynthesefragen (AO) *fixateur interne* device. In a prospective series of thoracolumbar "burst" fractures treated with indirect spinal decompression, Sjostrom et al. (57) showed that nearly 50% canal clearance could be achieved using pedicle screw instrumentation. This indirect reduction of the spinal canal was found to be less efficient in Denis type (57). Others have not found indirect reduction techniques to be as successful. Shono et al. reported that Harrington rod-sleeve combinations and the AO *fixateur interne* improved the initial canal compromise by only 12% and 18%, respectively (56).

Unfortunately, although it would seem to make intuitive sense to achieve complete canal clearance, it remains controversial as to what constitutes adequate decompression in patients with neurologic deficits. The extent to which canal encroachment is deemed to alter neurologic function significantly also varies at each vertebral level. Hashimoto et al. (33) have shown that neurologic impairment is probable with canal compromise of 35% at T-12, 45% at L-1, and 55% at L-2. Others have also found that canal encroachment of 50% at L-1 is associated with neurologic deficits (29,53,56,62). Therefore, if 50% reduction of canal compromise can be assumed on the basis of using indirect canal decompression via distraction instrumentation, it may then be possible to determine preoperatively which patients may benefit from this technique and which individuals may have significant residual canal fragments and inadequate decompression. However, Shono et al. (56) have shown that indirect reduction with posterior distraction techniques was unable to improve the canal clearance beyond the critical values of Hashimoto at the thoracolumbar junction, suggesting that neurologic impairment would persist.

Direct canal decompression can also be accomplished from a posterior approach via a transpedicular or posterolateral method. Both methods are safe and can be effective in the lumbar region below the level of the conus medullaris, especially if a large retropulsed fragment is lodged to one side of the canal adjacent to the pedicle. The transpedicular technique involves a unilateral laminotomy made at the level of the pedicle and the pedicle then is taken down with a high-speed burr. A reversed-angle curette or a special impactor is placed lateral and anterior to the dura to allow safe tamping of the retropulsed fragment (28,49). A defect should be developed in the posterior vertebral wall to allow the retropulsed fragments to be impacted into a reduced position. A bilateral approach may be necessary in selected cases. The cauda equina or exiting nerve roots can be gently retracted, but the spinal cord or conus should not be manipulated in this procedure. The posterolateral decompression technique frequently requires excision of the transverse process along with the pedicle. However, the decompression is then performed, similar to the technique previously described.

Each patient should be evaluated for documentation of canal clearance following posterior indirect or direct decompression, and that can be performed either intraoperatively or postoperatively. Intraoperative means of assessment of the patency of the spinal canal have been performed with ultrasound. Eismont et al. (23) have described the technique of intraoperative ultrasound in an attempt to prevent the complication of inadequate canal decompression. Using real-time ultrasonic images, visualization of the thecal sac and canal can be performed through a laminotomy or laminectomy without direct manipulation of the neural structures. A probe with surgical lubricant covered by a sterile plastic drape is immersed into the wound, which is filled with saline. The probe is then placed below the level of the fluid, and residual anterior compression by bone or disk material can be detected if present and further decompression is performed.

Alternatively, postoperative assessment of canal clearance can be performed with a CT scan, including axial and sagittally reconstructed images. Although artifact from the instrumentation can make the images difficult to interpret, the spinal canal can often be adequately visualized and the extent of decompression appreciated.

Primary anterior decompression is preferred if the retropulsed fragment is large and located in the midline in a patient with incomplete neurologic deficit or if the fracture occurs more than 2 weeks after the time of injury (7,30,35,42). Secondary anterior decompression should also be done if there is persistent canal compromise following posterior decompression based on imaging studies in a patient with residual neurologic deficits (4,11,53). The surgical approach is left sided to the thoracolumbar spine based on the ease of locating and manipulating it as compared to the inferior vena cava. A thoracoabdominal approach is used for exposure of the T10-12 vertebrae and a retroperitoneal approach for the first lumbar vertebra or more caudal. The spine is exposed one level cephalad and one level caudad to the injured segment. The segmental vessels are ligated at the midpoint of the vertebral bodies. The disk material and endplate cartilage of the cephalad and caudad level to the damaged vertebra are removed and a subtotal corpectomy performed. To prevent inadequate canal clearance, several key points must be remembered during anterior decompression. Initially, the patient must be properly positioned in lateral decubitus with the shoulders and pelvis stabilized in that the back is perpendicular to the floor. Maintaining the patient in the true lateral position allows proper orientation of the spinal canal. The decompression must be continued to the contralateral pedicle. This extent of the decompression can be extrapolated to the opposite side of the spinal cord or thecal sac and serve as an indication of canal patency without direct manipulation or visualization of the neural contents. Finally, the presence of a pulsating dural sac can also be a useful marker to assess the adequacy of canal decompression.

The incidence of inadequate canal decompression is unknown due to the several approaches and techniques currently applied to achieving canal patency. In addition, the degree of canal clearance that is required for neurologic recovery remains controversial. It is imperative that clinical correlation of the patient's postoperative neurologic status and imaging studies be performed to determine if insufficient canal clearance is present, although correlating this with symptomatic compression can be a difficult task.

DEVELOPMENT OF LATE PAIN/PARALYSIS

Patients who have sustained a thoracolumbar fracture with or without neurologic insult may continue to experience pain and late sequelae from several potential sources, including spinal deformity, residual neural compression, instrumentation failure or prominence, and central-type pain in complete spinal cord injuries. No reliable method is available to determine the exact source of late pain, and this problem can be challenging to the physician and the patient.

Significant pain may develop from spinal deformity after a surgically treated thoracolumbar fracture. The scope of abnormalities include posttraumatic kyphosis, posttraumatic scoliosis, and loss of lumbar lordosis. Posttraumatic deformities can alter the load presented to nearby facet joints and soft tissues. This may lead to pain and discomfort secondary to compensatory paraspinal musculature spasm in an attempt to maintain normal anatomic alignment (9). In addition, scoliotic deformities can lead to significant foraminal stenosis on the concavity of the curvature that can be a source of lumbar radicular pain. In the thoracic spine, intractable intercostal pain can also result from root compression along the concavity of the deformity.

Loss of lumbar lordosis can be a significant problem, as has been shown in "flat back" syndrome following posterior fusion for scoliosis (32,37). Patients with iatrogenic lumbar kyphotic deformity present with muscular pain in the upper back and lower cervical area, knee pain from compensatory flexion, an inability to stand erect, and gait abnormalities. The most effective treatment for the flat back syndrome is prevention. Distraction instrumentation in the lower lumbar spine should be avoided for this reason. Restoration of normal lordosis following trauma can be accomplished using transpedicular instrumentation in the lumbar spine spanning only one level above and below the fracture site. Treatment of established flat back syndrome is challenging and involves posterior lumbar corrective osteotomy with instrumentation and fusion.

Pain may also present from residual occult neural compression even in the absence of residual paraly-

sis. Patients with consistent pain, with or without an accompanying deformity or significant neural deficit, should be further evaluated, including a detailed neurologic examination and imaging studies. Bohlman et al. (8) reported on 45 patients who had chronic pain or neural deficit at an average of 4.5 years after thoracolumbar fracture. They noted improvement in pain in 41 patients, with complete relief in 30 and improved neurologic function in 21 of 25 patients with residual neural deficits following anterior decompression and fusion. Late treatment of chronic pain following thoracolumbar fractures has also been described by others. Transfeldt et al. (63) reported an 83% improvement in pain control following delayed anterior decompression.

Late pain related to posterior instrumentation can be a relatively common problem. Instrumentation dislodgment may present as hook dislodgment, hook-rod loss of fixation, or laminar fracture (22). Hook dislodgment is the most frequently reported complication of posterior instrumentation and is estimated to occur in 6% of patients (22). Hook pullout from beneath the lamina typically involves the proximal distraction hook and occurs during flexion and rotation bending. Hook-rod disengagement may occur, with excessive flexion at the most proximal hook site. Laminar fractures are more common when hooks are used in osteoporotic patients; when excessive laminar notching is present; when sharp hooks are used, especially at the sacrum; and during overdistraction (22). Methods of preventing these complications include proper hook placement and design, avoidance of excessive distraction, and proper rod contouring. In addition, the rod should span at least three vertebrae above the site of injury when using hooks to decrease the tendency of the upper hook to back out during flexion (51). The bifid hook has been found to be superior to plain or ribbed hooks in resisting laminar fracture during distraction and is also recommended (27). Additional stability of the hooks can be obtained by the use of sublaminar wires on the rods (12,29,47,59). The failure of hooks and rod dislodgment is becoming less common with the use of modern segmental instrumentation systems. Hooks for L-5 and sacral fixation tend to back out frequently; therefore, pedicle screw fixation is recommended at these levels to provide more reliable fixation (22). To prevent hook-rod disengagement, Edwards et al. (22) recommend that at least 1 cm of rod project beyond the hook.

Another problem that can arise from instrumentation is pain related to prominence of the implant, with development of overlying bursitis and skin problems. Proper contouring of the implant is important in this regard, especially in the thin patient.

Another source of pain that occurs in patients with complete spinal cord injuries is central-type pain. This pain is often poorly localized and associated with paresthesia or spasm. Rehabilitation, transcutaneous electrical stimulation (52), or rhizotomy may be helpful in selected cases.

POSTTRAUMATIC KYPHOSIS

Posttraumatic deformities may develop at the site of injury following conservative or surgical treatment of thoracolumbar fractures (40). Risk factors that may lead to progressive deformity include conservative treatment of unstable fractures, diminished bone mineral density, thoracolumbar junction fractures, iatrogenic instability, and problems related to instrumentation.

The Denis three-column classification of thoracolumbar fractures has allowed for greater understanding of what constitutes an unstable injury (18,19). Initial kyphosis of greater than 25 to 30 degrees or anterior compression greater than 40% to 50% is suggestive of posterior ligamentous and facet joint disruption (45). Studies have shown that burst fractures with greater than 50% collapse or greater than 20 degrees are prone to further deformity with conservative treatment (43). If conservative treatment is chosen for patients with an unstable fracture, prolonged bed rest for at least 8 weeks with a well-applied unilateral pantaloon cast is recommended, with careful radiographic follow-up.

Patients with a thoracolumbar fracture and significant osteoporosis are also at risk for late deformity. Diminished bone mineral density and strength can lead to further fracture collapse during consolidation and places hardware at risk for failure (15).

Fractures that occur at the thoracolumbar junction are at risk for delayed kyphotic deformity based on the biomechanical forces at this unique anatomic site. The thoracolumbar junction is a transition zone from the rigid thoracic spine and rib cage to the more mobile lumbar spine and is inherently subjected to greater forces. Careful observation and management by bracing or surgery are required for these injuries.

Iatrogenic instability can occur when patients with thoracolumbar fractures are treated with laminectomy alone (11,13,45,46,61). Surgical laminectomy removes any remaining posterior constraints and stability and can predispose to progressive kyphosis if not accompanied by arthrodesis and likely instrumentation. Laminectomy should be avoided in this group of patients.

Finally, posttraumatic kyphosis may develop from instrumentation failure as previously described. Distraction applied to the lumbar spine can lead to a flat back syndrome and significant sequelae. Pedicle screw instrumentation systems provide superior biomechanical constructs over distraction hook-rod constructs. However, segmental short pedicle screw and rod fusion of thoracolumbar injuries has been shown in one study to lead to early failure and progressive kyphosis (44). McLain et al. (44) used an early design Cotrel-Dubousset instrumentation system with pedicle screw-rod construct, one above and one below the fracture site. More rigid constructs can be obtained by using two-level pedicle screws above and one level pedicle screw and an infralaminar hook in the adjacent vertebral level below the fracture. If there is significant fracture comminution, restoration of the anterior column may be needed for a load-sharing construct.

When using pedicle screw systems for thoracolumbar fractures, the pedicle screw should be of the largest diameter and length possible and the rod-screw linkage must be rigid. The rod should be at least $^{1}/_{4}$ in. in diameter, and transverse linking with a rod or plate should be used to improve rotational stability of the construct. In anterior instrumented cases, meticulous strut fusion technique and use of modern rigid rod or plate constructs also provide improved stability. Use of rigid internal fixation, meticulous fusion techniques, and effective postoperative bracing prevent this complication of posttraumatic kyphosis. Pseudarthrosis can allow for excessive micromotion and eventual hardware fatigue and failure. A loss of instrumentation stability can lead to progressive deformity requiring revision surgery.

Recurrence of deformity is also possible after premature removal of instrumentation (32,34,48,67). It is also recommended that routine removal of hardware be avoided unless there is a specific indication to do so. The status of the fusion mass must be carefully determined before hardware removal.

Treatment of posttraumatic kyphosis is difficult at best. Most cases require a combined anterior and posterior approach or anterior fusion with instrumentation alone (36,41,43,54,64,65). Rarely, if the deformity is flexible, posterior instrumentation and fusion may be sufficient.

FAILURE OF FUSION

Surgical treatment of thoracolumbar fractures results in pseudarthrosis rates ranging from 2% to 10%

with posterior instrumentation and fusion (22). The nonunion rate is greater in the lumbosacral area as compared to the thoracolumbar region. It is likely that the newer, more rigid instrumentation systems will be associated with a lower pseudarthrosis rate.

The presence of pseudarthrosis is often difficult to detect clinically and radiographically. The patient may present with late-onset back pain, loss of correction, or hardware failure, including rod breakage or hook dislodgment. Oblique radiographs may be useful in detecting nonunion, as can CT scan axial images or tomograms.

At present, there is no substitute for meticulous decortication, facet joint excision, and placement of massive autogenous bone graft in enhancing fusion. Allograft bone should be used as a graft expander only in the posterior spine. Fusion rate can be augmented with stable constructs such as rigid instrumentation and postoperative bracing.

In treating a pseudarthrosis, the site should first be inspected for the presence of an occult or subclinical infection. Reexploration of the fusion site is not a simple procedure. Complete exposure and thorough removal of fibrous tissues are necessary. Autogenous bone graft should be packed into any available decorticated bleeding bone bed and additional stabilization added as well.

Pseudarthrosis may result after anterior grafting procedures (1). Graft dislodgment is largely prevented by careful attention to technical details (1,16). After the anterior procedure, a posterior fusion with compression instrumentation helps to further compress the graft and increase the fusion rate. An anterior instrumentation system can be used alternatively if it provides rigid fixation, thus allowing avoidance of a concomitant posterior procedure.

ADJACENT LEVEL DEGENERATION

Late-onset pain and discomfort may arise from the adjacent nonfused segments from several etiologies. Impingement of the adjacent normal facet joint from hardware can lead to pain and rapid degeneration. Pedicle screw instrumentation can be prominent and at the proximal nonfused facet joint should be inserted in a technique so as not to affect motion at that level. A more lateral starting point with "medialization" during screw placement may allow an unimpeded facet joint range. In addition, if it is noted, after insertion of the screw and associated longitudinal rod, that impingement may be a prob-

lem, screw washers should be placed to elevate the rod off the facet joint.

The development of a solid fusion may place increased load and stress onto the adjacent motion segments leading to accelerated degeneration. This so-called transition syndrome is more common in the highly mobile lumbar spine than in the thoracic spine (22). The risk of transition syndrome is increased when a fusion occurs in a malaligned position. If sagittal malalignment is not restored at the time of surgical intervention, a compensatory position is assumed by the adjacent vertebral levels to maintain a more "anatomic" position. The effect of the compensatory hyperextension in the lumbar spine for posttraumatic thoracic kyphosis is to increase the facet load at the uninjured levels, leading to acceleration of the degenerative cascade.

Although the concept of transition syndrome is controversial, studies have documented adjacent level breakdown in the clinical setting (39,55). Lee (39) reported on 18 patients in whom adjacent level degeneration developed at an average of 8.5 years after their initial fusion surgeries. Schlegel et al. (55) reported on a large series of 58 patients with adjacent segment breakdown. They identified 11 patients who had previously undergone thoracolumbar fusion who presented with late-onset back and leg pain. They found that significant loss of coronal and sagittal alignment was present in each patient and likely served as a predisposing risk factor for accelerated adjacent level pathology (55). It appears that proper instrumentation insertion and correction of deformity can serve to reduce the risk of this problem.

CONCLUSION

In summary, there is controversy as to the most appropriate treatment of thoracolumbar fractures. Nonetheless, complications associated with the surgical treatment of these injuries can be minimized in two ways: (a) The mechanism of injury, degree of canal compromise, and neurologic status must be clearly defined to render appropriate treatment, and (b) attention to surgical details can limit common complications, such as inadequate spinal canal decompression, posttraumatic spinal deformity, and pseudarthrosis. The management of the patient who is surgically treated for a thoracolumbar fracture with late-onset pain is challenging, as several etiologies are capable of causing variable symptoms that need to be evaluated in a systematic manner.

REFERENCES

1. Bauer R, Garfin S. Complications of surgery for lumbar stenosis. *Semin Spine Surg* 1993;5:123.

2. Bedbrook G. Spinal injuries with tetraplegia and paraplegia. *J Bone Joint Surg Br* 1979;61B:26.

3. Bedbrook G. Treatment of thoracolumbar dislocation and fractures with paraplegia. *Clin Orthop* 1975;27.

4. Benson D. Unstable thoracolumbar fractures with emphasis on the burst fractures. *Clin Orthop* 1988;230:14.

5. Bohlman H, Freehafer A, Dejak J. The results of treatment of acute injuries of the upper thoracic spine with paralysis. *J Bone Joint Surg Am* 1985;67A:360.

6. Bohlman H, Eismont F. Surgical techniques of anterior decompression and fusion for spinal cord injuries. *Clin Orthop* 1981;154:57.

7. Bohlman H. Treatment of fractures and dislocations of the thoracic and lumbar spine. *J Bone Joint Surg Am* 1985; 67A:165.

8. Bohlman H, Kirkpatrick J, Delamarter R, et al. Anterior decompression of late pain and paralysis after fracture of the thoracolumbar spine. *Clin Orthop* 1994;300:24.

9. Bolesta M, Bohlman H. Late sequelae of thoracolumbar fractures and fracture-dislocations—surgical treatment. In: Frymoyer J, ed. *The adult spine: principles and practice.* New York: Raven Press, 1991:1331–1352.

10. Bradford D, Akbarnia B, Winter R, et al. Surgical stabilization of fracture and fracture-dislocations of the thoracic spine. *Spine* 1977;2:185.

11. Bradford D, McBride G. Surgical management of thoracolumbar spine fractures with incomplete neurologic deficits. *Clin Orthop* 1987;218:201.

12. Bryant C, Sullivan J. Management of thoracic and lumbar spine fractures with Harrington distraction rods supplemented with segmental wiring. *Spine* 1983;8:532.

13. Burke D, Murray D. The management of thoracic and thoracolumbar injuries of the spine with neurologic involvement. *J Bone Joint Surg Br* 1976;58B:72.

14. Cain J, DeJong J, Dinenberg A, et al. Pathomechanical analysis of thoracolumbar burst fracture reduction. *Spine* 1993;18:1647.

15. Cogins M. Nonunions and malunions of thoracolumbar spine injuries. *Semin Spine Surg* 1995;7:137.

16. Cotler H, Cotler J, Stoloff A, et al. The use of autografts for vertebral body replacement of the thoracic and lumbar spine. *Spine* 1985;10:748.

17. Cotler J, Vernace J, Michalski J. The use of Harrington rods in thoracolumbar fractures. *Orthop Clin North Am* 1986;17:87.

18. Denis F. The three-column spine and its significance in the classification of acute thoracolumbar spine injuries. *Spine* 1983;8:817.

19. Denis F. Spinal instability as defined by the three-column spine concept in acute spinal trauma. *Clin Orthop* 1984;189:65.

20. Denis F, Armstrong G, Serals K, et al. Acute thoracolumbar burst fractures in the absence of neurological deficit: a comparison between operative and nonoperative treatment. *Clin Orthop* 1984;189:142.

21. Edwards C, Levine A. Early rod-sleeve stabilization of the injured thoracic and lumbar spine. *Orthop Clin North Am* 1986;17:121.

22. Edwards C, Boston H, Levine A, et al. Complications associated with posterior instrumentation for thoracolumbar injuries and their prevention. *Semin Spine Surg* 1993;5:108.

23. Eismont F, Green B, Berkowitz A, et al. The role of intraoperative ultrasonography in the treatment of thoracic and lumbar spine fractures. *Spine* 1984;9:782.

24. Erickson D, Leider L, Brown W. One-stage decompression-stabilization for thoracolumbar fractures. *Spine* 1977; 2:43.

25. Esses S, Botsford D, Kostuik J. Evaluation of surgical treatment for burst fractures. *Spine* 1990;15:667.

26. Frankel H, Hancock D, Hyslop G. The value of postural reduction in the initial management of closed injuries of the spine with paraplegia and tetraplegia. *Paraplegia* 1969;7:179.

27. Freedman L, Houghton G, Evans M. Cadaveric study comparing the stability of upper distraction hooks used in Harrington instrumentation. *Spine* 1986;11:579.

28. Garfin S, Mowery C, Guerra J, et al. Confirmation of the posterolateral technique to decompress and fuse thoracolumbar spine burst fractures. *Spine* 1985;10:218.

29. Gertzbein S, MacMichael D, Tile M. Harrington instrumentation as a method of fixation in fractures of the spine. *J Bone Joint Surg Br* 1982;64B:526.

30. Ghanayem A, Zdeblick T. Anterior instrumentation in the management of thoracolumbar burst fractures. *Clin Orthop* 1997;335:89.

31. Hardaker W, Cook W, Friedman A, et al. Bilateral transpedicular decompression and Harrington rod stabilization in the management of severe thoracolumbar burst fractures. *Spine* 1992;17:162.

32. Hasday C, Passoff T, Perry J. Gait abnormalities arising from iatrogenic loss of lumbar lordosis secondary to Harrington instrumentation in lumbar fractures. *Spine* 1983;8:501.

33. Hashimoto T, Kaneda K, Abumi K. Relationship between traumatic spinal canal stenosis and neurologic deficits in thoracolumbar burst fractures. *Spine* 1988;13:1268.

34. Jodoin A, Gillet P, Dupuis P, et al. Surgical treatment of post-traumatic kyphosis: a report of 16 cases. *Can J Surg* 1989;32:36.

35. Johnson J, Leatherman K, Holt R. Anterior decompression of the spinal cord for neurological deficit. *Spine* 1983;8:396.

36. Kostuik J, Matsusaki H. Anterior stabilization instrumentation and decompression for post-traumatic kyphosis. *Spine* 1989;14:379.

37. LaGrone M, Bradford D, Moe J, et al. Treatment of symptomatic flat back after spinal fusion. *J Bone Joint Surg Am* 1988;70A:569.

38. Larson S, Holst R, Hemmy D, et al. Lateral extracavitary approach to traumatic lesions of the thoracic and lumbar spine. *J Neurosurg* 1976;45:628.

39. Lee C. Accelerated degeneration of the segment adjacent to a lumbar fusion. *Spine* 1988;13:375.

40. Lindahl S, Willen J, Irstam L. Unstable thoracolumbar fractures. A comparative radiologic study of conservative treatment and Harrington instrumentation. *Acta Radiol Diagn* 1985;26:67.

41. Malcolm B, Bradford D, Winter R, et al. Post-traumatic kyphosis. *J Bone Joint Surg Am* 1981;63A:891–899.

42. McAfee P, Bohlman H, Yuan H. Anterior decompression of traumatic thoracolumbar fractures with incomplete neurological deficit using retroperitoneal approach. *J Bone Joint Surg Am* 1985;67A:89.

43. McAfee P, Yuan H, Lasda N. The unstable burst fracture. *Spine* 1982;7:365.

44. McLain R, Sparling E, Benson D. Early failure of short segment pedicle instrumentation for thoracolumbar fractures. *J Bone Joint Surg Am* 1993;2:162–167.

45. McEvoy R, Bradford D. The management of burst fractures of the thoracic and lumbar spine: experience in 53 patients. *Spine* 1985;10:631.

46. Morgan T, Wharton G, Austin G. The results of laminectomy in patients with incomplete spinal cord injuries. *Paraplegia* 1971;9:14.

47. Munson G, Satterlee C, Hammond S, et al. Experimental evaluation of Harrington rod fixation supplemented with sublaminar wires in stabilizing thoracolumbar fracture-dislocations. *Clin Orthop* 1984;189:97.

48. Myllunen P, Bostman O, Riska E. Recurrence of deformity after removal of Harrington's fixation of spine fracture. Seventy-six cases followed for two years. *Acta Orthop Scand* 1988;59:497.

49. Oro J, Watts C, Gaines R. Vertebral body impactor for posterior lateral decompression of thoracic and lumbar fractures. *J Neurosurg* 1989;70:285.

50. Osebold W, Weinstein S, Sprague B. Thoracolumbar spine fractures: results of treatment. *Spine* 1981;6:13.

51. Purcell G, Markolf K, Dawson E. Twelfth thoracic-first lumbar vertebral mechanical stability of fractures after Harrington-rod instrumentation. *J Bone Joint Surg Am* 1981; 63A:71.

52. Richardson R, Meyer P, Cerullo L. Transcutaneous electrical neurostimulation in musculoskeletal pain of acute spinal injuries. *Spine* 1980;4:42.

53. Riska E, Myllynen P, Bostman O. Anterolateral decompression for neural involvement in thoracolumbar fractures. *J Bone Joint Surg Br* 1987;69B:704.

54. Roberson J, Whitesides T. Surgical reconstruction of late post-traumatic thoracolumbar kyphosis. *Spine* 1985;10:307.

55. Schlegel J, Smith J, Schleusner R. Lumbar motion segment pathology adjacent to thoracolumbar, lumbar and lumbosacral fusions. *Spine* 1996;21:970.

56. Shono Y, McAfee P, Cunningham B. Experimental study of thoracolumbar burst fractures. A radiographic and biomechanical analysis of anterior and posterior instrumentation systems. *Spine* 1994;19:1711.

57. Sjostrom L, Karlstrom G, Pech P, et al. Indirect spinal canal decompression in burst fractures treated with pedicle screw instrumentation. *Spine* 1996;21:113.

58. Soreff J, Axdorf R, Bylund P, et al. Treatment of patients with unstable fractures of the thoracic and lumbar spine. *Acta Orthop Scand* 1982;53:369.

59. Sullivan J. Sublaminar wiring of Harrington distraction rods for unstable thoracolumbar spine fractures. *Clin Orthop* 1984;189:178.

60. Svensson O, Aaro S, Ohlen G. Harrington instrumentation for thoracic and lumbar vertebral fractures. *Acta Orthop Scand* 1984;55:38.

61. Tencer A, Allen B, Ferguson R. A biomechanical study of thoracolumbar spinal fractures with bone in the canal. The effect of laminectomy. *Spine* 1985;10:58.

62. Trafton P, Boyd C. Computed tomography of thoracic and lumbar spine injury. *J Trauma* 1984;24:506.

63. Transfeldt E, White D, Bradford D, et al. Delayed anterior decompression in patients with spinal cord and cauda equina injuries of the thoracolumbar spine. *Spine* 1990;15:953.

64. Weinstein J, Collalto P, Lehmann T. Long term follow-up of nonoperatively treated thoracolumbar spine fractures. *J Orthop Trauma* 1987;1:152.

65. Whitesides T, Shah S. On the management of unstable fractures of the thoracolumbar spine. *Spine* 1976;1:99.

66. Willen J, Lindblad S, Nordwall A. Unstable thoracolumbar fractures: a study by CT and conventional roentgenology of the reduction effect of Harrington instrumentation. *Spine* 1984;9:214.

67. Willen J, Lindahl S, Norwall A. Unstable thoracolumbar fractures: comparative clinical study of conservative treatment and Harrington instrumentation. *Spine* 1985;10:111.

LUMBAR SPINE: TUMOR

SCOTT C. WILSON AND THOMAS S. WHITECLOUD III

Cancer differs from other diagnoses that afflict the spine because the patient's life is always in question. If surgery for spinal metastatic disease does not safely alleviate pain, restore mechanical stability, and ensure neurologic function, the surgeon rarely has a second chance to correct the problem with further surgery. The patient's medical condition often deteriorates as a result of disease progression and makes further surgery medically contraindicated. Also, failure to control a primary sarcoma usually results in an inoperable local recurrence involving the entire operative area. Quite simply, most mistakes are buried. Therefore, the goal of this chapter is to outline the mistakes that must be avoided in the treatment of cancerous lesions of the lumbar spine, so that a "failed spine" can be prevented in the first place.

Metastatic carcinoma and multiple myeloma are more common than primary sarcoma or chordoma of the spine. Therefore, the majority of this chapter focuses on patients with metastatic or multifocal disease. Eighty percent of spinal metastases arise from primary carcinomas of the lung, breast, prostate, and kidney (29,33). The lumbar vertebrae are the most frequent locations of spinal metastases (6). It is also common for metastases to span more than one region of the spine (Table 1). Therefore, the lumbar spine should not be considered in isolation, and the entire spine of a cancer patient must be included in the preoperative evaluation. The principles that are discussed in this chapter are also applicable to the thoracic and cervical spine (please refer to the appropriate chapters within this book).

Hematogenous spread most often occurs via Batson's vertebral venous plexus (2,3,13). Tumor cells travel into the marrow of the vertebral bodies via the perforating vessels. Presumably, the frequency of metastatic involvement corresponds with the volume of red marrow within the vertebrae. Therefore, metastases occur in the anterior and middle columns of Denis (9) more frequently than in the posterior column. Barriers to prevention of local spread include the anterior longitudinal ligament, the posterior longitudinal ligament, the periosteum abutting the spinal canal, the ligamentum flavum, the periosteum of the lamina and spinous process,

the interspinous ligament, the supraspinous ligament, the cartilaginous endplate, and the anulus fibrosis. The posterior longitudinal ligament was found to be the weakest barrier to penetration (12).

Historically, surgery was performed primarily for metastasis presenting with spinal cord compression. These patients generally had more advanced disease and a more limited prognosis. The posterior approach was used routinely in concert with radiotherapy. Unfortunately, limited benefit was obtained due to the following: the inability to remove the entire tumor deposit and thus effectively decompress the neural elements, the problems with bleeding intraoperatively using a limited incision, and the mechanical instability that resulted if spinal instrumentation was not used (8,16). More recently, a more accurate appreciation of spine tumor pathophysiology has emerged. More effective neural decompression is accomplished with corpectomy using anterior and posterior approaches, and improved reconstructive options have dramatically improved the efficacy of spinal surgery (1,21,25). Also, because there are more effective treatments available for cancer patients today, they live longer with their disease. Therefore, surgery today has a much more important role in the management of patients with spinal metastases.

Anterior and middle column collapse in the lumbar spine results in kyphosis with retropulsion of material into the spinal canal and may cause cord, conus, or nerve root compression. Complete corpectomy is generally required for adequate neural decompression and prevention of future regrowth of the tumor. Anterior or retroperitoneal approaches are now used routinely for corpectomy and decompression of the neural canal. Excellent techniques for a posterior approach have also been described that can accomplish the same goals, and they are particularly useful in a frail individual who cannot tolerate a thoracotomy or abdominal approach to the lesion. If neurologic compromise is not present, more limited curettage of the tumor and anterior column reconstruction with or without posterior stabilization may be sufficient.

Reconstruction of bony defects after neural decompression using methylmethacrylate cement and Stein-

TABLE 1. SPINAL METASTASIS: AN OVERVIEW

Type	No. of Patients with Spine Metastases	Overall Patient No.	Overall Patient %	Cervical %	Thoracic %	Lumbar %	Sacral %
Pulmonary (2)	149	744	20	23	53	54	23
Breast (2)	114	844	14	18	46	61	28
Prostate (2)	59	146	40	49	71	6	41
Cervical (2)	46	379	12	7	20	57	46
Renal (2)	28	101	28	17	14	52	31
Gastrointestinal (2)	28	158	18	50	61	75	50
Melanoma (1)	114	7,010	1.6	18	58	49	49

mann's pins to serve as reinforcement rods was an early method of anterior reconstruction (18). This, in combination with Harrington rods posteriorly, represented one of the first advancements in the treatment of metastatic disease. Subsequently, corpectomy and reconstruction with anterior instrumentation were popularized by Arbit and Galicich (1), Kostuik et al. (21), and Onimus et al. (25). Today an even greater variety of reconstructive options are available. Examples of anterior fixation devices include the contoured anterior spinal plate, a low-profile plate designed for thoracic and lumbar spine fixation that provides multiple screw holes and is available in various lengths. The Z-plate is another anterior plate that allows dynamic compression. Kaneda's device provides anterior segmental fixation by using screws coupled to threaded rods that span the decompressed area. These devices, used in conjunction with titanium cages, structural allograft, or acrylic bone cement, can provide immediate stability. Titanium fixation devices are preferred to those made of steel because they create little scatter artifact on magnetic resonance imaging (MRI). Therefore, MRI can be more effectively used to monitor patients for postoperative tumor recurrence. What follows are six errors that may result in a failed spine and how to avoid these errors.

ONE: OPERATING WITHOUT A CORRECT DIAGNOSIS

Errors in diagnosis can result in an inappropriate decision to perform spine surgery and an incorrect choice of operative technique. Surgery should never be selected based on a presumptive diagnosis unless the patient has a previous history of cancer. Even in this situation, a confirmatory biopsy may be appropriate, depending on the clinical circumstances. Rare cases of second primary malignancies have been reported. For example, a radiation-induced sarcoma can occur in the radiation field of a previously irradiated tumor bed (20). Because the goals and techniques of surgery to treat primary ver-

sus metastatic disease are so profoundly different, a tissue diagnosis is the only way to avoid the mistake of performing an intralesional removal of a sarcoma that was thought to be a metastatic carcinoma. Sarcomas require a wide margin for effective local control. An intralesional procedure leaves tumor behind, contaminates the entire operative area, and greatly increases the risk of uncontrollable local recurrence. Therefore, a detailed history is important in identifying clinical clues that may indicate the need for biopsy.

Imaging the lumbar spine is best done with plain upright radiographs and good-quality MRI. These modalities provide an excellent way to assess the intraosseous and extraosseous extent of disease and to estimate the degree of mechanical compromise that has occurred. Computed tomography (CT) with fine cuts through the lesion can also be helpful in assessing the bony integrity of the vertebrae around the lesion and measuring the size of the pedicles for preoperative planning. CT myelography is reserved for situations in which there is a question of cord, conus, or nerve root impingement not elucidated by physical examination or MRI. MRI is also very helpful in identifying other lesions that are not apparent on plane radiographs or technetium bone scans (Fig. 1). Knowing

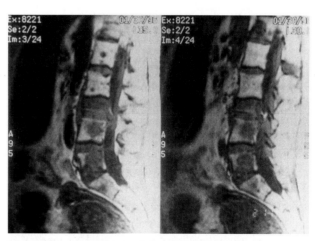

FIGURE 1. Sagittal T1-weighted magnetic resonance image of lumbosacral spine showing lesions of varying size in all of the lumbar vertebrae.

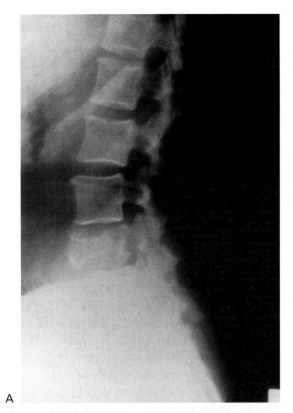

A

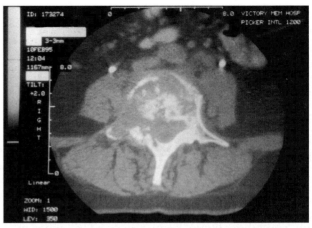

B

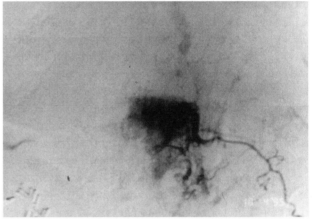

D

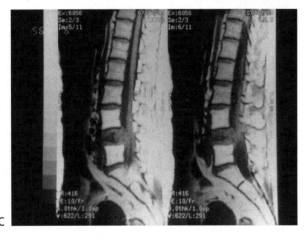

C

FIGURE 2. Renal cell metastasis of L-4 as seen on **(A)** plain film, **(B)** computed tomography, **(C)** sagittal T1-weighted magnetic resonance image, and **(D)** fluoroscopy showing embolization.

the full extent of disease within the spine is particularly helpful in preoperative planning and in planning the portals for radiation therapy.

Staging studies should include a contrast CT of the chest, abdomen, and pelvis and a total body bone scan (28). Also, prostate-specific antigen and serum and urine protein electrophoresis with immunoelectrophoresis can be very helpful in establishing the diagnosis for prostate cancer and multiple myeloma, respectively. Additionally, knowing the identity of the primary carcinoma may be very important preoperatively. For example, renal cell carcinoma is a particularly vascular tumor and should be preoperatively embolized immediately before surgery. This maneuver reduces the amount of intraoperative bleeding, which can otherwise be uncontrollable (Fig. 2).

TWO: INCORRECTLY ASSESSING THE OVERALL MEDICAL CONDITION OF A PATIENT WITH METASTATIC DISEASE WHEN CONSIDERING SPINAL SURGERY

Understanding the prognosis of a cancer patient is a difficult task that is very important in determining if he or she is healthy enough to withstand spinal surgery. Cancer patients experience not only the immediate effects of their disease but also a variety of associated problems as a result of the effects of the tumor and the consequences of treatment. For example, bone marrow depletion can occur from the systemic spread of the cancer or as a result of extensive radiotherapy to the skeleton. Anemia, leukocytopenia, and thrombocytopenia are common problems encountered in this setting. Cancer patients with a low total lymphocyte count have a suppressed immune system and a diminished capacity to fight perioperative bacteremia. They are also more likely to need red blood cell transfusions and, possibly, platelet transfusions during extensive surgery.

Cachexia is another common comorbidity of cancer and is associated with low albumin and total protein levels. These parameters identify nutritional depletion and indicate a poorer prognosis due to diminished wound-healing capacity and a compromised immune system.

When medical clearance is being obtained for general surgery, the examining physician should carefully evaluate cardiac function in patients who have received doxorubicin (Adriamycin) because of its cardiotoxic effects (7). Also, patients who received lung irradiation or bleomycin chemotherapy should undergo pulmonary function testing because they are at increased risk for compromised pulmonary function.

Another way of calculating perioperative risk is to determine the patient's physical performance status. Functional scales are helpful because treatment decisions are not dependent on attempting to calculate how long patients have to live (a very difficult educated guess that is often inaccurate) but rather how physically functional they are. Karnofsky developed a ten-point scale to measure physical performance, and subsequently, the Eastern Cooperative Oncology Group developed a simpler five-point scale, which is easy to use and important to understand (Table 2). Anyone with a poor performance status is unlikely to be a candidate for further conventional chemotherapy. Traditionally, a patient with a Karnofsky score of four or less is thought to be at much greater risk for development of side effects and therefore is a poor candidate for systemic chemotherapy. More simply, a patient who is too sick to get out of bed is too sick for chemotherapy. Therefore, the potential palliative benefits of chemotherapy are outweighed by potentially life-threatening complications of this treatment. The stresses of major spine surgery are comparable to those of a round of cytotoxic chemotherapy. Therefore, if the patient's performance status is too poor for medical intervention, the patient is also unlikely to be a good candidate for extensive spinal surgery. In patients with disease that is this debilitating, a palliative approach to care may be more appropriate. Narcotic analgesics and selective radiotherapy for bone lesions may still significantly improve the patient's quality of life with little risk of hastening death.

THREE: INCORRECTLY CHOOSING AN OPERATIVE PROCEDURE THAT IS NOT APPROPRIATELY MATCHED TO THE PATIENT'S PROGNOSIS

It is often very difficult to determine the prognosis of a patient with metastatic disease (31,34). Yet an estimation of the patient's expected life span helps in determining the type of operation that is most suited to balance the benefits with the risks of surgery. For example, a patient with an isolated metachronous

TABLE 2. CRITERIA FOR PERFORMANCE STATUS ON THE KARNOFSKY PERFORMANCE SCALE AND EASTERN COOPERATIVE ONCOLOGY GROUP PERFORMANCE SCALE

	Karnofsky Performance Scale		Eastern Cooperative Oncology Group Performance Scale
100	Normal; no complaints; no evidence of disease	0	Normal activity; asymptomatic
90	Able to carry on normal activity; minor signs or symptoms of disease	1	Symptomatic; fully ambulatory
80	Normal activity with effort; some signs or symptoms of disease	2	Symptomatic; in bed <50% of time
70	Cares for self; unable to carry on normal activity or to do active work	3	Symptomatic; in bed >50% of time; not bedridden
60	Requires occasional assistance but is able to care for most needs		
50	Requires considerable assistance and frequent medical care	4	100% bedridden
40	Disabled; requires special care and assistance	5	Dead
30	Severely disabled; hospitalization is indicated although death not imminent		
20	Very sick; hospitalization necessary; active supportive treatment is necessary		
10	Moribund, fatal processes progressing rapidly		
0	Dead		

Modified from Karnofsky DA, Abelmann WH, Craver LF, et al. The use of nitrogen mustards in the palliative treatment of carcinoma with particular reference to bronchogenic carcinoma. *Cancer* 1948;1:634–669.

TABLE 3. CLASSIFICATION OF SPINAL METASTASES

I. No significant neurologic or bone involvement
II. Involvement of bone without collapse or instability
III. Major neurologic involvement (sensory or motor) without significant involvement of bone
IV. Vertebral collapse with pain due to mechanical causes or instability but without significant neurologic involvement
V. Vertebral collapse or instability with major neurologic impairment

From Harrington KD. Metastatic disease of the spine. *J Bone Joint Surg Am* 1986;68A(7):1110–1115, with permission.

TABLE 4. EVALUATION SYSTEM FOR THE PROGNOSIS OF METASTATIC SPINE TUMORS

	Score
General condition (performance status)	
Poor (PS, 10–40%)	0
Moderate (PS, 50–70%)	1
Good (PS, 80–100%)	2
No. of extraspinal bone metastases foci	
≥3	0
1–2	1
0	2
No. of metastases	
≥3	0
1–2	1
0	2
Metastases to the major internal organs	
Unremovable	0
Removable	1
No metastases	2
Primary site of cancer	
Lung, stomach	0
Kidney, liver, uterus	1
Others, unidentified	—
Thyroid, prostate, breast	2
Rectum	—
Spinal cord palsy	
Complete	0
Incomplete	1
None	2
Total	12

PS, performance status.

renal cell metastasis may have a prognosis measured in years. A wide excision of this type of relatively radioresistant metastasis should be strongly considered to maximize the opportunity of obtaining durable local control. On the other hand, a patient with compression of the conus medullaris due to a large melanoma metastasis is more likely to have a life span measured in weeks. Surgical intervention plays a more selective role in this subset of patients with a much more guarded prognosis.

Several authors have created staging systems to better calculate prognosis in patients with metastatic carcinoma involving the spine. These studies have been useful in determining whether patients are appropriate candidates for spine surgery. The staging system of Harrington has been traditionally used to describe a metastatic spine lesion as mechanically stable or unstable and to identify associated neurologic compromise (17) (Table 3). Patients with metastatic lesions that were associated with mechanical compromise, neurologic deficit, or both, were considered good surgical candidates for corpectomy and decompression.

Tokuhashi et al. (35) proposed an evaluation system for prognosis of metastatic spine tumors. They reviewed the outcomes of 64 patients postoperatively and used six criteria, including general condition, the number of extraspinal bone metastases, the number of vertebral metastases, the number of metastases to the internal organs, the primary cancer site, and the severity of spinal cord palsy. Each parameter was graded from 0 to 2 to arrive at a total score between 0 and 12, as outlined in Table 4. Tokuhashi et al. concluded that an excisional operation (consisting of extensive curettage and reconstruction with methacrylate cement with or without a ceramic spacer and fixation hardware) was indicated for patients with a preoperative score of 9 or greater. Patients with a score of 5 or less had a more limited prognosis. Operative palliation to stabilize the spine with

instrumentation and decompress neural elements was preferred but without extensive tumor removal. Patients with a score of 6 to 8 were presumably handled on a case-by-case basis (35). Using their own patient database of 71 patients, Enkaoua et al. (10) validated Tokuhashi's staging system with one minor modification. Their data indicated that metastasis of unknown primary origin should be ranked 0, indicating a poorer prognosis (10).

Arbit and Galicich (1) reviewed 109 patients who underwent surgery to control spine metastases. They identified three adverse prognostic factors: cord compromise with a Frankel class of zero to three of five (0–3/5), primary disease arising in the lung or colon, and more than one vertebra involved. Perioperative mortality was 11% (1). Their conclusion was that patients with two or more risk factors should not undergo surgery.

As useful as these studies are to determine prognosis, they provide few guidelines as to the technique of surgery that is appropriate, based on the patient's prognosis. However, Tomita et al. (38) have taken the art of prognosis a step further by developing what they call a surgical strategy for spinal metastases that indicates the patient's prognosis and

Scoring System					Prognostic Score	Treatment Goal	Surgical Strategy
	Prognostic factors				2	Long-term local control	Wide or Marginal excision
Point	Primary tumor	Visceral mets.*	Bone mets.**		3		
1	slow growth (breast, thyroid, etc.)		solitary or isolated		4	Middle-term local control	Marginal or Intralesional excision
					5		
2	moderate growth (kidney, uterus, etc.)	treatable	multiple		6	Short-term palliation	Palliative surgery
					7		
4	rapid growth (lung, stomach, etc.)	un-treatable			8	Terminal care	Supportive care
					9		
					10		

FIGURE 3. Tomita's surgical strategy for spinal metastases (mets.). *No visceral mets. = 0 point. **Bone mets. including spinal mets. (From Tomita K, Kawahara N, Kobayashi T, et al. Surgical strategy for spinal metastases. *Spine* 2001;26 (3):298–306, with permission.)

the type of surgery that is most suited for a given prognosis (Fig. 3).

This system was developed by evaluating 67 patients with spine metastases and grading them according to the following three criteria: primary tumor location, presence of visceral metastases, and presence of bony metastases. A composite score ranged from 2 to 10. Patients with a score of 2 or 3 had a better prognosis, and long-term local control was recommended, indicating a wide or marginal excision. Patients with a score of 4 or 5 had an intermediate prognosis, and middle-term local procedures, including marginal or intralesional excision, were deemed most appropriate. Patients with a score of 6 or 7 had a poorer prognosis, and short-term palliative surgery such as instrumentation and simple decompression without tumor excision was recommended. Patients with scores of 8 through 10 had a very poor prognosis, with an average life expectancy of 5 months. These patients were thought to have limited potential benefits from surgery, with correspondingly prohibitive surgical risks. They did not undergo surgery but were given supportive hospice care.

FOUR: MISJUDGING THE TYPE AND EXTENT OF SURGICAL STABILIZATION THAT THE BONY LESIONS REQUIRE

Several factors must be considered in planning the extent of surgery: the location and amount of mechanical compromise of the vertebra, the presence or absence of spinal canal compromise, the presence of adjacent vertebral metastasis, and the quality of the remaining bone (Table 3). An excellent tumor staging system to describe the spine tumors was developed by Tomita et al. (37). Their system identifies the location of the lesion, the concurrence of fracture, and the presence of multiple lesions (37) (Fig. 4). The identification of metastatic lesions in adjacent vertebrae dictates the extent of fusion that is necessary for adequate stability, because pedicle screw or lamina hook fixation may be compromised by metastatic deposits in adjacent vertebrae. For example, a patient with metastatic breast cancer was found to have two separate lesions at L-2 and T-12. Significant collapse of the body was noted, requiring posterior instrumentation from T-6 to L-3 and anterior femoral allograft struts at L-2 and T-12 secured by a single spanning Kaneda plate (Fig. 5).

The quality of bone is dependent on several biological factors. Osteoporosis-like carcinoma is more often found in older patients. In patients who are debilitated by their cancer, secondary osteoporosis may occur in the form of Sudek's atrophy. Also, patients, particularly those with lung cancer, may have a paraneoplastic disorder whereby parathyroid hormone–related hormone is produced by tumor cells, resulting in hypercalcemia and loss of calcium from the bone. Prior exposure to therapeutic chemotherapy has been shown to decrease union rates in osteochondral allografts in a canine model (24) and in union rates of osteochondral and intercalary allografts in humans.

Cancer patients may have already received relatively high doses of radiation to the proposed operative area in an attempt to control the spine tumor. Spinal cord tolerance limits total doses to 4,500 rads, although

Intra-Compartmental	Extra-Compartmental	Multiple
Type 1 vertebral body	**Type 4** epidural ext.	**Type 7**
Type 2 pedicle extension	**Type 5** paravertebral ext.	
Type 3 body-lamina ext.	**Type 6** 2-3 vertebrae	

FIGURE 4. Tomita's classification of spinal tumors. (From Tomita K, Kawahara N, Kobayashi T, et al. Surgical strategy for spinal metastases. *Spine* 2001;26:298–306, with permission.)

spinal roots below the conus can safely withstand higher doses without injury. The total amount of radiation should be known for two reasons. First, it is important to know if additional radiation can be given after surgery, especially if the operation is intralesional and viable tumor is encountered. Second, it is important to decide if bone grafts should be avoided because of the diminished healing capacity of the local tissues. Cumulative radiation doses greater than 3,000 rads have been associated with compromised fracture healing in long bones (14). Because ionizing radiation causes fibrosis, diminishes the vascular supply of soft tissues, and causes bone to become hypocellular, thus reducing repair and remodeling capabilities (5,11,30,39), high doses can be expected to delay or inhibit the formation of bone graft fusion

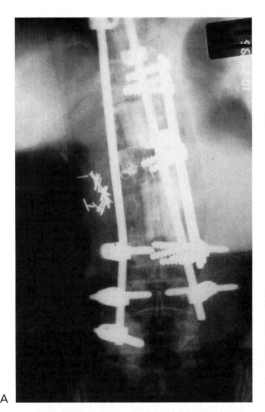
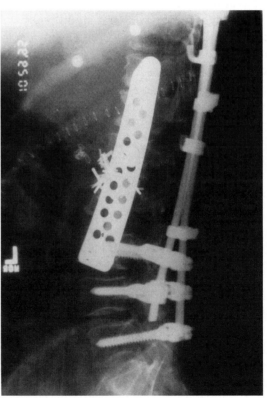

A   B

FIGURE 5. Example of L-2 and T-12 femoral strut allografts after corpectomies, with stabilization in front using a Kaneda plate and in back with segmental instrumentation with pedicle screws and sublaminar hooks. **A:** Anteroposterior view. **B:** Lateral view.

mass just as it interferes with fracture healing (15,19,23,26,27,40). Emery used a canine model to show that postoperative radiation inhibited bone graft incorporation in the spine. He recommended that radiation therapy be delayed for 6 weeks postoperatively to maximize the rate of bone graft incorporation (20). Otherwise, nonunion of the fusion site may occur, leading to mechanical failure.

FIVE: FAILING TO OBTAIN A WIDE MARGIN FOR PRIMARY MALIGNANT DISEASE

Primary sarcomas such as osteosarcoma and chondrosarcoma of the spine fortunately are very rare. For example, osteogenic sarcoma involves the spine in approximately 1.5% of cases, making for an incidence of 30 expected cases per year in the United States (20). Chordoma is another rare malignant neoplasm of bone found exclusively in the axial skeleton, preferring the cervical spine and sacrum. Chordoma of the lumbar spine is extremely rare and presents as a low-grade malignancy with a less frequent incidence of metastatic spread (4).

Sarcomas and chordomas require wide margins for effective local control to minimize the incidence of local recurrence. Obtaining wide margins without exposing the tumor is often a very challenging procedure. Piecemeal posterior vertebrectomy, for example, cannot be used to obtain wide margins because tumor is spilled into the operative field. Even if the tumor bed is free of residual tumor, intralesional exposure of the tumor contaminates the surgically exposed tissues with cancer cells. These seeds take root in the surrounding tissues and, in the vast majority of cases, grow to cause a local recurrence of the disease. An example of a failure to obtain wide margins of a primarily malignant disease is shown in Figure 6. This patient had a chordoma resected and had reconstruction using fibular strut graft anteriorly and Luque rod fixation with sublaminar wires posteriorly to create a fusion from T-10 to L-3. The stabilization was successful, but a wide marginal incision was not obtained. Ten years after surgery, the patient presented with a recurrence of the chordoma, and a wide excision was not possible. The patient underwent an intralesional debulking procedure, which relieved his symptoms of neural compression for a period of 3 years, only to have them recur. The MRI shown in Figure 6 (C and D) illustrates the most recent recurrence.

Techniques for total spondylectomy to obtain wide margins have been described by Magerl and Coscia

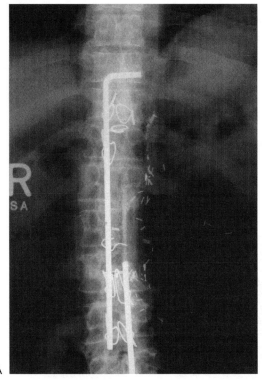
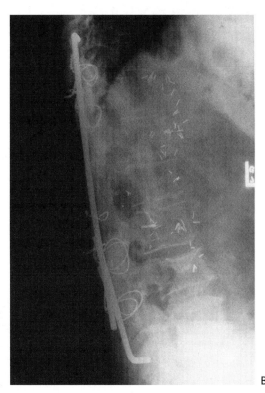

FIGURE 6. Example of a local recurrence of a primary chordoma of L-1. **A, B:** Plain films of the fusion of T-10 to L-3, with fibular strut at L-1 and Luque rods with sublaminar wires. (*continued*)

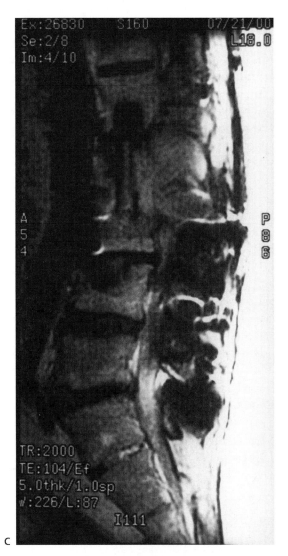

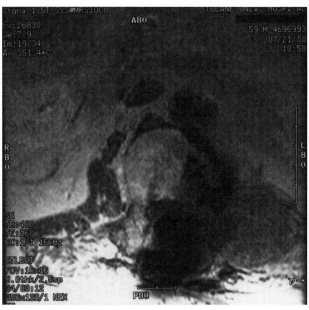

FIGURE 6. (*continued*) T2-weighted sagittal magnetic resonance image (MRI) **(C)** and T1-weighted axial MRI with gadolinium of L-1 **(D)**.

(22) and championed by Tomita et al. (36) (Fig. 7). Use of fine wire saws enables transection of the pedicles such that the posterior elements can be removed *en bloc*. Then the wire saws are passed anteriorly around the spine to cut through the disks above and below the tumor. A special retractor is used to prevent injury to the spinal cord and roots. The tumor is then removed by finger dissecting away the soft tissue anteriorly and rotating it laterally and posteriorly around the spinal cord. Posterior instrumentation with pedicle screws and interbody struts is used to create a stable construct.

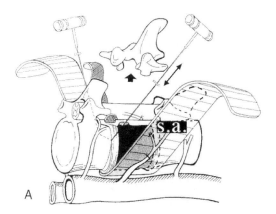

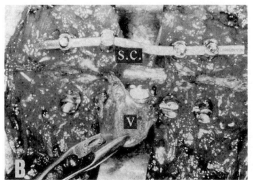

FIGURE 7. Tomita's technique for *en bloc* spondylectomy from a posterior approach. **A:** Spinal branch of segmental artery (s.a.) is ligated, and the nerve root is cut on one side. **B:** The affected vertebra (V) is carefully removed posterolaterally. s.c., spinal cord.

SIX: FAILING TO USE ADJUVANT TREATMENTS TO PREVENT DISEASE PROGRESSION IF INCOMPLETE EXCISION OF THE TUMOR IS PERFORMED

Most primary and metastatic cancers require multimodality treatment. Chondrosarcoma and chordoma are notable exceptions to this rule and are usually treated with surgery alone, unless they are deemed inoperable or microscopic residual tumor is left behind after attempted resection. Radiation therapy, chemotherapy, and hormonal therapy are usually required in addition to surgery for optimal management of cancerous lesions in the spine. Unlike trauma, which causes injury at a single point in time, cancer continues to grow and the amount of cumulative damage increases as time goes on. Therefore, if any cancer is left behind after surgery, it can continue to grow and form a local recurrence unless adjuvant treatments are used to control residual disease. Because radiotherapy is used for most metastatic lesions, this must be thought of as an integral part of the overall treatment plan. Close communication with the radiation oncologist is important to coordinate the overall effort to ensure local control of a patient's disease.

CONCLUSION

The surgeon rarely has an opportunity to correct a mistake resulting from erroneous surgery on tumors of the spinal vertebrae. Establishing the correct diagnosis before surgical treatment is essential. Determining the patient's medical eligibility for major surgery is critical in deciding whether surgical intervention is appropriate. Understanding the patient's overall prognosis is particularly important in deciding the optimal type of surgery to perform. Appreciating the biology of the tumor, the effects of adjuvant therapy on bone healing, and the extent of the tumor are also important factors to consider in selecting an appropriate surgical technique. It must be acknowledged that some patients with metastatic or primary disease are too advanced in their illness to be appropriate surgical candidates. They are best treated with supportive hospice care designed to palliate pain and preserve dignity. Regarding primary nonmetastatic malignant neoplasm of the spine, wide margins—as difficult as they may be to achieve—are necessary to ensure permanent local control of disease. The total *en bloc* spondylectomy described by Tomita is one technique

that can be used to accomplish this goal. Finally, adjuvant treatments must always be considered in the overall treatment plan. Radiotherapy, chemotherapy, and hormonal therapy are well-established modalities. Immunotherapy, such as the newly described monoclonal antibody treatment against HER2 in patients with metastatic breast cancer (32), is an emerging modality with promise for improving tumor control. Together, these adjuvants should work with surgery to improve the overall prognosis of patients with spinal malignancies by establishing durable local control, ensuring mechanical integrity of the spinal column, and maintaining neurologic function.

REFERENCES

1. Arbit E, Galicich JH. Vertebral body reconstruction with a modified Harrington rod distraction system for stabilization of the spine affected with metastatic disease. *J Neurosurg* 1995;83(4):617–620.
2. Batson OV. The function of vertebral veins and their role in the spread of metastases. 1940. *Clin Orthop* 1995;312:4–9.
3. Batson OV. The role of the vertebral veins in metastatic processes. *Ann Intern Med* 1942;16:38.
4. Bjornsson J, Wold LE, Ebersold MJ, et al. Chordoma of the mobile spine. A clinicopathologic analysis of 40 patients. *Cancer* 1993;71(3):735–740.
5. Bouchard JA, Koka A, Bensusan JS, et al. Effects of irradiation on posterior spinal fusions. A rabbit model. *Spine* 1994;19(16):1836–1841.
6. Brihaye J, Ectors P, Lemort M, et al. The management of spinal epidural metastases. *Adv Tech Stand Neurosurg* 1988;16:121–176.
7. Burchardt H, Glowczewskie FP Jr, Enneking WF. The effect of Adriamycin and methotrexate on the repair of segmental cortical autografts in dogs. *J Bone Joint Surg Am* 1983;65A(1):103–108.
8. Constans JP, de Divitiis E, Donzelli R, et al. Spinal metastases with neurological manifestations. Review of 600 cases. *J Neurosurg* 1983;59(1):111–118.
9. Denis F. The three column spine and its significance in the classification of acute thoracolumbar spinal injuries. *Spine* 1983;8(8):817–831.
10. Enkaoua EA, Doursounian L, Chatellier G, et al. Vertebral metastases: a critical appreciation of the preoperative prognostic Tokuhashi score in a series of 71 cases. *Spine* 1997;22(19):2293–2298.
11. Ergun H, Howland J. Postradiation atrophy of mature bone. *CRC Crit Rev Diagn Imaging* 1980;12(3):225–243.
12. Fujita T, Ueda Y, Kawahara N, et al. Local spread of metastatic vertebral tumors. A histologic study. *Spine* 1997;22(16):1905–1912.
13. Gainor BJ, Buchert P. Fracture healing in metastatic bone disease. *Clin Orthop* 1983;178:297–302.

14. Goodman AH, Serman MS. Post irradiation fractures of the femoral neck. *J Bone Joint Surg Am* 1963;45A(4):723–730.

15. Green N, French S, Rodriguez G, et al. Radiation-induced delayed union of fractures. *Radiology* 1969;93(3):635–641.

16. Hall AJ, Mackay NN. The results of laminectomy for compression of the cord or cauda equina by extradural malignant tumor. *J Bone Joint Surg Br* 1973;55B(3):497–505.

17. Harrington KD. Metastatic disease of the spine. *J Bone Joint Surg Am* 1986;68A(7):1110–1115.

18. Harrington KD. The use of methylmethacrylate for vertebral-body replacement and anterior stabilization of pathological fracture-dislocations of the spine due to metastatic malignant disease. *J Bone Joint Surg Am* 1981; 63A(1):36–46.

19. Howland WJ, Loeffler RK, Starchman DE, et al. Postirradiation atrophic changes of bone and related complications. *Radiology* 1975;117(3 Pt 1):677–685.

20. Huvos A. *Bone tumors: diagnosis, treatment, and prognosis,* 2nd ed. Philadelphia: WB Saunders, 1991:223–252.

21. Kostuik JP, Errico TJ, Gleason TF, et al. Spinal stabilization of vertebral column tumors. *Spine* 1988;13(3):250–256.

22. Magerl F, Coscia MF. Total posterior vertebrectomy of the thoracic or lumbar spine. *Clin Orthop* 1988;232:62–69.

23. Markbreiter LA, Pelker RR, Friedlaender GE, et al. The effect of radiation on the fracture repair process. A biomechanical evaluation of a closed fracture in a rat model. *J Orthop Res* 1989;7(2):178–183.

24. Mirra JM. *Bone tumors: clinical, radiologic, and pathologic correlations.* Philadelphia: Lea & Febiger, 1989:257.

25. Onimus M, Schraub S, Bertin D, et al. Surgical treatment of vertebral metastasis. *Spine* 1986;11(9):883–891.

26. Pelker RR, Friedlaender GE. The Nicolas Andry Award–1995. Fracture healing. Radiation induced alterations. *Clin Orthop* 1997;341:267–282.

27. Regen EM, Wilkins WE. The influence of roentgen irradiation on the rate of healing of fractures and the phosphatase activity of the callus of adult bone. *J Bone Joint Surg Am* 1936;18A(1):69–79.

28. Ruben P, Chen Y, Brosacchio RA. Staging and classification of the cancer and the host: a unified approach versus neotaxonomy. In: Perez CA, Brady LW, eds. *Principles and practice of radiation oncology,* 3rd ed. Philadelphia: Lippincott–Raven Publishers, 1998:213–229.

29. Schaberg J, Gainor BJ. A profile of metastatic carcinoma of the spine. *Spine* 1985;10(1):19–20.

30. Sengupta S, Prathap K. Radiation necrosis of the humerus. A report of three cases. *Acta Radiol Ther Phys Biol* 1973;12(4):313–320.

31. Sioutos PJ, Arbit E, Meshulam CF, et al. Spinal metastases from solid tumors. Analysis of factors affecting survival. *Cancer* 1995;76(8):1453–1459.

32. Slamon DJ, Leyland-Jones B, Shak S, et al. Use of chemotherapy plus a monoclonal antibody against HER2 for metastatic breast cancer that overexpresses HER2. *N Engl J Med* 2001;344(11):783–792.

33. Spiegel DA, Sampson JH, Richardson WJ, et al. Metastatic melanoma to the spine. Demographics, risk factors, and prognosis in 114 patients. *Spine* 1995;20(19):2141–2146.

34. Tatsui H, Onomura T, Morishita S, et al. Survival rates of patients with metastatic spinal cancer after scintigraphic detection of abnormal radioactive accumulation. *Spine* 1996;21(18):2143–2148.

35. Tokuhashi Y, Matsuzake H, Toriyama S, et al. Scoring system for the preoperative evaluation of metastatic spine tumor prognosis. *Spine* 1990;15(11):1110–1113.

36. Tomita K, Kawahara N, Baba H, et al. Total en bloc spondylectomy. A new surgical technique for primary malignant vertebral tumors. *Spine* 1997;22(3):324–333.

37. Tomita K, Kawahara N, Baba H, et al. Total en bloc spondylectomy for solitary spinal metastases. *Int Orthop* 1994;18(5):291–298.

38. Tomita K, Kawahara N, Kobayashi T, et al. Surgical strategy for spinal metastases. *Spine* 2001;26(3):298–306.

39. Woodard HQ. The influence of x-rays on the healing of fractures. *Health Phys* 1970;19(6):791–799.

40. Woodard HQ, Coley BL. The correlation of tissue dose and clinical response in irradiation of bone tumors and of normal bone. *AJR Am J Roentgenol* 1947;57(4):464–471.

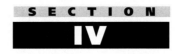

MANAGEMENT OF MISCELLANEOUS POSTOPERATIVE PROBLEMS

POSTOPERATIVE INFECTIONS AFTER SPINAL SURGERY: GENERAL PRINCIPLES

GREGORY D. CARLSON AND CAREY D. GORDEN

Postoperative spinal infections remain a serious cause of failed spine surgery. These complications prolong the normal course of postoperative healing and may lead to long-term pain and deformity. The additional expense involved in treating patients with deep postoperative spinal infections after lower back fusion may increase the total cost of care more than four times (10). Although the early wound infection presents with pain, purulent drainage, and wound dehiscence, infection of the disk space and spondylodiskitis may not be as readily recognized leading to increased morbidity and the need for prolonged care (59). Recognition of risk factors associated with deep postoperative infections may decrease the incidence of this problem in the wary surgeon's practice. This chapter defines perioperative risk factors that, if modified, may reduce the occurrence of surgical failure due to postoperative infections. Principles of medical and surgical treatment of the varying presentations of postoperative infection are discussed. The objective of this chapter is to provide the reader with an overview of the incidence of postoperative spinal infections, risk factors, diagnosis, preventative measures, and methods of treatment.

INCIDENCE

The use of perioperative antibiotics has decreased the rate of postoperative wound infections (72). However, postoperative infection rates for major spinal reconstructive surgery have not decreased substantially over the past decade. This may be attributable to increased implantation of spinal hardware, aging populations, and the modern surgeon's willingness to operate on patients with increased risk factors for infection.

Postoperative spinal infections have potentially serious consequences if not dealt with promptly and effectively. The rate of infection following a spinal surgery is dependent on the surgical procedure, region of the spine, and dorsal (posterior) or ventral (anterior) aspect of the procedure. Regardless of the spinal region, the most important anatomic determination of risk appears to be related to the approach. The anterior approach, which is less prone to infection, is largely advanced through relatively avascular tissue planes with less retraction of paraspinal muscular and devascularization of tissue (36,46,90).

Postoperative infection rates involving the cervical spine range from 0.1% to 3.0% (6,81). The anterior approach through an extensile approach has an extremely low incidence of infection that has led some authors to question the need for prophylactic antibiotic use in routine anterior cervical surgery (90). The addition of anterior hardware has not increased the incidence of postoperative infection (77).

The posterior cervical approach has a higher risk of infection, possibly because of more extensive tissue dissection and the close proximity to the hairline (77,87). Weiland and McAfee (85) reviewed 100 consecutive posterior cervical fusions using the triple-wire technique and reported no wound infections.

In a retrospective study of 1,247 patients who underwent posterior spinal instrumentation for treatment of adolescent idiopathic scoliosis, 22 patients (1.7%) experienced development of late infection, with a mean of 3.1 years after the initial procedure (14). One study showed the infection rate to be as little as 0.1% (83).

Infection rates associated with neuromuscular scoliosis tend to be higher. A study of neuromuscular scoliosis showed an 8.7% deep wound infection rate (79). Infection rates can run as high as 15% in patients with cerebral palsy (83). Infection rates may approach 50% in myelomeningocele spine surgery.

Surgery for spine metastases is associated with a complication rate of more than 10% (49). Exceptionally high rates of infection for spinal surgeries involving myelomeningoceles or paralytic scoliosis have been reported, as high as 57% in some studies (24).

Spinal operation via an anterior thoracic approach is becoming increasingly common. Postoperative infection rates for anterior thoracic procedures may be as high as 5% (52). This is quite variable, as noted by Naunheim et al. (52), who reported 126 anterior thoracotomy procedures with no superficial or deep wound infections. Minimally invasive spinal surgery with thoracoscopic assistance may increase superficial wound infections when compared to open procedures (28,48).

The reported incidence of infections following standard lumbar diskectomy is less than 1% (24). If the surgeon is experienced with the use of an operating microscope, the infection rate is similar to that of the open technique (47,55). Reported rates of infection after endoscopic diskectomy procedures are similar to those of the open technique (25).

The infection rate following laminectomy and fusion has been reported to be approximately 2% to 8% (24). Scoliosis fusions without metal have infection rates that are similar to those of lumbar laminectomy and fusion procedures. The addition of instrumentation to lumbar spinal fusions has substantially increased the rate of infection. The report of rates ranges from 0% to 13%, for an average of 7% (24).

MICROBIOLOGY

The microbiology of spinal infection is dominated by gram-positive cocci, represented by acute infectious presentations of *Staphylococcus aureus* and more indolent infections with *Staphylococcus epidermidis*. The incidence of gram-negative organisms causing postoperative infections is on the rise. Common organisms cultured from infected wounds postoperatively include *Enterococcus*, *Klebsiella*, *Escherichia coli*, *Proteus*, and *Pseudomonas*. Contamination of the surgical wound occurs during elective spine operation. However, most of the time normal skin flora do not cause an infection postoperatively. Most of the organisms that contaminate and eventually dominate an infection reside within the sebaceous glands and hair follicles (5). Therefore, preparation of the skin is crucial in preventing infections.

PREVENTION

Preoperative Management

Patient Factor

Identification of risk factors is paramount during presurgical planning to help ensure the best possible outcome for the patient. Care should be taken to minimize or eliminate potential factors. Well-known risk factors include malnutrition, obesity, poorly controlled diabetes, immunosuppression, steroid therapy, remote infections, and lengthy preoperative hospitalization.

Until recently, the nutritional status for patients undergoing elective spine surgery has largely been underemphasized. Without adequate patient nutrition, surgical wounds do not heal properly. Increased perioperative morbidity and mortality have been demonstrated in patients who are malnourished, especially the elderly population (78). It has been postulated that up to 25% of patients undergoing elective spine surgery are malnourished at the time of operation. These numbers may be higher in the elderly population (34).

The recommended preoperative assessment includes an adequate history and examination to identify malnutrition as well as laboratory testing. Recommended laboratory tests include serum albumin, transferrin, and total lymphocyte count. Other less commonly used tests include a skin anergy test and measurement of arm muscle circumference.

Improvement of nutritional parameters is mandatory to minimize postoperative spine infections. In a study of nutrition and complications associated with spinal surgery, deep wound infections developed in 11 of the 13 malnourished patients in the study. Due to the vital role that nutrition plays in wound healing and infection prevention, Klein et al. (34) suggest that patients with inadequate nutrition be supplemented before elective surgery.

Obesity has been described as a general risk factor for surgery. It may be a factor in greater blood loss and increased surgical time of the procedure (12). These patients are also more likely to have coexisting medical conditions, including hypertension, diabetes, and coronary artery disease.

Studies have indicated that diseases secondary to poorly controlled diabetes, such as cardiovascular disease, hypertension, and renal disease, also contribute significantly to postoperative spinal infections (38). Careful preoperative assessment and medical stabilization of chronic illnesses minimize the risk of postoperative infection.

Quite often, malnutrition, illness, and chemotherapy leave patients immunocompromised. It is important to note that not only do these individuals have a higher rate of infection after spine surgery than their nonimmunocompromised counterparts, but they are susceptible to a different group of pathogens (i.e., *Pseudomonas* and gram-negative bacteria) due to their diminished defense systems (9). Every attempt should be made to delay surgery until the patient's immune system can be stabilized.

Acute or chronic administration of steroids is often used in the patient who is preparing for spine surgery. Steroids pose additional risks for patients by disarming humoral and cellular immune responses, thus effectively decreasing signs and symptoms of inflammation (9). In patients who are undergoing surgery for spine metastases, there is a strong correlation between perioperative steroids and postoperative wound infections (49). Whenever possible, steroids should be discontinued before spine surgery.

During the preoperative evaluation, care should be taken to diagnose any remote or concomitant infections. Studies have shown that remote infections can triple the rate of postoperative infection (26). Nelson et al. (53) noted that seven patients with postoperative deep wound infections had positive urine cultures before surgery. On further analysis it was noted that cultures from the infected wound grew the same organism found in the preoperative urine cultures (53). Eradication of infectious foci before surgery is paramount in preventing infection. If surgical intervention is required in the face of possible concomitant colonization of frank infection, appropriate prophylactic antibiotics should be administered based on preoperative culture results.

Preoperative hospitalization exposes patients to more virulent and antibiotic-resistant hospital bacteria. Nosocomial bacteria migrate passively and may become a part of the patient's own flora, thereby increasing the incidence of postoperative infection. A study examining the correlation between length of preoperative hospitalization and incidence of postoperative infection showed that the rate of infection was approximately twice as high when compared with patients admitted 1 to 3 days before surgery (2). To decrease the incidence of postoperative infections, patients should be discharged to home and rescheduled on an elective basis. If this is not possible, hospital epidemiologic data should be used in choosing an appropriate prophylactic antibiotic regimen.

The preoperative surgical decision planning for anterior and posterior fusion and instrumentation has a profound effect on the outcome of an elective spinal operation. Anterior procedures combined with posterior fusion and instrumentation prolong operative time and increase the rate of infection. Staging of a procedure may give the patient time to handle the metabolic stresses of surgery adequately and keep the nutritional parameters well above normal. Because of the effect of malnutrition on infection rates, a study has demonstrated that patients undergoing staged spinal reconstruction benefit from total parenteral nutrition administered in the perioperative period (27).

Prophylactic Intravenous Antibiotics

Prophylactic intravenous antibiotics have significantly reduced the incidence of postoperative spinal infections (20,67,68,72,74). A retrospective study of 531 patients undergoing lumbar diskectomy showed that those who received prophylactic antibiotics had a postoperative infection rate of only 0.6%, versus 9.3% without prophylactic antibiotics (68). Many studies have reported a decreased incidence of infection in operations involving diskectomies, fusions, and instrumentations (24). The appropriate antibiotic regimen depends on microflora that are likely to be encountered. The most common prophylactic regimen in use is a first-generation cephalosporin, which covers the normal skin flora of gram-positive organisms. Perhaps the use and timing of antibiotic prophylaxis might be the most crucial part of preoperative management. A study of patients undergoing lumbar spine surgery reported an infection rate of 0.6%, in patients who received the initial dose of antibiotics before surgery, as opposed to 2.7% for those who received their first dose after surgery (68). To be effective, prophylactic antibiotics must penetrate the tissue in levels high enough to deter infection. Therapeutic doses of antibiotics must be in circulation within the system before surgery to prevent quantitative bacterial growth. Cefazolin, which is commonly used for surgical prophylaxis, may not adequately penetrate the intervertebral disk or cerebrospinal fluid (67). Higher concentrations of cefazolin were found within the cervical disk after 2-g prophylactic dosing, compared to the common 1-g regimen (63). Boscardin et al. (8) demonstrated that an intravenous bolus of cefazolin (2 g) produced the optimal level of intradiskal antibiotic levels 15 to 80 minutes after administration. Antibiotics should be administered 30 minutes before surgery and continued for 48 hours postoperatively for adequate microbial coverage. A study of patients who were given prophylactic cefazolin for longer than 48 hours postoperatively and then developed infections postoperatively found that these patients had bacteria of a more resistant nature (68).

If the patient is immunosuppressed or has been hospitalized preoperatively, a broad spectrum of antibiotics should be used to cover gram-positive as well as gram-negative microorganisms. Preoperative blood and urine cultures may help to identify potential pathogens.

Resistant strains of bacterial infections constitute a growing segment of spinal infections. The most common of these is methicillin-resistant staphylococcal (MRSA) infection. Klekamp et al. (35) noted that 16 of 35 spinal infections were secondary to MRSA infection. Significant risk factors for MRSA infection were lymphopenia, history of chronic infections, alcohol abuse, recent hospitalization, and prolonged postoperative wound drainage. Patients with MRSA infections were also somewhat less likely to have received vancomycin prophylaxis. The authors recommended that chemoprophylaxis with vancomycin should be targeted at patients with increased risk (35).

Intraoperative Prevention: Operating Room Protocol

Intraoperative risk factors can increase the incidence of spine infections if they are not recognized and properly addressed. The operating room is designed for a central sterile field with equipment and non-sterile items located along the periphery, thus enabling traffic to flow outward from the sterile field in an effort to reduce bacterial contamination (21). Movement in and out of the operating room should be kept to a minimum to decrease the number of airborne microbes (61). To prevent airborne contamination of the surgical field, the appropriate ventilation system should be used. Quebbeman (61) states that optimal ventilation can be achieved by changing the room air 20 to 25 times each hour using a HEPA filter, which removes 99.97% of particles and bacteria larger than 0.3 µm.

Adequate surgical attire and proper preoperative disinfection of the hands are necessary to minimize postoperative surgical infections from exogenous sources. The operating room attire should be made of nonlinting material, which must constitute an effective bacterial barrier (3). Hair is a source of bioparticular matter and should be covered with a bouffant-style cap. Facial hair should be covered with a full-faced surgical hood. Conversation should be kept to a minimum. Shoe covers can be useful in protecting shoes from blood yet have no proven efficacy in preventing the spread of infection (3,21).

Proper disinfection of the hands is necessary in reducing the number of transient contaminants and resistant flora. Of the three antibacterial compounds that are commonly used today—povidone-iodine (Betadine), chlorhexidine gluconate (Hibiclens), and hexachlorophene (Septisol foam)—a study has recommended chlorhexidine gluconate as the preferred antibacterial scrub compound because of its initial effectiveness, limited toxicity, and residual activity (45). The most effective length of time for hand scrubbing is debatable. A longer scrub may actually cause more damage to the skin, increasing bacterial overgrowth over time. Evidence suggests that a 120-second scrub that includes brushing of the fingertip and nail sufficiently disinfects the hands (40). Studies have shown the incidence of puncture holes during operations to be as high as 50% to 70% (3). As a part of universal precautions, the Centers for Disease Control and Prevention recommends double gloving as a standard practice.

Skin preparation should begin at the incision site and continue outward toward the periphery. The use of hexachlorophene is not recommended as a single agent due to its poor cleansing ability against gram-negative bacteria and potential central nervous system toxicity when absorbed through the skin (21). Several studies have shown chlorhexidine gluconate to be more effective in reducing skin flora than povidone-iodine (45). Alcohol, one of the oldest antiseptics, has been shown to be the most efficacious skin preparation agent (56). However, because of its drying effect on the skin and flammable nature, it has not gained widespread acceptance as a skin preparation agent. A study determining the efficacy of prepackaged sterile disposable prep sets has shown a consistently low infection rate of 0.7% to 0.9% (2). Removal of hair from the incision site increases the incidence of wound infection (45). If hair must be removed, it should be done immediately before surgery.

Sterile drapes are used to maintain the integrity of the sterile field. The drapes should cover the entire patient, leaving only the area of incision exposed. The efficacy of adherent plastic drapes is debatable and may increase the incidence of infections by providing a warm moist environment for bacteria to flourish and enter the wound from the edges of the plastic drape (26,61). Johnson et al. (31) demonstrated the superiority of iodophor-adherent drapes.

The surgeon controls several of the local factors that make the incision site a prime target for bacteria. Recognizing that it is virtually impossible to avoid all bacterial contamination within the wound, the surgeon's primary objective in preventing infections is to decrease the local risk factors. Tissue dissection should be performed in a manner that minimizes trauma to the area of dissection. Healthy tissue possesses considerable resistance to bacterial growth. Traumatized or dead tissue is limited in its capacity to resist bacterial growth, thereby leaving the area open to infection. Pressure and tension placed on the surrounding tissues decrease blood flow, in effect altering the surrounding physiology and leaving the area vulnerable to bacterial colonization. Sutures should be spaced evenly throughout the wound to distribute tension. Periodic loosening of the retractors allows tissue reperfusion, preventing necrosis (89). Periodic irrigation with saline prevents tissues from drying.

If used properly, electrocautery does not change the wound infection rate (50). Care should be taken to avoid excessive use, causing tissue necrosis. When closing, every effort should be made to achieve adequate hemostasis. A layered closure should be used to avoid any "dead spaces." Accumulation of blood and serum throughout the various layers of the wound results in seromas, hematomas, or "dead spaces" that promote bacterial growth associated with delayed wound healing (1). After lengthy spine procedures, wounds should be débrided of any devitalized tissue and irrigated with a topical antibiotic solution (24).

Increased duration of the surgical procedure is an intraoperative risk factor for infection (50). Increased blood loss may also be a factor (32). In a retrospective study of 850 spinal procedures, Wimmer et al. (90) identified high blood loss as an intraoperative risk factor for spine infection.

Indwelling catheters should be considered risk factors for infection. Central venous catheters have the highest rate of intravascular nosocomial infection. The most common source of bacterial invasion is from the skin surrounding the insertion site (16,26).

Catheter-associated urinary infections account for 40% of all nosocomial infections (26). Bacteriuria occurs in 1% to 5% of patients after short-term catheterization, and the number increases to 5% to 10% with long-term catheterization. Risks associated with catheterization are greater in the elderly or debilitated patient (26). Because of the high risk of infections associated with urinary catheters, placement should occur only when necessary and removal should follow at the earliest opportunity.

Postoperative Management

Increased postoperative drainage and seroma formation are associated with higher postoperative infection rates (32). Wound drains are commonly removed on the second postoperative day. If a seroma should form, needle aspiration can be attempted before open surgical drainage with closure over drainage tubes. Because of the high association between bacterial colonization of indwelling catheters, urinary

catheters should be removed at the earliest opportunity after surgery.

Iatrogenic factors such as bed rest and poor nutrition have been identified as risk factors for postsurgical patients. Bed rest and inactivity increase the loss of strength and muscle mass. Patient mobilization should be encouraged early after surgery to expedite healing. Nutritional support postoperatively is paramount to ensure expeditious wound healing. A study examining the effect of bathing after posterior spine surgery showed that prohibition of showering after the first few days postoperatively is unnecessary (13).

CLINICAL PRESENTATION

History

The presenting signs and symptoms associated with postoperative infection vary widely and depend on the microbial inoculation, host factors, and surgical procedure. Pain out of proportion to the normal postoperative course should be an immediate flag, raising concern.

Early awareness of a potential deep space infection is a crucial factor in the successful outcome of treatment. Patients with wound infections complain of increased pain. The pain is generally present at rest, out of proportion to the examination findings and not substantially improved with narcotics. Axial pain is most common; however, radicular pain may also be associated with postoperative spinal infections.

Postoperative cervical infections may present with headaches, trapezial or shoulder pain, torticollis, or dysphagia (6). In the lumbar spine, infections may present with abdominal pain, distention, hip symptoms (psoas abscess), and even contracture (39).

Constitutional symptoms are not always present during the initial stages of the infection. Low-grade fevers may be present in only 50% of patients. A complete evaluation of patients' genitourinary and respiratory systems should help eliminate other potential sources for bacterial seeding of the surgical wound. The immunocompromised patient who is at increased risk of infection may present late with a paucity of findings (9).

The wound should be examined for any drainage or erythema that is out of proportion to normal wound healing after surgery. The wound may appear erythematous and warm to the touch. Evidence of wound dehiscence with drainage may also be evidence of infection. However, lack of significant skin changes should not be misinterpreted. In late infections or postoperative diskitis, the wound may appear normal.

Postoperative wound infections can be categorized as either superficial or deep. An infection that does not penetrate the deep investing muscle fascia is considered superficial. With appropriate care these infections seldom develop into major complications (18). In actuality, the clinical differentiation between superficial and deep involvement can be elusive. Early surgical intervention should be entertained if there is any doubt as to the extent of the infection. In many cases determination of the depth of infectious penetration is made only after meticulous layer-by-layer dissection, irrigation, and débridement.

Onset

Postoperative spinal infections can be categorized as early, delayed, or late onset, based on the time to presentation after surgery. The most common presentation is early onset. Signs and symptoms of infection develop within the initial perioperative time period after surgery. The majority of these infections develop within the first 4 weeks after surgery and are typically associated with a virulent microbe such as *S. aureus* or a gram-negative organism such as *Enterococcus*.

The delayed-onset type of infection is classically represented by postoperative diskitis. Patients in whom this complication develops may have a routine initial perioperative course with normal-appearing wound healing. These patients have a perioperative course similar to that of the routine diskectomy patient with anticipated improvement in radicular symptoms. Usually, the patient returns weeks or months after surgery complaining of increasing low back pain, stiffness, or leg pain. He or she may have a history of constitutional symptoms, such as sweats, fever, or chills. The most common physical sign is paralumbar spasm, which may present with stiffness and scoliosis. Neurologic symptoms may mimic recurrent disk herniation or, more emergently, the possibility of epidural abscess and cauda equina syndrome (66). In many cases the wound has healed and may appear normal. The presence of swelling, erythema, or draining sinus should alert the practitioner of potential problems.

Jimenez-Mejias et al. (30) studied 31 cases of postoperative pyogenic spondylodiskitis (POS) and compared them with 72 cases of nonpostoperative pyogenic spondylodiskitis (NPOS). POS represented 30.1% of the patients with pyogenic spondylodiskitis. The onset of symptoms occurred an average of 28 days after surgery. Predisposing factors were less frequent in POS than in NPOS cases. Neurologic complications and inflammatory signs in the spine were more frequent with POS than with NPOS. Coagulase-negative *Staphylococcus* and anaerobic bacteria were seen more frequently with POS than with NPOS. Percutaneous bone biopsies yielded the etiology in 66.7% of cases, open bone biopsies in 100%, blood cultures in 55.6%, and cultures of adjacent foci in 94.4%. Eleven patients (35.5%) were cured with antimicrobial treatment, but surgical treatment was necessary in 64.5%. No relapses or deaths were recorded. Seventeen patients (54.8%) had severe functional sequelae, which were associated with inflammatory signs in the spine, higher levels of leukocytosis, higher erythrocyte sedimentation rates (ESR), and paravertebral abscesses (30).

Late-onset infections describe conditions of indolent microbial contamination of tissue most commonly associated with retained hardware that present months or years after surgery without preceding breakdown of overlying skin in the majority of cases (14,22,62,64,65,79,84). As the late infection may present in the course of workup for a failed spinal surgery, these infections are usually diagnosed at the time of hardware removal. Although Robertson and Taylor (69) described late infections complicating scoliosis surgery after Dwyer anterior instrumentation, the majority of these infections involve posterior spinal instrumentation and have been most commonly described after deformity surgery. Microbes are low-virulence skin organisms, including *Propionibacterium acnes*, *S. epidermidis*, and rare coagulase-negative *Staphylococcus* species (14,64,84).

Heggeness et al. (23) argued for a hematogenous origin of infection in a series of six late spinal infections. In all cases, there was a delay of at least 10 months between surgery and the clinical development of sepsis. In five of the six cases, a distant focus of infection could be identified (23). However, because late infections involve microbes that commonly colonize the skin, this has led investigators to postulate intraoperative seeding that remained subclinical for an extended period (64,84).

Epidural Abscesses

Epidural abscesses in the spinal column occur infrequently, and early diagnosis is often difficult.

Baker et al. (4) found that 16% of epidural abscesses were due to postoperative infection. One study indicated a rate of two cases per 10,000 per year, with the peak age incidence occurring in the sixth or seventh decade of life (44). The most important factor in the diagnosis is heightened awareness. Mortality can exceed 20% due to rapid evolution of the disease (44).

Although rare, there is a typical clinical presentation associated with postoperative epidural abscess. A 10-year prospective study of spinal epidural abscesses showed that patients may present with back pain, progressive neurologic deficit, low-grade fever, nuchal rigidity, radicular pain, weakness of an extremity, sensory deficit, bladder or bowel dysfunction, and frank paralysis (15,66). Most cases of epidural abscesses occur in the posterior area of the epidural space where more areolar tissue is present (18). Yet, a recent study showed an equal occurrence of anterior and posterior spinal epidural abscesses (15).

Patients with epidural abscesses present with elevated erythrocyte formation and high peripheral white blood cell counts. Sixty percent also have positive blood cultures (44). One study suggested that a lumbar puncture to obtain cerebrospinal fluid for analysis is warranted because 13% of patients with spinal epidural abscesses also have meningitis (4). Yet, another study advises caution when deciding to withdraw cerebrospinal fluid because of the risk of spreading the infection to the intrathecal compartment (44).

DIAGNOSIS

Laboratory Findings

Diskitis after microdiskectomy is frequently missed or detected late because of misinterpretation of postoperative complaints and examinations. The white blood cell count may be deceptively low in the patient with suspected postoperative infection. Schultz and Assheuer (76) prospectively examined 31 patients after routine single level diskectomies. From the first to tenth postoperative day, C-reactive protein (CRP) and ESR were found to be less than 2.5 µg/mL and less than 45 mm per hour, respectively. Bircher et al. (7) demonstrated a maximum rise in ESR within the first postoperative week followed by a steady decline over the next 6 weeks. In contrast, patients with postoperative wound sepsis or diskitis demonstrated elevated values (7,59,76).

CRP, thought to be a more specific test for septic inflammation, peaks around the second postoperative day and normalizes in 1 to 2 weeks (76).

Imaging

Early plain radiographic studies are of mixed value in the diagnosis of spinal infection. Intervertebral joint space narrowing may be an early sign of septic change; however, these changes may also be associated with routine diskectomy. Initial bony changes take place 3 to 4 weeks after the initial infection develops. Nielsen et al. (54) demonstrated that the mean time from operation to first radiologic lesions was 2.0 months, from operation to maximal lesions 4.0 months, and to the first radiologic sign of healing 5.5 months. The earliest lesion was blurring of the endplate or minor destructions, leading to cavitation of the vertebral body. Follow-up showed a significantly higher incidence of decrease in disk height, intercorporal fusion, and major osteophytes in the diskitis group (54).

Technetium-99 bone scans are more sensitive than plain radiographs in demonstrating early changes seen in postoperative spinal infections. However, radionuclide imaging is frequently positive after diskectomy, and there is a significant incidence of false-negative studies in documented cases of postoperative diskitis (60,80).

Magnetic resonance imaging (MRI) is the diagnostic imaging modality of choice to identify suppurative changes in the spine (42). It is emerging as the most sensitive and specific modality for early detection of pyogenic and nonpyogenic infections and their complications, as well as in follow-up evaluation. Degenerative disk disease, seronegative spondyloarthropathies, and spondyloarthropathy associated with long-term hemodialysis may mimic the imaging abnormalities of infective spondylitis (70).

A study of infections demonstrated the superiority of enhanced MRI with gadolinium in comparison to noncontrast MRI in delineating an epidural abscess. Interventional MRI without contrast shows a diffuse encasement of the subarachnoid space. MRI enhanced with gadolinium presents with linear enhancement surrounding unenhanced pus (73). Contrast-enhanced MRI is a valuable tool for diagnosing multilevel abscesses and can help in documenting treatment response to antibiotics.

The MRI appearance of intervertebral diskitis is decreased signal intensity in the marrow spaces adjacent to the endplate and in the disk space on T1-weighted images. The normal definition between the disk space and the vertebral body is lost. On T2-weighted images, there is an increase in the signal within the disk (51) (Fig. 1).

The benefits of MRI include early recognition of changes 3 to 5 days after the onset of infection, no need for ionizing radiation, and the advantages of morphologic definition of bone, disk, and neurologic structures. Recurrent disk herniations and epidural abscess formation can be ruled out in the patient with neurologic findings. The relative ease of obtaining the MRI study in most centers plus the added benefit of sequential evaluation of response to treatment make

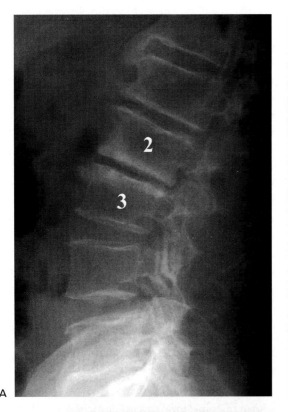

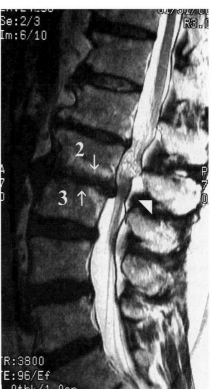

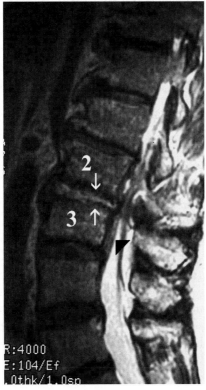

FIGURE 1. A 75-year-old diabetic man admitted to the hospital with severe unremitting back pain 5 days after epidural steroid injection for lumbar stenosis. The patient failed to respond to intravenous antibiotics and was treated with open débridement. **A:** Lateral lumbar radiograph demonstrates L2-3 spondylosis. **B:** T2-weighted magnetic resonance image (MRI) 3 months before epidural injections, notable for severe lumbar stenosis at L2-3. Disk space at L2-3 has normal dark signal consistent with degenerative spondylosis. **C:** T2-weighted MRI 1 week after epidural injection demonstrates high signal intensity within L2-3 disk space, consistent with diskitis.

MRI the imaging study of choice. Contrast enhancement allows for the definition of peripherally enhancing epidural or psoas abscess (17).

Differentiating early postoperative MRI changes from those of septic diskitis continues to be a challenge. Grane et al. (19) were unable to distinguish typical postoperative MRI changes in a series of uninfected patients compared retrospectively to patients with diskitis. They determined that suspicion of septic postoperative diskitis should be confirmed by MRI, serum CRP, and disk aspiration. MRI alone was not reliable as the sole method for distinguishing septic from symptomatic aseptic diskitis in the early postoperative stage (19) (Fig. 2).

Aspiration/Biopsy

Wound aspiration has a limited role in determining the presence of an immediate postoperative wound infection. The decision to initiate treatment should be based on previously described signs and symptoms that deviate from the normal postoperative course. A low-grade fever or leukocytosis may be present; however, the absence of these findings should not be mistaken for normal wound healing in the patient with suspicious symptoms. In the presence of a defined swelling or fluctuance, local aspiration may provide information for early identification through Gram's stain and culture. However, a negative aspiration should not discourage the surgeon from pursuing an aggressive management. If sufficient suspicion is aroused, early surgical exploration and débridement should be instituted, particularly in the presence of possible infected hardware. Aggressive surgical intervention allows the preservation of hardware in the majority of cases (29,78,82,83). To treat a patient with antibiotics alone, without appropriate surgical débridement, is to risk long-term problems, including persistent osteomyelitis, pseudarthrosis, and spinal instability (86).

In the case of possible postoperative spondylodiskitis, CT-guided biopsy may yield an organism for appropriate antibiotic regimen. Because of the relatively low morbidity associated with the procedure, percutaneous biopsy should be attempted before starting antibiotic therapy. Percutaneous bone biopsies yield the etiology in approximately two-thirds of cases, compared to nearly 100% yield with open bone biopsies (30). Early treatment is of the utmost impor-

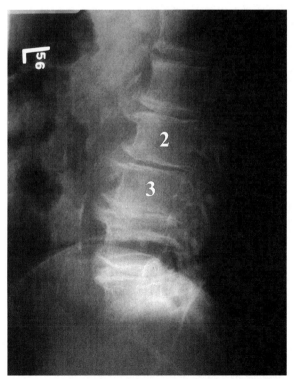 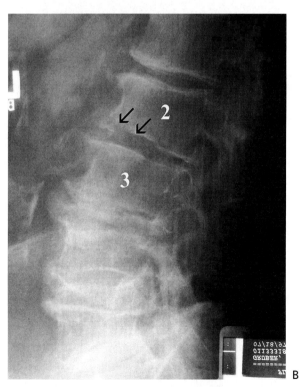

FIGURE 2. An 85-year-old man treated with L3-5 lumbar laminectomy for severe stenosis. His postoperative course was marked with increasing back pain. Because of his cardiac pacemaker, early magnetic resonance imaging was not possible. The patient responded medically to intravenous antibiotics; however, late deformity and instability hampered recovery. **A:** Preoperative lateral lumbar radiograph with spondylosis. L-2 and L-3 vertebrae are marked for comparison. **B:** Postoperative radiograph with rarefaction and early osseous collapse (*black arrows*) at the interior endplate of L-2 vertebrae. (*continued*)

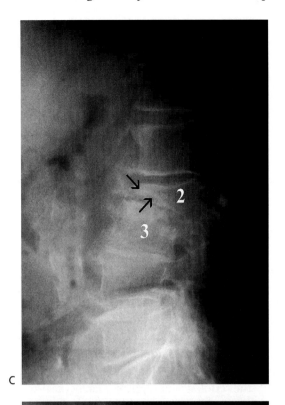

C

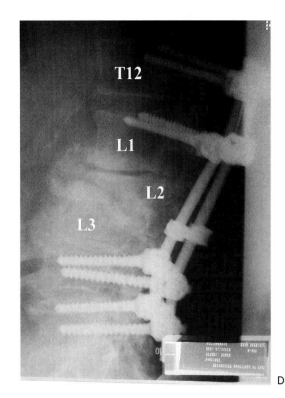

D

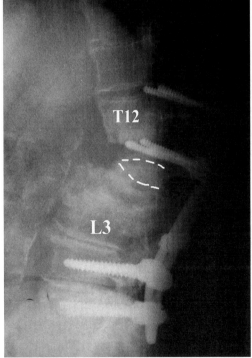

E

FIGURE 2. (*continued*) C: Late postoperative radiograph demonstrating L-2 collapse and local kyphosis. Black arrows show region of progressive bone loss of L-2 body. **D:** Because of the age and poor health of the patient, posterior *in situ* instrumentation and fusion were performed. One-month postoperative x-ray showing loss of proximal screw fixation with early pullout. **E:** Osteomyelitis of T-12 to L-3 vertebrae, progressive kyphotic collapse with loss of proximal fusion. Anterior bone destruction of T-12 is visible. Dashed lines show collapse of L-1 vertebrae.

tance and should not be prolonged for lack of biopsy information availability. Studies have demonstrated that early broad-spectrum antibiotic therapy is efficacious in the majority of cases, regardless of whether the offending organism has been identified (59).

Anterior intervertebral débridement is frequently necessary for chronic infection or evidence of abscess formation or in patients who do not respond to medical management. New percutaneous approaches appear to provide similar benefits of surgical débridement and abscess decompression as traditional open procedures (57).

DIFFERENTIAL DIAGNOSIS

The differential diagnosis of a potential spine infection demands consideration of a full spectrum of disease processes. The decision to treat a postoperative wound condition as superficial and amenable to medical management should be undertaken with caution. Back pain out of proportion to the expected clinical course should lead to the consideration of diskitis, which can be difficult to diagnose. CRP, ESR, and temperature elevation in conjunction with back pain should lead to early treatment. Retrodiskal diskitis can be treated conservatively, whereas retrodiskal abscesses require surgical intervention (76).

Epidural abscess formation after spinal surgery is rare as an isolated entity. Lowell et al. (41) reported an increased incidence of epidural abscess after microdiskectomy in patients who received intraoperative methylprednisolone injection in the epidural operative region. Iatrogenic inoculation of the epidural space may precipitate infection. The use of an epidural catheter for anesthesia may predispose to epidural abscess (75). Epidural abscess may complicate spondylodiskitis. This becomes an important differential diagnosis in the individual with signs of infection, increasing back pain, and neurologic findings. Contrast-enhanced MRI is the study of choice to delineate enhancement surrounding unenhanced pus and to document a decrease in abscess size associated with response to therapy (37,73). Early surgical decompression in combination with parenteral antibiotics is the treatment of choice, as the prognosis for recovery is directly associated with the medical and neurologic preoperative condition of the patient (33).

TREATMENT

Medical Management

Bed rest, immobilization, and antibiotic therapy remain the primary modalities for postoperative diskitis management. Postacchini et al. (59) noted that close postoperative observation permitted early detection of intervertebral diskitis. They demonstrated that in patients treated early, average 8 days after surgery versus 31 days, symptomatic recovery occurred earlier, average 1.8 months compared to 3.9 months. Patients treated early required a shorter duration of parenteral therapy, mean 41 days for relief of symptoms, compared to a mean of 62 days in the late group. In this series ESR was always higher than 70, needle biopsy did not affect the length of therapy, and osseous changes developed in only 3 of the 12 patients (59). The recommended duration for parenteral therapy ranges from 2 to 6 weeks. However, this should be determined based on the patient's symptomatic and inflammatory response to therapy. A multidisciplinary approach with infectious disease consultation is recommended (24,30).

Surgical Management

Postoperative Diskitis

Prompt surgical management should proceed in those patients with failure to respond to medical treatment, neurologic compromise, or documented epidural abscess. Severe intractable back pain should signal failure to respond to therapy. Postoperative sepsis associated with disk space infection warrants urgent surgical débridement.

The surgical approach varies depending on the disease entity. Generally, the anterior approach is advocated for spondylodiskitis. However, in the early postsurgical period after diskectomy, a posterior reexploration is advantageous and allows simultaneous nerve root decompression and removal of recurrent disk fragments. In chronic cases, the anterior approach is frequently necessary, allowing for débridement of bone involvement, decompression of paraspinal abscesses, and appropriate stabilization if needed. The goals of intervertebral débridement and soft tissue decompression can be addressed through traditional open approaches or minimally invasive techniques (57).

The prognosis for patients with spondylodiskitis is generally good (60,76). Risk factors for poor outcomes include multiple medical problems, prior spinal surgery, and MRSA staphylococci (66).

Spinal Wound Infection

In the presumed postoperative spinal wound infection, there is very little room for medical management. Short of addressing a possible superficial suture inflammation, surgical débridement should be instituted early. Isolation of the infecting organisms is maximized by obtaining tissue or aspirate before instituting antibiotic therapy. However, this should not meaningfully delay the start of broad-spectrum antibiotic therapy. Delay in appropriately aggressive surgical management in the case of a deep space infection may result in prolonged morbidity and poor functional outcome. In the presence of hardware, any sign of potential wound dehiscence, prolonged or recurrent drainage, or induration with erythema should be dealt with in an expedient surgical manner.

Thalgott et al. (82) defined parameters of response to therapy based on the presence of a single organism versus multiple organism contamination, presence of myonecrosis, and individual patients' immune response or physiology, including traditional factors of immune deficiency as well as cigarette smoking. Response to therapy was best in single organism infections in the immunocompetent host that did not smoke. Multiple organism infections with myonecrosis were exceedingly difficult to manage and portended a poor outcome. Smoking was associated with slow response to therapy and poor prognosis (82).

Picada et al. (58) analyzed a series of 817 instrumented lumbar fusions to examine the necessity of hardware removal for the successful treatment of spine infections. Deep wound infections developed in 3.2% (n = 26) of the patients; 24 of these patients achieved a clean closed wound without the removal of instrumentation (58). Early diagnosis; surgical débridement; primary or secondary closure, or both; and adequate antibiotic coverage should be sufficient in treating postoperative spine infections, thereby allowing the instrumentation to remain in place in the majority of cases.

The technique of surgical reexploration should follow a thorough sequential fashion. To avoid potential deep space contamination, each tissue layer should be irrigated and débridement performed before the deeper layer is opened. A deep subfascial exploration should be performed in all cases. In the event of significant myonecrosis, débridement of all necrotic tissue is recommended. Conservative resection of compromised tissue on the initial débridement with open wound packing may preserve posterior coverage. Every effort should be made to retain autologous bone graft. One should remove all other devitalized tissue such as dural barriers or fat grafts. Hardware should be retained for spinal stability. In the event of a late postoperative infection, hardware removal, soft tissue débridement, and antibiotics, first parenterally administered followed by an oral course, should clear the infection (14,23,64,90,91).

Primary wound closure facilitates local wound care and overall nursing requirements. If the patient is septic, one should consider open drainage. In most cases the medical condition of the patient is stable and closure of fascia facilitates hardware coverage. Primary fascial closure prevents retraction of the paraspinal muscle; however, excessive suture tension in the face of borderline tissue may lead to progressive tissue loss. Suction-irrigation systems allow for ease of patient care and maintenance of normal fascial tension. These systems are recommended for multiorganism infections and may be accompanied with multiple débridements to obtain final wound healing (82). The surgeon should be ready to return to the operating room for repeat débridement in 3 to 5 days, depending on the patient's response to therapy.

Postoperative infections after back operations can produce complex wounds with myonecrosis, deep dead space, and exposed orthopedic hardware, bone, and dura. The most common site of wounds requiring plastic surgical intervention in the neurologically intact patient is the posterior thoracic region. In spinal cord–injured patients, the most common site is the lumbosacral area (71). In wounds that involve the mid to upper thoracic spine, the latissimus dorsi muscle or musculocutaneous flaps can be rotated. Lower midline wounds, especially in the thoracolumbar region, may require more complex means of coverage. These include reversed latissimus dorsi flaps, free flaps, extended intercostal flaps, or fasciocutaneous rotation flaps. Some authors advocate raising the paraspinous muscle flaps for a simple means of wound and hardware coverage (43). In the low back the superior gluteal muscle flap is a reasonable flap to fill deep dead space and has some advantages over free flaps (88).

The long-term outcomes of postoperative spinal infection have not been well documented. Disagreement and difficulty have surrounded the assessment and comparison of outcomes. Postoperative spinal infection can prolong a patient's recovery from spinal surgery and exacerbate symptoms of lower back pain. Calderone et al. (11) suggested that outcome with postoperative infections is similar to that of other patients with low back pain undergoing fusion without postoperative infectious complications.

Pseudarthrosis after postoperative wound infection is a recognized factor contributing to poor clinical outcomes after spinal fusion. The pseudarthrosis rate after infection in the lumbar spine may approach 38%. Risk factors that may adversely affect arthrodesis after successful débridement include female sex, the use of allograft bone, and extension of the fusion mass to the sacrum (86). Poor long-term outcomes are associated with arachnoiditis, progressive deformity, spinal instability, and pseudarthrosis.

REFERENCES

1. Altemeier WA, Burke JF, Pruitt BAJ, et al. The influence of operating techniques on the rate of wound infection. In: Altemeier WA, Burke JF, Pruitt BAJ, et al., eds. *Manual on control of infection in surgical patients.* Philadelphia: JB Lippincott Co, 1984.
2. Altemeier WA, Burke JF, Pruitt BAJ, et al. Preoperative preparation of the patient. In: Altemeier WA, Burke JF, Pruitt BAJ, et al., eds. *Manual on control of infection in sur-*

gical patients. Philadelphia: JB Lippincott Co, 1984:71–93.

3. Altemeier WA, Burke JF, Pruitt BAJ, et al. Preparation of the operating team and supporting personnel. In: Altemeier WA, Burke JF, Pruitt BAJ, et al., eds. *Manual on control of infection in surgical patients.* Philadelphia: JB Lippincott Co, 1984:95–110.

4. Baker AS, Ojemann RG, Swartz MN. Spinal epidural abscess. *N Engl J Med* 1975;293:463–468.

5. Baxby D, Woodroffe RC. The location of bacteria in skin. *J Appl Bacteriol* 1965;28(2):316–321.

6. Bertalanffy H, Eggert HR. Complications of anterior cervical discectomy without fusion in 450 consecutive patients. *Acta Neurochir (Wien)* 1989;99(1–2):41–50.

7. Bircher M, Tasker T, Crawshaw C, et al. Discitis following lumbar surgery. *Spine* 1988;13:98–102.

8. Boscardin JB, Ringus JC, Feingold DJ, et al. Human intradiscal levels with cefazolin. *Spine* 17[6 Suppl]:S145–S148.

9. Broner FA, Garland DE, Zigler JE. Spinal infections in the immunocompromised host. *Orthop Clin North Am* 1996;27(1):37–46.

10. Calderone RR, Garland DE, Capen DA, et al. Cost of medical care for postoperative spinal infections. *Orthop Clin North Am* 1996;27(1):171–182.

11. Calderone RR, Thomas JC Jr, Haye W, et al. Outcome assessment in spinal infections. *Orthop Clin North Am* 1996;27(1):201–205.

12. Capen DA, Calderone RR, Green A. Perioperative risk factors for wound infections after lower back fusions. *Orthop Clin North Am* 1996;27(1):83–86.

13. Carragee EJ, Vittum DW. Wound care after posterior spinal surgery. Does early bathing affect the rate of wound complications? *Spine* 1996;21(18):2160–2162.

14. Clark CE, Shufflebarger HL. Late-developing infection in instrumented idiopathic scoliosis. *Spine* 1999;24(18):1909–1912.

15. Darouiche RO, Hamill RJ, Greenberg SB, et al. Bacterial spinal epidural abscess. Review of 43 cases and literature survey. *Medicine (Baltimore)* 1992;71(6):369–385.

16. Dellinger EP. Perioperative infection. In: Meakins JL, ed. *Surgical infections: diagnosis and treatment.* New York: Scientific American Medicine, 1994:217–234.

17. Friedmand DP, Hills JR. Cervical epidural spinal infection: MR imaging characteristics. *AJR Am J Roentgenol* 1994;163(3):699–704.

18. Gepstein R, Eismont FJ. Postoperative spine infections. In: Garfin SR, ed. *Complications of spine surgery.* Baltimore: Williams & Wilkins, 1989:302–322.

19. Grane P, Josephsson A, Seferlis A, et al. Septic and aseptic post-operative discitis in the lumbar spine—evaluation by MR imaging. *Acta Radiol* 1998;39(2):108–115.

20. Guiboux JP, Ahlgren B, Patti JE, et al. The role of prophylactic antibiotics in spinal instrumentation. A rabbit model. *Spine* 1998;23(6):653–656.

21. Hardin WD, Nichols RL. Aseptic technique in the operating room. In: Fry DE, ed. *Surgical infections.* Boston: Little, Brown & Company, 1995:109–117.

22. Hatch RS, Sturm PF, Wellborn CC. Late complication after single-rod instrumentation. *Spine* 1998;23(13):1503–1505.

23. Heggeness MH, Esses SI, Errico T, et al. Late infection of spinal instrumentation by hematogenous seeding. *Spine* 1993;18(4):492–496.

24. Heller J, Levine M. Postoperative infections of the spine. *Semin Spine Surg* 1996;8:105–114.

25. Hermantin F, Peters T, Quartararo L, et al. A prospective, randomized study comparing the results of open discectomy with those of video-assisted arthroscopic microdiscectomy. *J Bone Joint Surg Am* 1999;81:958–965.

26. Howard RJ. Surgical infections. In: Schwartz SI, Shires GT, Spencer FC, eds. *Principles of surgery,* 6th ed. New York: McGraw-Hill, 1994:145–173.

27. Hu SS, Fontaine F, Kelly B, et al. Nutritional depletion in staged spinal reconstructive surgery. The effect of total parenteral nutrition. *Spine* 1998;23(12):1401–1405.

28. Huang TJ, Hsu RW, Sum CW, et al. Complications in thoracoscopic spinal surgery: a study of 90 consecutive patients. *Surg Endosc* 1999;13(4):346–350.

29. Ido K, Shimizu K, Nakayama Y, et al. Suction/irrigation for deep wound infection after spinal instrumentation: a case study. *Eur Spine J* 1996;5(5):345–349.

30. Jimenez-Mejias ME, de Dios Colmenero J, Sanchez-Lora FJ, et al. Postoperative spondylodiskitis: etiology, clinical findings, prognosis, and comparison with nonoperative pyogenic spondylodiskitis. *Clin Infect Dis* 1999;29(2):339–345.

31. Johnson DH, Fairclough JA, Brown EM. Rate of bacterial recolonization of the skin after preparation: four methods compared. *Br J Surg* 1978;74:64.

32. Kayvanfar JF, Capen DA, Thomas JC. Wound infections after instrumented postero-lateral adult lumbar spine fusions. American Academy of Orthopaedic Surgeons Annual Meeting, Orlando, FL, 1995.

33. Khanna RK, Malik GM, Rock JP, et al. Spinal epidural abscess: evaluation of factors influencing outcome. *Neurosurgery* 1996;39(5):958–964.

34. Klein JD, Hey LA, Yu CS, et al. Perioperative nutrition and postoperative complications in patients undergoing spinal surgery. *Spine* 1996;21(22):2676–2682.

35. Klekamp J, Spengler DM, McNamara MJ, et al. Risk factors associated with methicillin-resistant staphylococcal wound infection after spinal surgery. *J Spinal Disord* 1999;12(3):187–191.

36. Kuslich SD, Ulstrom CL, Griffith SL, et al. The Bagby and Kuslich method of lumbar interbody fusion. History, techniques, and 2-year follow-up results of a United States prospective, multicenter trial [see comments]. *Spine* 1998;23(11):1267–1278; discussion, 1279.

37. Lang IM, Hughes DG, Jenkins JP, et al. MR imaging appearances of cervical epidural abscess. *Clin Radiol* 1995;50(7):466–471.

38. Lawrie GM, Morris GC Jr, Glaeser DH. Influence of diabetes mellitus on the results of coronary bypass surgery. Follow-up of 212 diabetic patients ten to 15 years after surgery. *JAMA* 1986;256(21):2967–2971.

39. Lestini W, Bell G. Spinal infection: patient evaluation. *Semin Spine Surg* 1996;8(2):81–94.

40. Lowbury EJL, Lilly HA, Bull JP. Methods for disinfection of hands and operation sites. *Br Med J* 1964;2:531.

41. Lowell TD, Errico TJ, Eskenazi MS. Use of epidural steroids after discectomy may predispose to infection. *Spine* 2000;25(4):516–519.

42. Maiuri F, Iaconetta G, Gallicchio B, et al. Spondylodiscitis. Clinical and magnetic resonance diagnosis. *Spine* 1997;22(15):1741–1746.

43. Manstein ME, Manstein CH, Manstein G. Paraspinous muscle flaps. *Ann Plast Surg* 1998;40(5):458–462.

44. Martin RJ, Yuan HA. Neurosurgical care of spinal epidural, subdural and intramedullary abscess and arachnoiditis. *Orthop Clin North Am* 1996;27(1):125–136.

45. Masterson BJ. Skin preparation. In: Meakins JL, ed. *Surgical infections: diagnosis and treatment.* New York: Scientific American Medicine, 1994:119–125.

46. McAfee PC. Complications of anterior approaches to the thoracolumbar spine. Emphasis on Kaneda instrumentation. *Clin Orthop* 1993;306:110–119.

47. McCulloch J. Focus issue on lumbar disc herniation: macro- and microdiscectomy. *Spine* 1996;21:45S–56S.

48. McDonnell MF, Glassman SD, Dimar JR II, et al. Perioperative complications of anterior procedures on the spine. *J Bone Joint Surg Am* 1996;78(6):839–847.

49. McPhee IB, Williams RP, Swanson CE. Factors influencing wound healing after surgery for metastatic disease of the spine. *Spine* 1998;23(6):726–732; discussion, 732–733.

50. Meakins JL. Guidelines for prevention of surgical site infection. In: Meakins JL, ed. *Surgical infections: diagnosis and treatment.* New York: Scientific American Medicine, 1994:127–138.

51. Modic M, Feiglin D, Piraino D, et al. Vertebral osteomyelitis: assessment using MR. *Radiology* 1985;157:157–166.

52. Naunheim KS, Barnett MG, Crandall DG, et al. Anterior exposure of the thoracic spine [see comments]. *Ann Thorac Surg* 1994;57(6):1436–1439.

53. Nelson CL, Green TG, Porter RA, et al. One day versus seven days of preventive antibiotic therapy in orthopaedic surgery. *Clinical Orthop* 1983;176:258–263.

54. Nielsen VA, Iversen E, Ahlgren P. Postoperative discitis. Radiology of progress and healing. *Acta Radiol* 1990;31(6):559–563.

55. Onik G, Kambin P, Chang M. Minimally invasive disk surgery. Nucleotomy versus fragmentectomy. *Spine* 1997;22:827–830.

56. Osler T. Antiseptics in surgery. In: Fry DE, ed. *Surgical infections.* Boston: Little, Brown & Company, 1995:119–125.

57. Parker LM, McAfee PC, Fedder IL, et al. Minimally invasive surgical techniques to treat spine infections. *Orthop Clin North Am* 1996;27(1):183–199.

58. Picada R, Winter RB, Lonstein JE, et al. Postoperative deep wound infection in adults after posterior lumbo-sacral spine fusion with instrumentation: incidence and management. *J Spinal Disord* 2000;13(1):42–45.

59. Postacchini F, Cinotti G, Perugia D. Post-operative intervertebral discitis. Evaluation of 12 cases and study of ESR in the normal postoperative period. *Ital J Orthop Traumatol* 1993;19(1):57–69.

60. Puranen J, Makela J, Lahde S. Postoperative intervertebral discitis. *Acta Orthop Scand* 1984;55:461–465.

61. Quebbeman EJ. Preparing the operating room. In: Meakins JL, ed. *Surgical infections: diagnosis and treatment.* New York: Scientific American Medicine, 1994:107–118.

62. Ramirez N, Richards BS, Warren PD, et al. Complications after posterior spinal fusion in Duchenne's muscular dystrophy. *J Pediatr Orthop* 1997;17(1):109–114.

63. Rhoten RL, Murphy MA, Kalfas IH, et al. Antibiotic penetration into cervical discs. *Neurosurgery* 1995;37(3):418–421.

64. Richards BS. Delayed infections following posterior spinal instrumentation for the treatment of idiopathic scoliosis. *J Bone Joint Surg Am* 1995;77(4):524–529.

65. Richards BS, Herring JA, Johnston CE, et al. Treatment of adolescent idiopathic scoliosis using Texas Scottish Rite Hospital instrumentation. *Spine* 1994;19(14):1598–1605.

66. Rigamonti D, Liem L, Sampath P, et al. Spinal epidural abscess: contemporary trends in etiology, evaluation, and management. *Surg Neurol* 1999;52(2):189–196; discussion, 197.

67. Riley LH III. Prophylactic antibiotics for spine surgery: description of a regimen and its rationale. *J South Orthop Assoc* 1998;7(3):212–217.

68. Rimoldi RL, Haye W. The use of antibiotics for wound prophylaxis in spinal surgery. *Orthop Clin North Am* 1996;27(1):47–52.

69. Robertson PA, Taylor TK. Late presentation of infection as a complication of Dwyer anterior spinal instrumentation. *J Spinal Disord* 1993;6(3):256–259.

70. Rothman MI, Zoarski GH. Imaging basis of disc space infection. *Semin Ultrasound CT MR* 1993;14(6):437–445.

71. Rubayi S. Wound management in spinal infection. *Orthop Clin North Am* 1996;27(1):137–153.

72. Rubinstein E, Findler G, Amit P, et al. Perioperative prophylactic cephazolin in spinal surgery. A double-blind placebo-controlled trial. *J Bone Joint Surg Br* 1994;76(1):99–102.

73. Sadato N, Numaguchi Y, Rigamonti D, et al. Spinal epidural abscess with gadolinium-enhanced MRI: serial follow-up studies and clinical correlations. *Neuroradiology* 1994;36(1):44–48.

74. Sapico FL. Microbiology and antimicrobial therapy of spinal infections. *Orthop Clin North Am* 1996;27(1):9–13.

75. Sarubbi FA, Vasquez JE. Spinal epidural abscess associated with the use of temporary epidural catheters: report of two cases and review. *Clin Infect Dis* 1997;25(5):1155–1158.

76. Schulitz KP, Assheuer J. Discitis after procedures on the intervertebral disc. *Spine* 1994;19(10):1172–1177.

77. Shapiro SA, Snyder W. Spinal instrumentation with a low complication rate. *Surg Neurol* 1997;48(6):566–574.

78. Stambough JL, Beringer D. Postoperative wound infections complicating adult spine surgery. *J Spinal Disord* 1992;5(3):277–285.

79. Szoke G, Lipton G, Miller F, et al. Wound infection after spinal fusion in children with cerebral palsy. *J Pediatr Orthop* 1998;18(6):727–733.

80. Szypryt E, Hardy J, Hinton C, et al. A comparison between magnetic resonance imaging and scintigraphic bone imaging in the diagnosis of disc space infection in an animal model. *Spine* 1988;13:1042–1048.

81. Tew JM Jr, Mayfield FH. Complications of surgery of the anterior cervical spine. *Clin Neurosurg* 1976;23:424–434.

82. Thalgott JS, Cotler HB, Sasso RC, et al. Postoperative infections in spinal implants. Classification and analysis—a multicenter study. *Spine* 1991;16(8):981–984.

83. Theiss SM, Lonstein JE, Winter RB. Wound infections in reconstructive spine surgery. *Orthop Clin North Am* 1996;27(1):105–110.

84. Viola RW, King HA, Adler SM, et al. Delayed infection after elective spinal instrumentation and fusion. A retrospective analysis of eight cases. *Spine* 1997;22(20):2444–2450; discussion, 2450–2451.

85. Weiland D, McAfee P. Posterior cervical fusion with triple-wire strut graft technique: one hundred consecutive patients. *J Spinal Disord* 1991;4:15–21.

86. Weiss LE, Vaccaro AR, Scuderi G, et al. Pseudarthrosis after postoperative wound infection in the lumbar spine. *J Spinal Disord* 1997;10(6):482–487.

87. Wellman BJ, Follett KA, Traynelis VC. Complications of posterior articular mass plate fixation of the subaxial cervical spine in 43 consecutive patients. *Spine* 1998;23(2):193–200.

88. Wendt JR, Gardner VO, White JI. Treatment of complex postoperative lumbosacral wounds in nonparalyzed patients. *Plast Reconstr Surg* 1998;101(5):1248–1253; discussion, 1254.

89. Whitecloud TS, Butler JC, Cohen JL. Complications with the variable spinal plating system. *Spine* 1989;14:472–476.

90. Wimmer C, Gluch H, Franzreb M, Ogon M. Predisposing factors for infection in spine surgery: a survey of 850 spinal procedures. *J Spinal Disord* 1998;11(2):124–128.

91. Wimmer C, Nogler M, Frischhut B. Influence of antibiotics on infection in spinal surgery: a prospective study of 110 patients. *J Spinal Disord* 1998;11(6):498–500.

POSTOPERATIVE CERVICAL SPINE INFECTIONS

SANFORD E. EMERY AND JOHN J. ORO

Because of the region-specific anatomy, infections of the cervical spine can be disastrous for the patient and the surgeon. The presence of the spinal cord in the canal predisposes to paralysis from space-occupying lesions of the vertebral column. The structural design of the neck allows for support of a 10- to 12-lb head and at the same time allows for substantial range of motion. Because no adjunct supporting structures such as the ribcage are present, however, if the inherent anatomic structures of the cervical spine are compromised by infection, instability can easily occur. Any instability or deformity can then pose a threat to the neural structures. Cervical spine infections thus require prompt recognition and management.

Goals of treatment for cervical spine infections, whether *de novo* or in the postoperative setting, are (a) clearance of the infection, (b) decompression of the neural elements if needed, and (c) stabilization of the spine with correction of deformity if necessary. Surgical treatment depends on the need for identification of an organism, neurologic status, and issues of stability and deformity.

POSTERIOR INFECTIONS

Posterior infection of the cervical spine is most appropriately termed an *epidural abscess*. To be clear semantically, one should refer to this as a *dorsal epidural abscess*; this helps clarify it from the clinical entity of diskitis or vertebral osteomyelitis, in which there is anterior column destruction with or without anterior purulence. Rarely, pus may track around dorsally from an anterior column source, but a true dorsal epidural infection without any anterior involvement may develop (Fig. 1). Spontaneous dorsal epidural abscesses are probably spread hematogenously from another focus, and it is unknown why a given infection may lodge in this anatomic site. Fortunately, dorsal epidural abscesses are relatively uncommon (1,3). After an invasive procedure such as epidural steroid injection, an epidural abscess can certainly occur. As with any surgery, there is some risk of a postoperative infection following posterior decompression or fusion procedures in the cervi-

cal spine. For a patient who is status post multilevel laminectomy, the risk of any cord compression with a postoperative infection is much less, because the epidural space is already unroofed; however, after a large laminectomy, if the posterior wound abscess creates enough pressure, neurologic deficit could occur. This situation would demand immediate débridement. If the patient had not needed stabilization after a laminectomy or laminoplasty, it is unlikely that an early postoperative wound infection would require any additional stabilization considerations, because the inherent ligamentous and bony structures would be intact. Posterior instrumentation and fusion procedures, such as are done with lateral mass plating, have some risk of postoperative infection, although, again, this is very low (6,8). If this occurs, management would consist of irrigation and débridement, possibly with more than one trip back to the operating room. As with other areas of the spine, if the internal fixation is providing stability, it should be left in place, and the success rate of clearing an infection without removing well-fixed instrumentation should be quite high (11).

Infections after epidural steroid injections are more likely to lead to cord compromise, given the confines of the epidural space. If dorsal epidural infection is producing cord compression and neurologic deficit, it is necessary to decompress this surgically. This requires a laminectomy over the appropriate levels as determined by preoperative studies.

Decisions must be made at the time of surgery regarding the amount of decompression needed to relieve the spinal cord and débride the abscess versus potential destabilization of the spine with varying amounts of removal of the posterior elements. Postoperative immobilization needs to be determined on a case-by-case basis, but if there is no anterior column involvement, a soft collar would typically be appropriate.

ANTERIOR INFECTIONS

Infections following anterior cervical spine procedures are fortunately rare. The soft tissues of the neck are quite

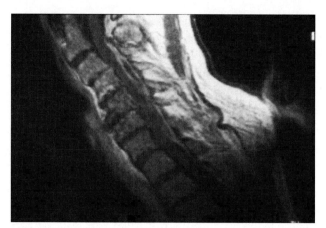

FIGURE 1. Lateral magnetic resonance image showing a dorsal mass compressing the thecal sac and spinal cord. This was treated with a posterior laminectomy, and frank purulence was débrided over several levels.

vascular, and superficial wound infections are unusual; thus, deep postoperative infections of the spine are also uncommon. One diagnostic procedure that carries a risk of infection is diskography (2,12). Diskitis is a known possible complication of performing diskograms, with seeding of the disk from skin flora or more likely from esophageal injury. The esophagus lies directly anterior to the vertebrae and can be easily punctured with a needle if great care is not taken. This is a procedure that should only be done by individuals trained in the technique to minimize complications. If a postdiskography diskitis develops, it may take days or weeks to manifest. Typically, the patient would present with increasing neck

pain. Systemic symptoms such as fever and chills are typically uncommon. Plain radiographs may show some changes in the disk, with narrowing and initially endplate rarefaction followed by later sclerosis. Typically, this would occur on both sides of the disk. The diagnosis should be confirmed with magnetic resonance imaging (MRI), which is usually diagnostic. Specific antibiotic treatment requires obtaining an organism from the infected site. This brings up the issue of needle biopsy versus open biopsy in the anterior cervical spine. In this scenario, because the infection was caused by a needle after diskography, these authors favor open biopsy with débridement and fusion. An adequate débridement back to healthy subchondral or cancellous bone followed by autogenous iliac crest bone grafting should be successful in clearing the infection with appropriate antibiotic support. Use of allograft in this setting would not be recommended unless there were no alternatives. A recent study demonstrated that immediate internal fixation to treat infection in the cervical spine was successful in creating stability and did not result in persistent infection (10). Postoperative care would be similar to a patient having an anterior cervical diskectomy and fusion, with the exception of the adjunct intravenous antibiotic treatment.

Consultation with the infectious disease service is recommended. Typically, diskitis or vertebral osteomyelitis is treated with 6 weeks of intravenous antibiotics followed by a course of oral antibiotics for anywhere from 1 to 3 months. Host considerations

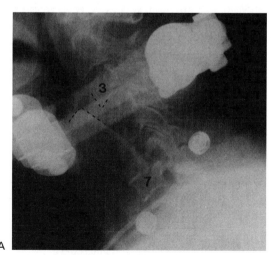
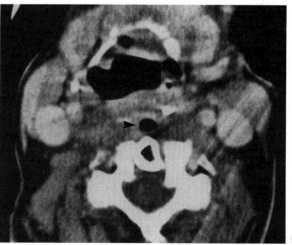

FIGURE 2. An 81-year-old woman with cervical myelopathy had a three-level anterior corpectomy and autogenous iliac strut graft from C-3 to C-7. **A:** Lateral radiograph showing displacement of the cephalad and of the graft anteriorly. This occurred early in the postoperative course, and a revision procedure was performed using a fibula strut graft. **B:** Subsequent to revision strut grafting operation, an abscess developed where the original iliac strut displaced and eroded into the esophagus. Note the air pocket in the abscess (*arrow*) anterior to the fibula strut seen in cross section. The abscess was successfully treated with open irrigation, débridement, intravenous antibiotics, and halo vest immobilization. (From Bridwell KH, DeWald RL, eds. *The textbook of spinal surgery*, 2nd ed. Philadelphia: Lippincott–Raven Publishers, 1997:1432, with permission.)

such as the quality of the patient's immune status need to be considered in tailoring an antibiotic regimen for a given individual.

Postoperative infection in the anterior cervical spine can also occur following diskectomy and fusion procedures or corpectomy and strut graft procedures (7,9). If a graft displaces anteriorly, there is some risk of esophageal erosion (Fig. 2). This can result in an abscess formation or severe infection tracking distally, causing a severe infection called *mediastinitis*. Symptoms of postoperative infection would typically include increasing pain, with possible swallowing problems and other systemic signs of infection. A contained abscess may not manifest as wound drainage. Swelling may or may not be present on examination. Any suspicion of postoperative infection should be evaluated with laboratory investigations such as complete blood count, sedimentation rate, and C-reactive protein. These last two values may be elevated postoperatively but can still be useful as baseline information.

Computed tomography or MRI evaluation may show an abscess or air from infection (Fig. 2). This requires open operative débridement. If the operative area can be adequately débrided and the strut graft is in place with early healing and stable fixation, the graft can be left in place (5). Severe infections or compromised host factors may warrant removal of the graft and maintenance of the patient in traction until another débridement or two can be performed every 48 hours. Operative débridement plus antibiotics should be able to control the infection such that another strut graft, preferably using autogenous bone, can be placed for stability and ultimate arthrodesis (4). Halo vest immobilization or even posterior stabilization with internal fixation would be generally recommended in this situation. Any identifiable injury to the esophagus that may have caused the infection would need to be repaired, and consultation with the otolaryngology or general surgery service would be appropriate. Esophageal injuries need to be protected with nasogastric suction and intravenous hyperalimentation until the esophagus is healed to avoid esophageal fistulae.

CONCLUSION

Postoperative or postprocedural infections of the cervical spine are best managed with early diagnosis, aggressive antibiotic therapy, and often open surgical débridement. Because these types of infection are rare, the spine surgeon must be diligent to maintain a high index of suspicion in patients who have increasing pain postoperatively or other signs or symptoms discussed in this chapter. Diagnostic modalities should include laboratory investigation and radiographic imaging, particularly MRI. Goals of treatment are to clear the infection, decompress the spinal cord if needed, and maintain or create stability with the use of anterior or posterior arthrodesis techniques, or both.

REFERENCES

1. Baker AS, Ojemann RG, Swartz MN, et al. Spinal epidural abscess. *N Engl J Med* 1975;293:463–468.
2. Connor PM, Darden BV. Cervical discography complications and clinical efficacy. *Spine* 1993;18:2035–2038.
3. Danner RL, Hartman BJ. Update on spinal epidural abscess: 35 cases and review of the literature. *Rev Infect Dis* 1987;9:265–274.
4. Dietze DD Jr, Fessler RG, Jacob RP. Primary reconstruction for spinal infections. *J Neurosurg* 1997;86:981–989.
5. Emery SE, Chan DPK, Woodward HR. Treatment of hematogenous pyogenic vertebral osteomyelitis with anterior debridement and primary bone grafting. *Spine* 1989;14:284–291.
6. Heller JG, Silcox DH III, Sutterlin CE III. Complications of posterior cervical plating. *Spine* 1995;20:2442–2448.
7. Kelly MF, Spiegel J, Rizzo KA, et al. Delayed pharyngoesophageal perforation: a complication of anterior spine surgery. *Ann Otol Rhinol Laryngol* 1991;100:201–205.
8. Levi ADO, Dickman CA, Sonntag VKH. Management of postoperative infections after spinal instrumentation. *J Neurosurg* 1997;86:975–980.
9. Newhouse KE, Lindsey RW, Clark CR, et al. Esophageal perforation following anterior cervical spine surgery. *Spine* 1989;14:1051–1053.
10. Rezai AR, Woo HH, Errico TJ, et al. Contemporary management of spinal osteomyelitis. *Neurosurgery* 1999;44(5):1018–1025.
11. Thalgott JS, Cotler HB, Sasso RC, et al. Postoperative infections in spinal implants: classification and analysis—a multi-center study. *Spine* 1991;16:981–984.
12. Zeidman SM, Thompson K, Ducker TB. Complications of cervical discography: analysis of 4400 diagnostic disc injections. *Neurosurgery* 1995;37:414–417.

POSTOPERATIVE THORACIC AND LUMBAR SPINE INFECTIONS

JOHN G. HELLER AND MITCHELL F. REITER

Wound infections are an inevitable risk of surgery. Despite optimal patient health, the best sterile technique, and judicious use of antibiotics, some percentage of patients experience a postoperative infection. When such a complication occurs, the surgeon must do his or her best to diagnose the problem in a timely fashion and take appropriate steps to eradicate the infection while accounting for the unique issues that may accompany a spinal problem. Delays in diagnosis and inadequate treatment tend to compound the therapeutic challenges. Although admittedly the authors' prejudice, postoperative spinal infections are not problems that can be handled with medical treatment alone.

Substantial suspicion of an infection begets surgical intervention that facilitates timely and accurate diagnosis as well as initiates treatment. Half-hearted intervention risks inadequate treatment and potentially increases the patient's risk of morbidity, whereas decisive and well-planned intervention should yield a higher probability of eliminating the infection and minimizing the comorbidity associated with it.

INCIDENCE AND PREVENTION

A postoperative infection can be a devastating complication that significantly adds to the cost and morbidity of an operation. The relative risk and consequences of this difficult problem can be reduced through careful preoperative patient assessment, intraoperative attention to detail, and postoperative diligence. The likely incidence of postoperative infection cannot be easily quantified. Available information supports the notion that the relative risk of infection is proportional to the magnitude of the procedure undertaken, with additional allowances made for unique comorbid conditions of the patient. If one looks at the risk of infection as a spectrum, the laminotomy/diskectomy would be at the low end of the scale. With timely administration of prophylactic antibiotics, the likelihood of postoperative diskitis should be approximately 0.5% (37,60).

As the scale of the anatomic dissection increases, so does the risk of infection. If one adds a fusion, the incidence of infection increases to roughly 2%, with published reports ranging from 1% to 5% (42,47). Procedures that use spinal instrumentation appear to engender greater risk of infection. Reports of rates approaching 5% have been published, but the authors' experience suggests that this might be an overly pessimistic estimate (23,24,28,35). Whether this is due to the instrumentation itself or to the added time and dissection needed to place the construct is not fully known. Anterior thoracic and lumbar fusion procedures have a lower reported rate of wound infection, approximately half when compared to posterior fusions (13). In any event, the specific risk is not the point. What one must take away from the discussion is the notion that larger-scale undertakings beget greater risks, including infection. Furthermore, if the patient and surgeon should be so unlucky as to have to face such a complication, its potential consequences are also magnified in proportion to the scale of the surgical procedure.

Many host factors have been noted as risk factors for postoperative spinal infections. Clearly, conditions that impair a host's immune status or wound healing can predispose them to infection. Perhaps the leading cause of such impairment is malnutrition. Either preoperatively or in the postoperative period, nutritional deficiency has been shown to be highly associated with lumbar wound infection (14,31,63). Klein et al. (32) demonstrated that 25% of 114 patients undergoing elective lumbar fusion were found to be malnourished preoperatively and that 11 of the 13 infectious complications occurred in the malnourished group. Serum albumin of less than 3.5 and a total lymphocyte count of less than 1,500 are both markers of malnutrition. Obesity, another form of malnutrition, also conveys a relative risk of infection. Whether this is due to nutritional factors alone is unclear, because obesity generally increases operative time and adds significantly to the volume of the wound that is poorly vascularized.

Subcutaneous fat necrosis can also cause abnormal amounts of postoperative wound drainage, which delays sealing of the wound to external sources of inoculation. Diabetes mellitus, especially when poorly controlled, increases one's relative risk of infection (62). Patients with myelodysplasia and cerebral palsy are prone to an increased risk of infection, presumably due to chronic urinary tract colonization and poor tissue quality at the surgical site (64). Immunocompromised patients, including those with acquired immunodeficiency syndrome or those receiving medications such as steroids (rheumatoid arthritis) or chemotherapy also face a greater possibility of infection. Coexistent infections, such as pneumonia, urinary tract infection, or skin ulcers, can produce a bacteremic state that may seed a wound after surgery (7). Also, there are those who believe that nicotine use conveys an independent risk of infection. Whether or not this is true, its use certainly compromises a host's ability to eradicate the infection, as shown by Thalgott et al. (65). Although it has not been well established, local irradiation impairs wound healing and may convey an independent risk of infection because of a diminished local blood supply (43). However, when such wounds experience healing problems, it may be difficult to distinguish between a wound dehiscence that is colonized and an infected wound that has dehisced. Finally, the length of preoperative hospitalization increases the rate of wound complications (72). Cruse and Foord (9) reported a doubling of the wound infection rate for each week a patient was hospitalized before surgery.

Knowledge of these host risk factors predisposing toward wound infections can help the surgeon minimize the likelihood of this dreaded complication. If the opportunity presents itself, the surgeon must make every effort preoperatively to reduce the patient's relative risk of a wound infection. Sadly, one does not always have the luxury of time, because patients can present with emergent conditions, the treatment of which must proceed in full recognition of the unsavory circumstances in which they arise. In such cases, the surgeon is well advised to educate the patient and family about the relative risks that they face given the medical circumstances. On the other hand, elective surgery allows for full consideration of the medical history. Correctable conditions must be identified and corrected preoperatively, whenever possible or practical. Glucose control should be optimized in diabetics. Patients should be screened preoperatively for malnutrition and, when possible, corrective measures taken (29). Smokers should be strongly encouraged to quit before surgery. This measure pays dividends in numerous ways, not the least of which might apply to infection rates. The authors attempt to educate their patients about the adverse role that tobacco products play in wound healing, fusion success, pulmonary complications, deep venous thrombosis, and the like. We have also found the use of urine assays for nicotine metabolites to be useful in ensuring patient compliance.

Coexistent infections must be identified and treated before the patient is subjected to nonemergent surgery. When this is not practical, appropriate cultures should be obtained before operation, and the choice of prophylactic antibiotics should be adjusted to account for likely pathogens. Treatment of the coexisting infection is then completed perioperatively, as suggested by the culture and sensitivity data. In patients who are hospitalized preoperatively for a prolonged period, consideration should be given to discharging them for a period of time to allow the reestablishment of normal skin flora before spinal surgery, provided that their condition affords such a window in time.

Many intraoperative variables play a role in predisposing a patient to infectious complications. Because of the number of confounding variables, it is extremely difficult to prove with certainty the efficacy of any one operative technique at lowering the infection rate; however, common sense and some time-tested principles of surgery lead to some recommendations. Other than sterile technique, the simplest measure to prevent wound infections is the proper use of prophylactic antibiotics (57). For elective cases in normal hosts, a first-generation cephalosporin should be given 30 to 60 minutes before the incision (19,52). Some authors have proposed different antibiotic regimens based primarily on experimental evidence that shows poor penetration of the intervertebral disk and cerebrospinal fluid by some first-generation cephalosporins; however, excellent clinical results have been shown with routine use of first-generation cephalosporins (51). Their administration is continued for 24 hours postoperatively. Lengthier courses of antibiotics, such as those that pay homage to the myth of continuing antibiotics "until the drains are out," have no basis in science.

Minimizing operating room traffic, using laminar flow air systems, and decreasing the length of the procedure may also help reduce ambient colony counts and thus the bacterial inoculum in the wound. Attention to the time-honored teachings of Halsted, including the gentle handling of tissues and débridement of devitalized tissue, is crucial. A final inspection should be made before closure to ensure good hemostasis and adequate removal of necrotic material. Frequent irrigation with bactericidal antibiotics as well as the intermittent release of surgical retractor to minimize muscle ischemia has been found to be helpful (3,54,58). Layered closures help obliterate dead space, and closed-suction drainage systems help prevent the formation of seromas and hematomas. Such fluid collections can predispose to infection through continued wound drainage and by furnishing an iron-rich environment that functions as an ideal culture medium for bacteria. A series by Lowell et al. (39) also demonstrated a substantially higher rate of postoperative infection in patients who received epidural methylprednisolone at the conclusion of lumbar diskectomy procedures.

Finally, this discussion must include a word about foreign bodies. Virtually any foreign body can convey some incremental risk of infection. Although it would be ludicrous to think that spinal procedures should proceed without them, one should consider that materials such as bone wax, Gelfoam, polymethylmethacrylate, and metallic implants can serve as a locus minoris resistentiae for an inoculum, thus contributing to the risk of infection (25).

CLASSIFICATION AND DIAGNOSIS

The point of any classification scheme is to facilitate treatment, establish a prognosis, aid in further research, or any combination thereof. In the case of the spine, various authorities have sought to distinguish wound infections as either superficial or deep, early or late, or acute or chronic (16). Although descriptive, these terms tend not to be very useful in the management of the problem. More recently, Thalgott et al. (65) provided an analysis of postoperative spinal wound infections that was shown to correlate with complexity of treatment and prognosis. They borrowed from Cierny's approach to classification and management of appendicular osteomyelitis. They classified spine wound infections based on the severity of the infection and the nature of the host. The infections were stratified into three subgroups determined by two factors: the location (superficial vs. deep) and the microbiologic diagnosis (single organism vs. polymicrobial). The hosts were also subdivided into three groups based on their systemic defenses, metabolic capabilities, and local tissue health (65).

Superficial infections generally occur in the acute postoperative period; that is to say, one will observe them within the first 2 weeks of surgery. Whether they constitute an "early" infection is a matter of semantics.

They are generally characterized by erythema, wound drainage, local edema, tenderness, and possibly fluctuance. The patient may complain of increased local pain. Low-grade fevers can be observed, as well as diaphoresis. Laboratory tests may be misleadingly normal, but one may also observe a mild leukocytosis. The C-reactive protein (CRP) and erythrocyte sedimentation rates (ESR) are elevated; however, in interpreting postoperative CRP and ESR values one must keep in mind that both values are elevated after surgery. The ESR typically peaks 5 days postoperatively, with its magnitude of elevation being proportional to the extent of the operation performed, and returns to normal over a period of approximately 6 weeks. The CRP, on the other hand, typically peaks within 2 days and returns to baseline over 5 to 14 days. Thus, the CRP is a more valuable test in the early postoperative period (53,67). An important cautionary note is in order. A "superficial" infection may only be the tip of a dangerous and deceptive iceberg, as it often coexists with a deep wound infection. This possibility and its implications for treatment should always be carefully considered (21).

Deep infections can be difficult to diagnose. The wound often appears deceptively normal. Thus, delay in diagnosis is common, and it therefore serves little purpose to try to distinguish them as early or late. Patients typically complain of pain that is greater than expected for the postoperative course, a general sense of illness, and often anorexia. Diaphoresis is common, especially at night. Patients may or may not manifest a febrile response (26). The authors have encountered a number of patients with extensive suppurative deep infections without any observable fever (22). The surgeon is admonished to be particularly suspicious in the case of a compromised host, such as a malnourished, diabetic, or elderly patient. Also, one should keep in mind that, in this day of more liberal use of postoperative oral narcotics, an escalating drug requirement may not reflect either physiologic tolerance or drug-seeking behavior. More than one patient has been discovered to have a deep wound infection with vertebral osteomyelitis after having had a spinal cord stimulator or narcotic pump, or both, implanted (40) (Fig. 1). The white blood cell count, CRP, and ESR all tend to be somewhat higher than with superficial infections. A normal white blood cell count, as with the absence of fever, does not preclude the presence of a deep wound infection (36).

Late wound infections do exist; however, they are distinctly unusual. The authors suggest that this designation be reserved for the type of infection

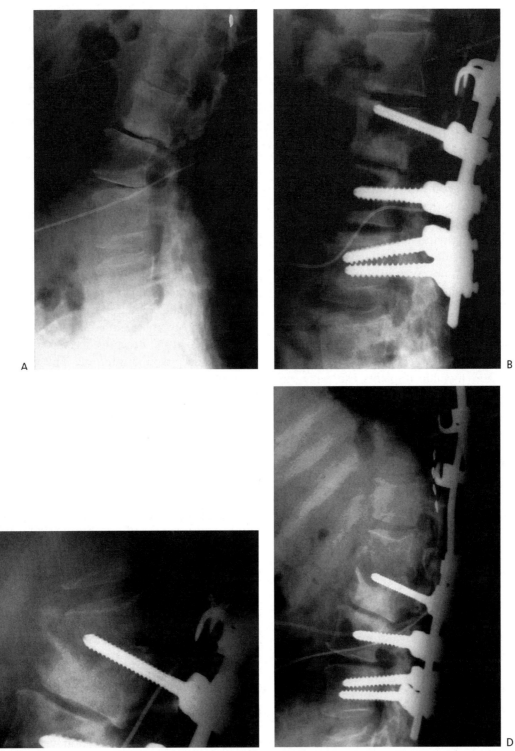

FIGURE 1. This 58-year-old woman presented to another institution with complaints of increasing back pain and new neurogenic claudication, which was refractory to medical care. Her surgeon diagnosed her with suprajacent segmental degeneration and lumbar stenosis above an old lumbar decompression and fusion **(A)** (lateral preoperative radiograph). A revision posterior lumbar decompression with a segmental instrumentation and fusion was attempted from L-1 to L-4 **(B)** (lateral radiograph shortly after surgery). The patient complained of increasing discomfort perioperatively. A lateral radiograph taken some months later **(C)** was misinterpreted as demonstrating a junctional fracture secondary to osteoporosis. Note the loss of disk space height and endplate destruction with segmental collapse and kyphosis, all of which imply intervertebral osteomyelitis and diskitis. The surgeon subsequently performed an extension of her instrumentation and fusion to T-9 **(D)**. (*continued*)

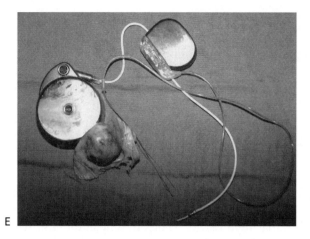

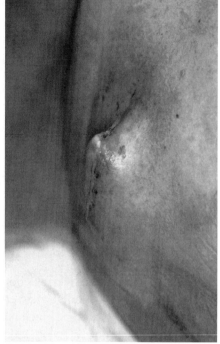

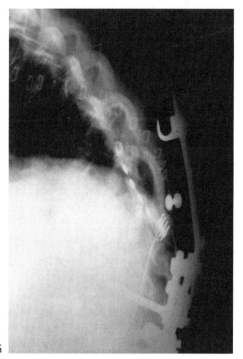

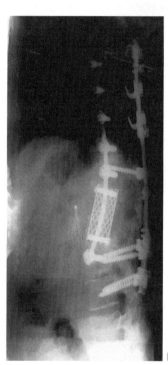

FIGURE 1. (*continued*) The procedure was complicated by a wound "dehiscence," drainage, and eventually loss of fixation of the superior hooks. This was managed with a débridement, partial implant removal, and latissimus dorsi flap. By the time that the patient presented to the authors for treatment, her pain was being managed with an implantable spinal cord stimulator and an indwelling narcotic pump **(E)** (devices retrieved at surgery). Inspection of her torso suggested displaced implants eroding the suture line of the myocutaneous flap **(F)**, which was readily appreciated on her sitting lateral radiograph **(G)**. She was treated in stages, beginning with complete removal of all implants and an extensive wound débridement, as well as extensive culturing of the tissues removed. While correcting her profound malnutrition, a staged reconstruction was performed **(H)** that included anterior corpectomies of T-12 and L-1 with a reconstruction, fusion, and instrumentation from T-7 to L-2 using a mixture of autologous iliac bone graft and morcellized fresh frozen cancellous allograft bone. This was followed soon thereafter by a definitive posterior segmental instrumentation and fusion (T-7 to L-3) with posterior iliac crest autograft. She was treated with intravenous antistaphylococcal therapy for 6 weeks. The infection was eradicated and all levels of the fusion healed.

described by Viola et al. (68). Analogous to the arthroplasty that presents with an infection long after implantation, these infections present more than a year after their surgery, and sometimes many years later. Whether they represent hematogenous seeding following a bacteremia or activation of a latent bacterial inoculum is a matter of conjecture. They are usually associated with spinal implants, with or without a nonunion. They are readily managed with implant removal, débridement, and a suitable course of intravenous antibiotics. If a pseudarthrosis is found at the time of débridement and the spine is clinically stable, repair of the fusion should await eradication of the infection. If the pseudarthrosis is determined to be asymptomatic, no additional treatment may be necessary other than observation over time.

Thalgott's classification of postoperative infection has proved most instructive. This is a modernized version of the "seed and soil" concept of infection. Like Cierny's work with treating long bone infections, this classification accounts for what is causing the infection, the host in which it arises, and the quality of the local tissues. The host is classified as (a) nonsmoker with a normal medical history, (b) local or systemic illnesses (e.g., diabetes) and/or a smoker, or (c) immunocompromised, with severe malnutrition or an Injury Severity Score greater than 18 in the case of a trauma victim. The infectious processes were classified into groups: I, single organisms with either superficial or deep involvement; II, multiple organisms with deep involvement; and III, single or multiple organisms with extensive local myonecrosis. In the authors' retrospective review, it happened that these subgroups tended to correlate with one another; that is to say, 62% of group I infections involved type A hosts and no type C hosts. Group II infections were not observed in type A hosts, whereas 75% of the hosts were type B and 25% were type C. Group III infections, as one might expect, occurred exclusively in type C patients. Thalgott's analysis also highlighted a sobering correlation between the infection group and the course of treatment. Twelve of 13 group I infections were readily managed with one débridement, 4 weeks of antibiotics, and a mean hospital stay of 14 days. Of group II infections, 75% were sterilized after three débridements, with either primary or delayed wound closure, 6 weeks of antibiotics, and a mean hospitalization of 32 days. As one might imagine, group III infections fared the worst. Successful treatment required a mean of six operations, flap closure of the wound, 12 weeks of antibiotics, and a mean inpatient stay of 78 days. Not surprisingly, the mean direct inpatient costs of treating the wound infections were

$42,000, $128,000, and $437,000 for groups I, II, and III, respectively (65).

The contribution of this analysis should not be underestimated. When a wound infection occurs, the treating physicians have a framework with which they can analyze the magnitude of the problem that they and the patient face. The treatment plan should then take into account all of the relevant variables, with each being recognized and addressed prospectively. Early and aggressive management of systemic illness, nutritional needs, and local wound environment usually leads to a successful outcome in less time than that reported by Thalgott. The authors warn against dismissing an infection as "superficial" and embarking on half-hearted, local treatment. This is essentially a diagnosis of exclusion, as the frequency of coexistent deep infection is high. Failure to recognize the deep process may condemn a patient to a more protracted course of illness and treatment (10).

With the possible exception of diskitis following a laminotomy/diskectomy, imaging modalities are of little use in the prompt diagnosis of a postoperative spinal wound infection. Magnetic resonance imaging (MRI) has a high sensitivity and specificity for diagnosing postoperative diskitis. However, it has proved unreliable in distinguishing, by either signal characteristics or morphology, the difference between benign postoperative fluid collections and an abscess (30,55). Therefore, in a clinical setting that is suspicious for a wound infection, technology cannot help the surgeon distinguish between a hematoma or an epidural collection of pus. Surgical exploration not only answers the question but initiates effective treatment.

Anterior spinal wound infections have received little attention because of their relatively small numbers. However, computed tomography (CT) or MRI may provide a clue if retroperitoneal or intrathoracic fluid collections are identified. Guided aspiration or surgical exploration, or both, may be necessary to distinguish between loculated pleural effusions and empyemas (Fig. 2) or between lymphoceles and paralumbar abscesses (Fig. 3). When the presentation is more delayed, secondary changes may be more apparent radiographically. Although one would wish to diagnose the infection before the radiographic hallmarks of intervertebral diskitis and osteomyelitis occur, plain radiographic, CT, and MRI changes become important in mapping the extent of involvement of the anterior and posterior vertebral elements, as well as the surrounding tissues (48). CT-guided biopsies can provide a microbiological diagnosis in selected cases (2). A negative culture, however, does not exclude the diagnosis, because the false-negative

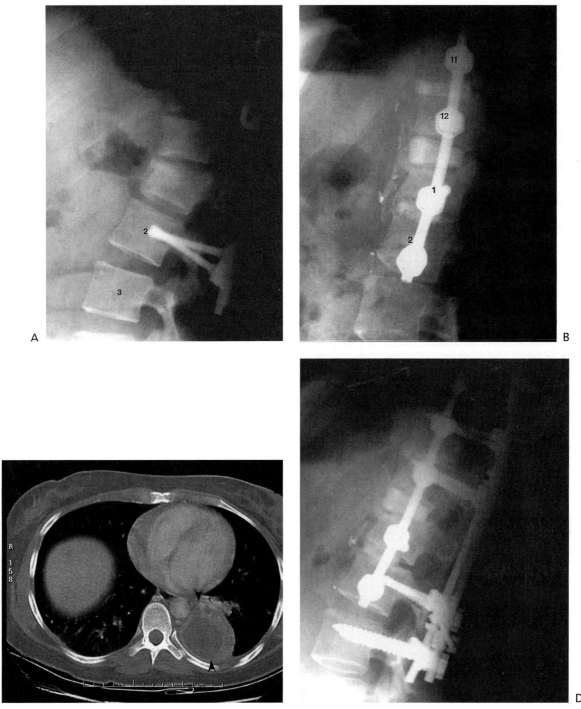

FIGURE 2. A 35-year-old woman sustained an L-1 burst fracture in an automobile accident that was initially treated elsewhere with a complete L-1 laminectomy and L1-2 facetectomy, followed by the instrumentation and fusion shown in **(A)**. Ultimately, a nonunion was diagnosed and treatment attempted, with removal of her posterior implants, then an anterior realignment and multilevel instrumentation and fusion from T-10 to L-2 **(B)**. Within the first month of surgery the patient gave increasing but nonspecific complaints of back and abdominal pain, anorexia, fevers, chills, and urinary frequency. Her urinary tract infection was diagnosed. The symptoms rapidly improved during the week that she received antibiotics, only to return and worsen after their cessation. A subsequent CT scan of the chest and abdomen demonstrated a loculated empyema that proved to be associated with a deep wound infection **(C)** (*arrowheads*). She underwent extensive irrigation and débridement through a repeat thoracotomy; then a staged posterior segmental instrumentation and fusion **(D)** was performed as she was receiving a 3-month course of intravenous antibiotics. At latest follow-up, the infection had resolved and the posterior fusion had healed.

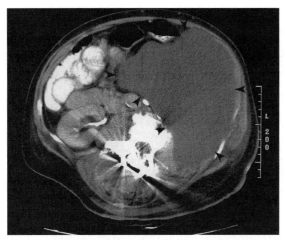

FIGURE 3. A sterile lymphocele developed in this patient after a combined anterior-posterior instrumentation and fusion for progressive lumbar scoliosis in adulthood. Clinically, she complained of abdominal pain and anorexia. In contrast to a patient with an infection, however, she had no fevers, sweats, chills, or malaise. The computed tomography scan clearly demonstrates the lymphocele (*arrowheads*). Note that there is little, if any, inflammatory reaction around, in contrast to the empyema in Figure 2C. Nonetheless, the fluid collection was aspirated and cultured to ensure that it was sterile before treatment.

rate will be at least 20%. These biopsies are especially unreliable if the patient has been treated with antibiotics. Deep wound aspiration is recommended by some but may miss a more localized infection of a seroma or hematoma. Ultrasonography has been found to be incapable of distinguishing an abscess from other fluid collections but may be useful in guiding aspiration of suspicious wounds (34). Nuclear medicine studies in the acute postoperative period have not been found useful. Although they may play a greater role in the diagnosis of delayed infections, they still have an unacceptably high false-negative rate (44,49,70). At present, the authors believe that there is still no substitute for early operative exploration of a suspected postoperative wound infection.

TREATMENT

The diagnosis or suspicion of a postoperative spinal wound infection begets aggressive management. The goals of treatment are to (a) eradicate the infection while maintaining or improving the patient's medical state, (b) obtain a stable physiologic wound closure, (c) restore or maintain the mechanical integrity of the affected spinal motion segments, and (d) promote bone graft healing or repair nonunions where necessary (65). Inadequate measures such as treatment with antibiotics alone or in conjunction with bedside suture

removal and local dressing changes are mentioned only to be condemned. Although one might "get away with" this approach, such a course of action imposes a noteworthy clinical risk of allowing a more extensive infection to become established. The authors recommend that patients should be taken to the operating room, where the wound can be thoroughly explored, cultured, irrigated, and débrided under sterile conditions. Although this approach may occasionally result in the operative drainage of a sterile seroma, it is believed that the benefits of early surgical intervention exceed the risks of delay, particularly in the presence of metallic implants, bone graft, and exposed dura (5,42).

Legitimate debate continues in regard to wound management in one circumstance. Some would argue that acute postoperative diskitis can be managed medically, provided that the pathogen can be identified via percutaneous aspiration. To be clear, medical management would consist of immobilization and appropriately administered antibiotics such that adequate serum levels are maintained. The latter is typically bed rest at the outset, followed later by an appropriately fitted orthosis. Response to treatment is monitored on the basis of the patient's symptoms, which should improve rapidly, and serial CRP and ESR values. The authors concede this option provided that the primary complaint is back pain, that there is no wound drainage, that the patient remains neurologically normal from presentation through the course of the treatment, and that the clinical response is rapid. Medical treatment should be abandoned in favor of surgery if the above conditions are not present or if the patient's condition deteriorates clinically. Such a medical treatment plan also warrants close clinical follow-up. Unfortunately, if an epidural abscess evolves, the complaint remains back pain until late in the evolution of the problem. The onset of paralysis is rapid and can proceed with little warning. When treating this complication, one should be sure to educate the patient and family of the downside risks and what symptoms to watch for. If there has been sufficient delay in diagnosis such that radiographic evidence of vertebral osteomyelitis is present, the authors would argue against medical therapy alone (Fig. 4).

The operative management of a spinal wound infection proceeds in a stepwise fashion. The subcutaneous plane is explored and cultured first. Dermal margins are excised if necessary, and any necrotic tissue is débrided. To minimize the amount of coagulation required to achieve hemostasis in hyperemic dermis, it is recommended that the dermis be infiltrated with dilute epinephrine solution (1:100,000 to 1:500,000) and be allowed to blanch before opening the wound. The wound is copiously irrigated using pulsatile lavage with antibiotic solution that is effective against gram-positive as well as gram-negative organisms. Once the superficial layer has been rendered surgically "clean," the fascia is opened so that the full depth of the wound can be explored. Some authors propose that, if the deep fascia appears intact and uninfected, one may aspirate the deep wound and only open the deep fascia if a Gram's stain reveals evidence of deep infection (18). However, as mentioned previously, the likelihood of a coexistent deep wound infection is sufficiently high that the authors believe the deep layers should be explored. Culture, débridement, and irrigation of the deep wound are performed. Antibiotics can be administered once the deep cultures have been obtained. Initially, broad-spectrum coverage is recommended, which can be tailored to the culture and sensitivity data when available. Meticulous débridement of all devitalized tissue is mandatory. Loose bone graft fragments, Gelfoam, fat grafts, or other nonessential materials should be removed. Adherent bone graft should be left in place (42).

The issue of whether the instrumentation needs to be removed continues to be a source of controversy. This typically arises when medical consultants who are unfamiliar with the unique issues of spinal infections extrapolate recommendations based on outdated information from the treatment of long bone osteomyelitis. This specific point has been addressed in several studies with unanimous findings. For spinal wounds in particular, the notion that antibiotic treatment may be incapable of eradicating the infection in the presence of hardware is a myth with no basis in fact (8,12). Independent of the fact that numerous authors have demonstrated a high likelihood of eliminating infection in the presence of well-fixed spinal implants, removal of such implants in some cases would invite potentially catastrophic damage on the patient because of segmental instability (1,35,46,47,65,71). Especially in an age of readily available titanium implants, which appear more infection "resistant" than stainless steel, not only should well-fixed implants be left in place, but it might be appropriate to replace loose implants with an alternative method of fixation. Glassman et al. (18) demonstrated at a minimum of 1-year follow-

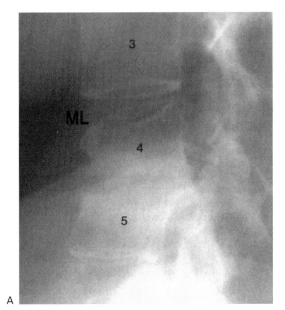
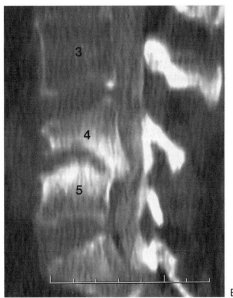

FIGURE 4. A 43-year-old morbidly obese woman was initially treated for a lumbar disk herniation with an L4-5 diskectomy. She had initial pain relief, but then progressively worsening lower back pain developed. Six months after the index surgery, the patient underwent a repeat diskectomy and noninstrumented posterior L4-5 intertransverse fusion with autogenous iliac crest bone graft. After this procedure her back pain continued to worsen, and imaging studies reportedly revealed evidence of diskitis/osteomyelitis. She was then treated with a posterior incision and drainage, at which time the cultures grew *Candida albicans* and the patient was placed on oral fluconazole (Diflucan). She continued to have incapacitating low back pain, but she remained free of any symptoms of neural compression. When she presented to our institution, her lateral lumbar x-ray **(A)** demonstrated advanced disk space and endplate destruction consistent with vertebral osteomyelitis. The sagittal reformations of her myelogram computed tomography (CT) scan **(B)** illustrate the degree of bone involvement, as well as the dense reactive bone surrounding the infection. (*continued*)

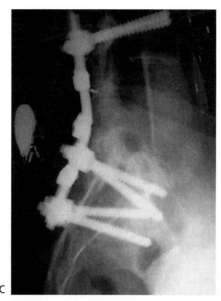
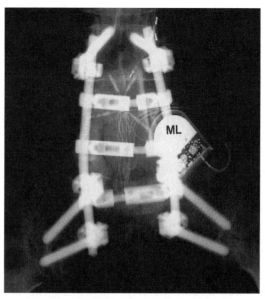

C   D

FIGURE 4. (continued) This case demonstrates a complex postoperative lumbar spine infection that includes extensive anterior vertebral body destruction due to osteomyelitis. It is also unusual because of the fungal organism. Management issues are all the more difficult due to multiple previous surgeries and morbid obesity. Indications for surgical treatment included (a) failure of medical treatment, (b) intractable pain, (c) extensive anterior bony involvement with osteomyelitis, and (d) a kyphotic deformity with segmental instability. An anterior débridement and strut grafting were deemed essential. Unfortunately, a reformatted CT scan with sagittal and coronal reconstructions revealed that the bony involvement was too extensive to allow for preservation of the L-4 or L-5 bodies. The strength of the residual portions was judged inadequate to support the strut grafts, and sufficient bone would not remain for adequate posterior segmental fixation.

A transperitoneal approach was made to perform corpectomies of L-4 and L-5, followed by placement of a strut graft fashioned from a fresh frozen distal femoral allograft from L-3 to the sacrum. The plan was to proceed with a same-day posterior procedure, but the anterior surgery was very long and prudence dictated staging the posterior reconstruction. Three days later the posterior L-3 to S-2 instrumented fusion was carried out with autogenous iliac crest bone graft and implantation of a bone growth stimulator **(C, D)**. The surgeries were followed by 6 weeks of parenteral amphotericin B while at strict bed rest in a nursing home. This was followed by an extended course of oral fluconazole. Subcutaneous injections of low-molecular-weight heparin supplemented the protection offered by the patient's prophylactic vena cava filter. Pneumatic compression devices were not practical given the size of her legs. At latest follow-up (2 years), her x-rays and CT scans demonstrated circumferential graft healing. Her infection has not recurred. Unfortunately, noteworthy pain complaints persist.

This case demonstrates several important points. First, a higher index of suspicion following the patient's failed initial surgeries may have allowed earlier detection of the infection. Additionally, the inadequate posterior débridement followed by an excessively long course of observation on oral antibiotics allowed the destructive process to continue. Had she been treated earlier in the disease process, it is likely that an anterior L4-5 débridement and grafting could have been performed, followed by a single segment posterior instrumentation and fusion. (From Ludwig SC, Kowalski JM, Heller JG. Post-operative spinal wound infections. In: Vaccaro AR, ed. *Masters' cases: spine surgery.* New York: Thieme Medical Publishers, 2000:220–228, with permission.)

up elimination of infection in all 19 patients in his series, with preservation of the hardware. Picada et al. (47) were able to achieve sterile wounds in 24 of 26 patients without removing their lumbar fixation. Wimmer et al. (71) achieved the same results in all of their 14 patients with internal fixation (71).

True late wound infections that occur once the wounds and fusions have long since healed represent a unique circumstance. It is unclear whether these infections are due to hematogenous seeding or late activa-tion of a hardware inoculation that occurred during implantation (20). In either case, these wound infections behave differently than acute infections, and their treatment must be adjusted accordingly. Most studies on delayed infection have found a high incidence of low-virulence pathogens such as diphtheroids, *Propionibacterium acnes*, and *Staphylococcus epidermidis* (59,68).

Operative cultures should be held for longer periods of time in these cases to allow slower-growing organisms to develop, and low-virulence organisms should not be dismissed as contaminants. Authors have also reported finding the instrumentation covered with a glycocalyx, consisting of an exopolysaccharide that inhibits host defenses. Most studies of late infections have demonstrated high cure rates with removal of the instrumentation as part of the treatment (50). Admittedly, none of these studies on delayed infection treated their patients with preservation of the hardware. In light of the fact that stability and achieving fusion are usually no longer an issue in late cases, we currently recommend removal of instrumentation for infections that present in a delayed manner. Additionally, several authors have reported high pseudarthrosis rates in the presence of delayed infections, including five of eight patients in the study by Viola et al. (68), and hardware removal facilitates exploration of the fusion mass. Symptomatic nonunions can usually await treatment until the infection has been eradicated.

Once the entire wound has been thoroughly irrigated and débrided, the issues of wound closure, drainage, and need for future operative débridements must be addressed. Primary closure of wounds is favored when possible. Although many studies have reported success with packing the wounds open, followed by delayed primary closure, initial closure over closed-suction drains reduces protein losses, lessens the risk of superinfection, and prevents local soft tissue retraction (11). A layered surgical closure lessens dead space. Some authors have reported success with suction irrigation systems for the first few postoperative days; however, the benefits of this labor-intensive method are unclear and somewhat controversial (15,66). We often recommend a routine second-look irrigation and débridement within 48 to 72 hours. An exception would be Thalgott's type I case, which has exhibited a good clinical response and is growing a relatively susceptible organism (65). Types II and III mandate a second débridement. At the second look a new set of cultures should be obtained and the wound carefully assessed. Patients should be returned for operative débridements at 48- to 72-hour intervals until operative cultures are negative, the wound appears healthy, and no additional necrotic material is encountered. Drains are typically left in place for 3 to 5 days after final débridement. Glassman et al. (18) reported good success with temporary placement of antibiotic impregnated polymethylmethacrylate beads in those cases in which significant dead space remains after débridement. Unfortunately, this strategy obliges the patient to an N+1 surgery for final bead removal.

Soft tissue coverage in the spine can be a problem in cases with extensive myonecrosis and in certain situa-

tions such as the multiply operated or irradiated spine. Muscle flaps have been found to be a valuable adjunct in managing complex spine wounds (27,33,61). Flap coverage facilitates wound healing by providing vascularized tissue to reduce dead space, enhance local oxygen delivery, and facilitate antibiotic delivery. The latissimus muscle has a dual blood supply that allows it to be medially or laterally based, rotated, advanced, or reversed as a turnover flap for coverage of complex thoracic or lumbar wounds. Trapezial flaps cause more disability than latissimus flaps, but the muscle can also be rotated, advanced, or turned over for use in cervical or thoracic cases. A technique in which bilateral paraspinal muscle flaps are elevated and advanced has been shown to be very effective in covering complex thoracic and lumbar wounds (41). Lower lumbar and sacral wounds may best be covered with a gluteal flap (56,69). Other proven options include omental or rectus abdominis flaps and the use of tissue expanders (17,45). Proper planning and implementation of these techniques are critical. We recommend early plastic surgical consultation in any case in which wound closure may be troublesome. One may be well advised to have a plastic surgeon inspect the wound at the initial débridement so that the need for a flap can be assessed and the appropriate options considered. This is especially true if the presence of vertebral osteomyelitis requires an anterior surgical procedure, as one would not wish to harm either a rectus abdominis or latissimus dorsi muscle that would otherwise have been a useful local flap.

Until now this discussion has essentially dealt with the management of posterior spinal wounds. However, not all infections occur after posterior operations. Fortunately, anterior spinal wound infections are less common, because repeated access to the anterior thoracic and lumbar regions is more problematic. If deep posterior lumbar wounds are difficult to recognize, the point warrants additional emphasis in regard to anterior infections. The treatment principles are the same, but one is advised to recruit the assistance of either a vascular or thoracic surgeon to assist with the exposure and débridement of the retroperitoneum or thoracic cavity. Due to the complexity of the exposure and its associated morbidity, one is a bit less likely to pursue repeated débridements. Fortunately, dead space and hypovascularity are less of a problem anteriorly.

Anterior surgery may also be indicated when a posterior wound infection has progressed to include vertebral osteomyelitis. This is usually appreciated on plain radiographs, especially when they are compared to ones made preoperatively. MRI is quite sensitive to intraosseous edema or inflammatory response but tends to overestimate the degree of osseous involvement. Reformatted CT scans are very useful in defining the degree of bone destruction and any cystic cavitation adjacent to the vertebral endplates and in defining the margin of reactive bone around the infection. These images are essential to planning the degree of anterior débridement and reconstruction that are required to eliminate the anterior component of the process (Fig. 4B).

Anterior fusions may also be the salvage procedure of choice when pursuing a fusion in the wake of a posterior infection. From the thoracic spine down to about L-4, one might be able to achieve a single stage anterior interbody fusion(s) and instrumentation as a stand-alone procedure. When doing so we recommend combining the mechanical strength of interbody allografts or cages with a liberal quantity of autogenous iliac bone because of the latter's osteogenic potential. Due to the limited bone available from the anterior ilium, it may be necessary to harvest the posterior iliac crest before making the anterior exposure.

Unfortunately, the reconstructive options are not quite as simple when the process extends to the lumbosacral junction (Fig. 4). As there is no reasonable anterior method of fixation that extends to the pelvis, the surgeon is usually relying on posterior methods of fixation in pursuit of an anterior fusion. This can be quite a challenge, but some advantages may be exploited. Generally speaking, the previous pedicle and alar screw holes can be reused. CT scans made after implant removal will determine their suitability. The trick is to have screws of proper dimensions available and to have polymethylmethacrylate available as a grout for the screws if the fit is not secure enough. Assuming that one has one iliac crest left to harvest, we suggest using it for the anterior fusion where the local environment is more favorable. Once stable posterior fixation is achieved and the infection is under control, the anterior débridement and reconstruction proceeds. This may be done as a single stage provided that the débridement is adequate. To be sure, the exposure will be hazardous, because the normal tissue planes have been obliterated by paravertebral inflammation. The skills of a vascular surgeon will be substantially challenged during the exposure. The tendency is not to débride enough. To avoid this trap, be sure the exposure and the débridement are extensive enough. As miserable as the experience can be, one only wants to have to do this once. Although there are no data to substantiate it, we recommend placing a prophylactic vena cava filter before such a sequence of procedures. This is especially true when

an anterior operation will involve considerable manipulation of the great vessels. As the patients who require these staged procedures are generally type III cases, and all too often obese diabetic patients, we sometimes have kept them at bed rest in a nursing home for 6 to 12 weeks before allowing them up for household ambulation. If they are better hosts with a body habitus that affords satisfactory bracing, we are more liberal with early household activity. Community activity and physical rehabilitation should await radiographic and CT evidence of graft healing, which is typically apparent within 6 months. All the while they should be monitored with serial CRP, ESR, and white blood cell count to ensure eradication of the infection. These values are followed for at least 6 months after all medical treatment has been stopped to monitor for any recrudescence of infection.

Once a stable wound environment has been achieved, patients should be continued on appropriate intravenous antibiotics for at least 6 weeks in cases of wound infections involving bone grafts or spinal implants, or both. Superficial wound infections, deep wound infections in the absence of bone grafts or implants (e.g., lumbar laminectomy for stenosis), and uncomplicated intervertebral diskitis can be treated for shorter periods of time based on the surgeon's judgment. Postoperative management should include aggressive treatment of any coexistent medical conditions. Malnutrition must be avoided and judicious use of nasal or percutaneous gastrostomy tubes or even hyperalimentation should be considered. An appropriate bed needs to be ordered based on the patient's condition. In patients with spinal cord injuries and those who are not being mobilized, an air-fluidized bed can minimize pressure and mechanical interference with wound healing. This may be especially true for patients who have been reconstructed with a muscle flap (56).

The effect of postoperative thoracic or lumbar wound infection on long-term outcome is not fully known. Calderone et al. (6) compared 15 patients with and without wound infections and found no difference in late outcome between the groups, but both groups in their study did poorly. Wound infections clearly increase the incidence of pseudarthrosis. In a series of more than 700 patients, 64 of whom sustained a wound infection, Lonstein et al. (38) found a pseudarthrosis rate of 29% among those with the infections. This was threefold greater than the overall nonunion rate for the entire study group (38). As noted earlier, late wound infections may be at risk for pseudarthroses, but the consequences of failed fusion in these patients is less clear, as is the need to pursue a union. Finally, the cost of treating postoperative thoracic and lumbar wound infections must be considered. As shown by Thalgott et al. (65), the need for additional surgeries, prolonged hospitalization, and intravenous antibiotics all combine to make these infections an extremely costly event. Calderone et al. (4) also found that a postoperative wound infection typically increased the cost of treatment by greater than fourfold. This can place an excessive burden on the health care industry and is further reason why continued efforts should be focused on prevention; thus, when encountered, this complication must be treated aggressively and definitively. The authors believe that lessons learned from earlier investigations can prepare spinal surgeons to reduce the risk of wound infections, diagnose them earlier, and treat them in a more considered and systematic fashion such that the overall physical and monetary cost to the patient will be reduced.

REFERENCES

1. Abbey DM, Turner DM, Warson JS, et al. Treatment of post-operative wound infections following spinal fusion with instrumentation. *J Spinal Disord* 1995;8(4):278–283.
2. Babu NV, Titus VT, Chittaranjan S, et al. Computed tomographically guided biopsy of the spine. *Spine* 1994; 19(21):2436–2442.
3. Benjamin JB, Volz RG. Efficacy of a topical antibiotic irrigant in decreasing or eliminating bacterial contamination in surgical wounds. *Clin Orthop* 1984;(184):114–117.
4. Calderone RR, Garland DE, Capen DA, et al. Cost of medical care for post-operative spinal infections. *Orthop Clin North Am* 1996:27(1):171–182.
5. Calderone RR, Larsen JM. Overview and classification of spinal infections. *Orthop Clin North Am* 1996;27(1):1–8.
6. Calderone RR, Thomas JC Jr, Haye W, et al. Outcome assessment in spinal infections. *Orthop Clin North Am* 1996;27(1):201–205.
7. Capen DA, Calderone RR, Green A. Perioperative risk factors for wound infections after lower back fusions. *Orthop Clin North Am* 1996;27(1):83–86.
8. Carragee EJ. Instrumentation of the infected and unstable spine: a review of 17 cases from the thoracic and lumbar spine with pyogenic infections. *J Spinal Disord* 1997;10(4):317–324.
9. Cruse PJ, Foord R. A five-year prospective study of 23,649 surgical wounds. *Arch Surg* 1973;107(2):206–210.
10. Currier BL, Heller JG, Eismont FJ. Cervical spinal infections. In: Clark CR, ed. *The cervical spine*. Philadelphia: Lippincott–Raven Publishers, 1998:659–690.
11. Dernbach PD, Gomez H, Hahn J. Primary closure of infected spinal wounds. *Neurosurgery* 1990;26(4):707–709.
12. Dietze DD Jr, Fessler RG, Jacob RP. Primary reconstruction for spinal infections. *J Neurosurg* 1997;86(6):981–989.
13. Faciszewski T, Winter RB, Lonstein JE, et al. The surgical and medical perioperative complications of anterior spinal fusion surgery in the thoracic and lumbar spine in adults. A review of 1223 procedures. *Spine* 1995;20(14):1592–1599.
14. Garfin S, Vaccaro A, eds. *Orthopaedic knowledge update: spine.* Rosemont, IL: American Academy of Orthopaedic Surgeons, 1997:267–270.
15. Garrido E, Rosenwasser RH. Experience with the suction-irrigation technique in the management of spinal epidural infection. *Neurosurgery* 1983;12(6):678–679.
16. Gepstein R, Eismont FJ. Post-operative spine infections. In: Garfin SR, ed. *Complications of spine surgery.* Baltimore: Williams & Wilkins, 1989:302–322.
17. Giordano PA, Griffet J, Argenson C. Pedicled greater omentum transferred to the spine in a case of post-operative infection. *Plast Reconstr Surg* 1994;93(7):1508–1511.
18. Glassman SD, Dimar JR, Puno RM, et al. Salvage of instrumental lumbar fusions complicated by surgical wound infection. *Spine* 1996;21(18):2163–2169.
19. Guiboux JP, Ahlgren B, Patti JE, et al. The role of prophylactic antibiotics in spinal instrumentation. A rabbit model. *Spine* 1998;23(6):653–656.
20. Heggeness MH, Esses SI, Errico T, et al. Late infection of spinal instrumentation by hematogenous seeding. *Spine* 1993;18(4):492–496.
21. Heller JG. Infections of the cervical spine. In: An HS, ed. *Surgery of the cervical spine.* London: Martin-Dunitz, 1994:335–356.
22. Heller JG. Spinal infections. In: Kasser JR, ed. *Orthopaedic knowledge update 5.* Chicago: American Academy of Orthopaedic Surgeons, 1996:643–656.
23. Heller JG, Garfin SR. Post-operative infection of the spine. *Semin Spine Surg* 1990;2(2):268–282.
24. Heller JG, Levine MJ. Post-operative infection of the spine. *Semin Spine Surg* 1996:8(2):105–114.
25. Heller JG, Massie BS, Abitbol JJ, et al. Post-operative spinal wound infection. *Clin Orthop* 1992;284:99–108.
26. Herkowitz H, ed. *Rothman-Simeone the spine*, 4th ed. Vol 2. Philadelphia: WB Saunders, 1999:1671.
27. Hochberg J, Ardenghy M, Yuen J, et al. Muscle and musculocutaneous flap coverage of exposed spinal fusion devices. *Plast Reconstr Surg* 1998;102(2):385–389; discussion, 390–392.
28. Hodges SD, Humphreys SC, Eck JC, et al. Low postoperative infection rates with instrumented lumbar fusion. *South Med J* 1998;91(12):1132–1136.
29. Hu SS, Fontaine F, Kelly B, et al. Nutritional depletion in staged spinal reconstructive surgery. Effect of total parenteral nutrition. *Spine* 1998;23(12):1401–1405.
30. Hueftle MG, Modic MT, Ross JS, et al. Lumbar spine: post-operative MR imaging with Gd-DTPA. *Radiology* 1988;167(3):817–824.

31. Klein JD, Garfin SR. Nutritional status in the patient with spinal infection. *Orthop Clin North Am* 1996;27(1):33–36.

32. Klein JD, Hey LA, Yu CS, et al. Perioperative nutrition and post-operative complications in patients undergoing spinal surgery. *Spine* 1996;21(22):2676–2682.

33. Klink BK, Thurman RT, Wittpenn GP, et al. Muscle flap closure for salvage of complex back wounds. *Spine* 1994;19(13):1467–1470.

34. Korge A, Fischer R, Kluger P, et al. The importance of sonography in the diagnosis of septic complications following spinal surgery. *Eur Spine J* 1994;3(6):303–307.

35. Levi AD, Dickman CA, Sonntag VK. Management of post-operative infections after spinal instrumentation. *J Neurosurg* 1997;86(6):975–980.

36. Levine MJ, Heller JG. Spinal infections. In: Garfin SR, Vaccaro AR, eds. *Orthopaedic knowledge update: spine.* Philadelphia: Lippincott–Raven Publishers, 1997:657–690.

37. Lindholm TS, Pylkkanen P. Discitis following removal of intervertebral disc. *Spine* 1982;7(6):618–622.

38. Lonstein J, Winter R, Moe J, et al. Wound infection with Harrington instrumentation and spine fusion for scoliosis. *Clin Orthop* 1973;96:222–233.

39. Lowell TD, Errico TJ, Eskenazi MS. Use of epidural steroids after discectomy may predispose to infection. *Spine* 2000;25(4):516–519.

40. Ludwig SC, Kowalski JM, Heller JG. Post-operative spinal wound infections. In: Vaccaro AR, ed. *Masters' cases: spine surgery.* New York: Thieme Medical Publishers, 2000;220–228.

41. Manstein ME, Manstein CH, Manstein G. Paraspinous muscle flaps. *Ann Plast Surg* 1998;40(5):458–462.

42. Massie JB, Heller JG, Abitbol JJ, et al. Post-operative posterior spinal wound infections. *Clin Orthop* 1992;284:99–108.

43. McPhee IB, Williams RP, Swanson CE. Factors influencing wound healing after surgery for metastatic disease of the spine. *Spine* 1998;23(6):726–732; discussion, 732–733.

44. Palestro CJ. Radionuclide imaging after skeletal interventional procedures. *Semin Nucl Med* 1995;25(1):3–14.

45. Paonessa KJ, Hostnik WJ, Zide BM. Use of tissue expanders for wound closure of spinal infections or dehiscence. *Orthop Clin North Am* 1996;27(1):155–170.

46. Perry JW, Montgomerie JZ, Swank S, et al. Wound infections following spinal fusion with posterior segmental spinal instrumentation. *Clin Infect Dis* 1997;24(4):558–561.

47. Picada R, Winter RB, Lonstein JE, et al. Post-operative deep wound infection in adults after posterior lumbosacral spine fusion with instrumentation: incidence and management. *J Spinal Disord* 2000;13(1):42–45.

48. Reiter MF, Heller JG. Spinal infections. In: Morris PJ, Wood WC, eds. *The Oxford textbook of surgery,* 2nd ed. Oxford: Oxford University Press, 2000:3127–3132.

49. Reuland P, Winker KH, Heuchert T, et al. Detection of infection in post-operative orthopedic patients with technetium-99m–labeled monoclonal antibodies against granulocytes. *J Nucl Med* 1991;32(12):2209–2214.

50. Richards BS. Delayed infections following posterior spinal instrumentation for the treatment of idiopathic scoliosis. *J Bone Joint Surg Am* 1995;77(4):524–529.

51. Riley LHR. Prophylactic antibiotics for spine surgery: description of a regimen and its rationale. *J South Orthop Assoc* 1998;7(3):212–217.

52. Rimoldi RL, Haye W. The use of antibiotics for wound prophylaxis in spinal surgery. *Orthop Clin North Am* 1996;27(1):47–52.

53. Rosahl SK, Gharabaghi A, Zink PM, et al. Monitoring of blood parameters following anterior cervical fusion. *J Neurosurg* 2000;92[2 Suppl]:169–174.

54. Rosenstein BD, Wilson FC, Funderburk CH. The use of bacitracin irrigation to prevent infection in post-operative skeletal wounds. An experimental study. *J Bone Joint Surg Am* 1989;71(3):427–430.

55. Ross JS, Masaryk TJ, Modic MT, et al. Lumbar spine: post-operative assessment with surface-coil MR imaging. *Radiology* 1987;164(3):851–860.

56. Rubayi S. Wound management in spinal infection. *Orthop Clin North Am* 1996;27(1):137–153.

57. Rubinstein E, Findler G, Amit P, et al. Perioperative prophylactic cephazolin in spinal surgery. A double-blind placebo-controlled trial. *J Bone Joint Surg Br* 1994;76(1):99–102.

58. Savitz SI, Savitz MH, Goldstein HB, et al. Topical irrigation with polymyxin and bacitracin for spinal surgery. *Surg Neurol* 1998;50(3):208–212.

59. Schofferman L, Zucherman J, Schofferman J, et al. Diphtheroids and associated infections as a cause of failed instrument stabilization procedures in the lumbar spine. *Spine* 1991;16(3):356–358.

60. Schulitz KP, Assheuer J. Discitis after procedures on the intervertebral disc. *Spine* 1994;19(10):1172–1177.

61. Shektman A, Granick MS, Solomon MP, et al. Management of infected laminectomy wounds. *Neurosurgery* 1994;35(2):307–309; discussion, 309.

62. Simpson JM, Silveri CP, Balderston RA, et al. The results of operations on the lumbar spine in patients who have diabetes mellitus. *J Bone Joint Surg Am* 1993;75(12):1823–1829.

63. Stambough JL, Beringer D. Post-operative wound infections complicating adult spine surgery. *J Spinal Disord* 1992;5(3):277–285.

64. Szoke G, Lipton G, Miller F, et al. Wound infection after spinal fusion in children with cerebral palsy. *J Pediatr Orthop* 1998;18(6):727–733.

65. Thalgott JS, Cotler HB, Sasso RC, et al. Post-operative infections in spinal implants. Classification and analysis—a multicenter study. *Spine* 1991;16(8):981–984.

66. Theiss SM, Lonstein JE, Winter RB. Wound infections in reconstructive spine surgery. *Orthop Clin North Am* 1996;27(1):105–110.

67. Thelander U, Larsson S. Quantitation of C-reactive protein levels and erythrocyte sedimentation rate after spinal surgery. *Spine* 1992;17(4):400–404.

68. Viola RW, King HA, Adler SM, et al. Delayed infection after elective spinal instrumentation and fusion. A retrospective analysis of eight cases. *Spine* 1997;22(20):2444–2450; discussion, 2450–2451.

69. Wendt JR, Gardner VO, White JI. Treatment of complex post-operative lumbosacral wounds in nonparalyzed patients. *Plast Reconstr Surg* 1998;101(5):1248–1253; discussion, 1254.

70. Whalen JL, Brown ML, McLeod R, et al. Limitations of indium leukocyte imaging for the diagnosis of spine infections. *Spine* 1991;16(2):193–197.

71. Wimmer C, Gluch H. Management of post-operative wound infection in posterior spinal fusion with instrumentation. *J Spinal Disord* 1996;9(6):505–508.

72. Wimmer C, Gluch H, Franzreb M, et al. Predisposing factors for infection in spine surgery: a survey of 850 spinal procedures. *J Spinal Disord* 1998;11(2):124–128.

MISCELLANEOUS POSTOPERATIVE COMPLICATIONS OF SPINAL SURGERY

GREGORY M. SASSMANNSHAUSEN, PERRY A. BALL, AND WILLIAM A. ABDU

DURAL TEARS, CEREBROSPINAL FLUID LEAKS, AND PSEUDOMENINGOCELE

Modern techniques of spinal instrumentation and an increased prevalence of high-energy spinal trauma have led to a corresponding increase in surgical intervention for patients who previously would not be considered surgical candidates. As the tools for spine surgery have become more powerful, the potential for injury to the patient also increases. With this comes an increased potential for complications, ranging from wound infections to hardware failure and nonunion. However, traumatic dural tears, incidental unintended durotomies, and subsequent cerebrospinal fluid (CSF) leaks are potential complications that the spine surgeon may cause or encounter, posing a significant challenge. Although generally straightforward to treat initially, the potentially devastating sequelae from mismanagement necessitate that the surgeon understands the prevention, diagnosis, and treatment of these complications early on.

INCIDENCE

The incidence of dural tears and CSF leaks following spine or neck surgery has been reported in many studies (1,15,18,30,32,54,58,61,62,72). However, the rate is probably underreported due to the lack of associated morbidity with most tears (32). Reported incidence of dural tears or CSF leaks after cervical spine surgery ranges from 0 to 25% (2,54,61,62,81,82). In a multicenter review of elective cervical diskectomy, the reported incidence of dural tears or CSF fistula was 0.03% of 10,416 cases (54). In reviewing eight large cervical spine surgery series, Keiper and Stambough (32) reported the combined incidence of dural laceration as 0.84%.

The reported incidence after lumbar spine surgery, which exceeds that of cervical spine surgery, ranges from 0.11% to as high as 13% (12,30,51,58,61,65).

Turner et al. (72) attempted a metaanalysis of 74 articles relevant to spinal stenosis surgery and reported that the mean incidence of dural laceration was 5.91%, with a maximum reported incidence of 27.27%.

Revision surgery proves to increase the incidence of dural injury. The frequency sharply rises with the extent of scarring and adhesions from successive procedures. The rate of CSF leaks in revision surgery is approximately 1 in 6 (78). Of 857 cases of spinal stenosis surgery over 20 years, Epstein and Epstein (15) reported a 4.6% incidence of CSF fistula at first operation and an increased incidence of 9.8% at second procedures.

In cases of thoracolumbar or lumbar fractures, the incidence again exceeds those secondary to elective cervical or lumbar surgery. Cammisa et al. (8) found dural tears in 37% of patients with a lumbar burst fracture. These patients all had a preoperative neurologic deficit and an associated laminar fracture. They reported that the presence of a preoperative neurologic deficit and an associated laminar fracture was a sensitive and specific predictor of dural laceration and entrapment of neural elements. Keenen et al. (31) also reported a 7.7% incidence of dural tears in surgically treated patients with burst fractures; this increased to 25% in lumbar burst fractures. These findings were supported by Hardaker et al. (23) in a series reporting a 15% incidence of dural lacerations after severe thoracolumbar burst fractures that required surgical stabilization.

ETIOLOGY

Although dural lacerations may result from direct trauma, the most common cause is iatrogenic during spinal surgery. Important factors that appear to be significant in leading to iatrogenic dural injuries involve the surgeon, the operative technique, and the patient population. These may include the experience of the surgeon and a failure to attend to the basic principles of modern surgery. The use of high-speed drills or placement of hooks, sublaminar wires, or pedicle screws has also been implicated in leading to an increased incidence (18,81). Previous spinal surgery increases the likelihood of developing dural injuries as well (15). Patients who undergo anterior cervical decompression due to ossification of the posterior longitudinal ligament and subsequent cervical myelopathy are at an increased risk of developing an iatrogenic dural tear caused by the potential absence of dura adjacent to the ossified part of the posterior longitudinal ligament (62,81).

Although less common, dural injuries may result from either direct or indirect trauma to the spine. Most leaks that result from indirect trauma to the dura or cord are not of consequence unless the patient undergoes a surgical procedure. However, if the patient undergoes a surgical procedure that unroofs the bony and ligamentous structures, the bone and soft tissue along with any blood clot removed may allow the leak to develop (40).

As previously mentioned, there is an association between burst fractures and concomitant dural lacerations. This is particularly true for lumbar burst fractures with involvement of the lamina and the presence of a neurologic deficit (8,31). In thoracolumbar burst fractures with incomplete neurologic deficits from retropulsed bone, canal impingement exceeding 50% results in at least 90% of such patients having dural tears (8). Therefore, in cases of thoracolumbar or lumbar fractures with a large amount of displacement, a dural tear must be considered a complicating factor of the injury and must be considered in the surgical approach if surgical treatment is indicated.

PREVENTION

The best and easiest way to manage complications is prevention. The surgeon must make adequate preoperative plans, particularly if pursuing reoperation or planned stabilization after trauma, as anatomy may be distorted or the dura may be thinned and scarred. While performing the procedure, the surgeon must hold to the basic principles of surgery, including adequate exposure, lighting, and identification of known structures. Care must be taken not to tear or pull tissues with instruments but rather to place the foot plate of the Kerrison perpendicular to the bone or soft tissue and to make a "clean cut" (40). An elevator can also be placed underneath bony edges to assess for the absence or presence of adhesions of the dura to adjacent structures. While the dura is exposed, it can be covered with a cottonoid or adequately retracted to

prevent inadvertent injury from instruments or pieces of bone. Extreme care must be taken when using the power drill. It should be used in the medial to lateral direction so that if slippage does occur, it is less likely to injure the underlying dura and cord (32).

In the case of reoperation, the dissection should begin from normal tissue and then proceed to the area of scar, as normal planes may be established and assist with identifying the dura and surrounding structures. By starting laterally at the facets and working medially, the lateral aspect of the canal may be identified along with the nerve roots, and any bony or ligamentous decompression can be carried out, thus increasing visualization. This is generally easier than starting medially and working laterally. The midline dorsal scar does not need to be removed from the dura or nerve roots unless it is tethering and causing traction (40).

In the preoperative planning stage, plain radiographs, computed tomography (CT) scans, and magnetic resonance imaging (MRI) scans must be carefully reviewed for the presence of spina bifida occulta, particularly in patients with spondylolisthesis. This can routinely be overlooked. However, an unfortunate slip through the bifid vertebra with a periosteal elevator, retractor, or osteotome may cause extensive damage to the dura, nerve root, or neural tissue (40). Careful attention to bony defects seen in preoperative imaging studies in those with prior surgery is also critical to prevent dural injury.

Local wound drains have been implicated as another potential source leading to CSF fistulae. The drain removes the blood present in the wound, which acts as a patch and also acts to tamponade the leak by increasing the pressure in the wound. The drain creates a tract from the wound to the skin after it is removed, which allows for the potential development of a dural-cutaneous fistula and possible sequelae (14,32,40). However, this tenet has been challenged by Wang et al. (76), who, in their study, used closed-suction drainage during wound closure, found that this did not increase the chance of developing a persistent spinal fluid leak, and concluded that a closed-drainage system can be used in the presence of a dural repair.

DIAGNOSIS

Diagnosis of a dural tear or CSF leak is easiest to make at the time of injury in the operating room and is usually obvious. Intraoperatively, clear fluid emanating from the wound must always raise the suspicion that there is dural injury with concomitant CSF leaking. Surgical intervention of a spinal burst fracture, particularly if a neurologic deficit exists, mandates that the surgeon closely evaluate the dura intraoperatively, as concomitant dural injury is likely. Recognition of the dural tear before wound closure is the single most important factor in reducing risk to the patient.

If the wound is not diagnosed in the operating room and is closed, symptoms may develop from the CSF leak. Classic symptoms include headache that worsens with standing and possible nausea, vomiting, and photophobia. Drainage of clear fluid from the wound should again raise suspicion. The CSF may be reabsorbed by the surrounding tissues and collect in the subcutaneous tissues; subsequently, a palpable mass and swelling around the wound may be seen and felt (1). Therefore, in a patient with symptoms of a dural tear, a careful physical examination looking for these signs must be performed.

If signs and symptoms are consistent with a CSF leak, imaging studies may assist with the diagnosis. MRI is the study of choice, with interest directed toward the surrounding soft tissues that demonstrate fluid excess of what would be expected after a surgical procedure (40). Other diagnostic studies include contrast myelography, which may show extravasation. Radioiodinated or technetium-labeled serum albumin scans, again looking for extravasation, have been described but are not routinely used (17,78).

TREATMENT

Because most dural tears are iatrogenic, most are discovered intraoperatively if careful assessment is undertaken. Once a leak is identified, further bony resection may be necessary to appreciate the location and extent of the tear. If discovered intraoperatively, it should be closed primarily if possible. The goal of closure is a watertight seal. All dural tears must be closed without compromising intraluminal diameter (40). Eismont et al. (14) have put forth six basic principles in dural tear closures:

1. The operative field must be unobstructed, dry, and well exposed.
2. Dural nonabsorbable suture of a 6-0 or 7-0 gauge with a tapered or reverse cutting needle is used in either a simple or running-locking stitch.
3. All repairs should be tested by using the reverse Trendelenburg's position and Valsalva maneuver.
4. Paraspinous muscles and overlying fascia should be closed in two layers with nonabsorbable suture used in a watertight fashion.

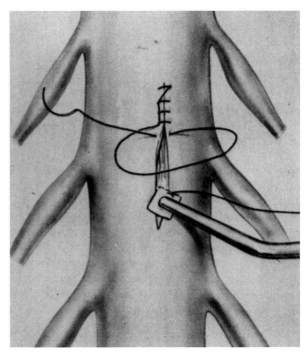

FIGURE 1. Dural repair using a running-locking dural suture on a reverse cutting needle. (From Eismont FJ, Wiesel SW, Rothman RH. The dural repair using a running-locking dural suture on a reverse cutting needle. *J Bone Joint Surg Am* 1981;63:1132–1136, with permission.)

5. Drains should not be used.
6. Bed rest in the supine position should be maintained for 72 to 96 hours after repair.

The interrupted or running stitch should be 1/16 in. from the edge of the dura on each side and approximately 1/8 in. apart (40) (Fig. 1). Care must be taken to be sure that a nerve root is not caught in the suture, making a benign complication into a serious problem (44). A piece of muscle or fat can be sewn over the dural repair in an attempt to increase the watertight closure (Fig. 2). If the seal still is not watertight, fibrin glue is applied, followed by another layer of fascia, and then a final layer of fibrin is placed on top to create a "fibrin sandwich" graft (59). These are again tested with a patient Valsalva or the reverse Trendelenburg's position.

Unfortunately, dural tears exist that are either too large or have macerated edges that do not allow for primary closure while maintaining adequate intraluminal diameter or place excessive pressure on the underlying neural tissue. This is often the case in trauma-related tears. In this circumstance, a patch graft of fascia lata or muscle tissue should be used for best closure. Because of reported cases of transmission of Creutzfeldt-Jakob disease by cadaveric grafts, allograft dura should be used only as a last resort (68,79). After initial anchoring stitches are applied, a

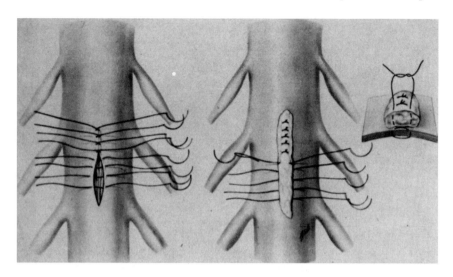

FIGURE 2. Muscle, fascia, or fat can be sewn over the dural tear to achieve a watertight closure. (From Eismont FJ, Wiesel SW, Rothman RH. The dural repair using a running-locking dural suture on a reverse cutting needle. *J Bone Joint Surg Am* 1981;63:1132–1136, with permission.)

simple technique with initial stitch placed from the graft to the dura is recommended (14) (Fig. 3).

When tears occur laterally along the nerve root or in areas that are not exposed secondary to the passage of wires for internal fixation, a small piece of muscle or Gelfoam can be used as a patch in the general area. Defects repaired with suture or muscle alone tend to leak at pressurization levels within the physiologic range, whereas those supplemented with tissue adhesives failed at higher pressurization rates (7). The addition of fibrin glue to the Gelfoam or muscle has

been shown to be a highly effective adjunctive means of assisting dural closure (7,59).

Lateral or ventral tears that are too large for simple patching or not amenable to suturing provide a difficult challenge. Mayfield and Korakawa (41) described a technique of repairing such tears. A median durotomy is made and a plug of fat is passed using a transdural approach placing the suture from central to lateral. The fat is then pulled through to create a seal (Fig. 4). If the dural tear is less than 2 to 3 mm long, the fat plug can be anchored nicely. If the tear is

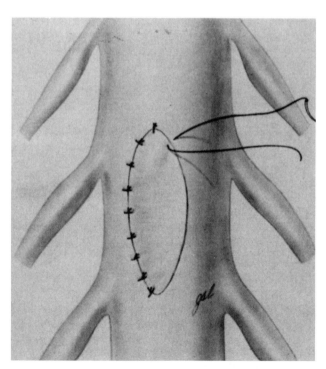

FIGURE 3. If dural material is inadequate to allow closure, a free fascia graft should be secured to the margins of the tear and possibly reinforced with fibrin glue. (From Eismont FJ, Wiesel SW, Rothman RH. The dural repair using a running-locking dural suture on a reverse cutting needle. *J Bone Joint Surg Am* 1981;63:1132–1136, with permission.)

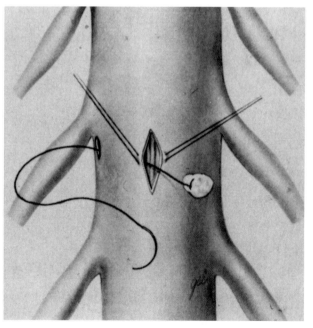

FIGURE 4. For dural tears that are inaccessible for direct primary closure, a transdural approach can be used to pull a small piece of fat or muscle into the defect through a median durotomy. The median durotomy is then closed in a standard fashion. (From Eismont FJ, Wiesel SW, Rothman RH. The dural repair using a running-locking dural suture on a reverse cutting needle. *J Bone Joint Surg Am* 1981;63:1132–1136, with permission.)

longer than 2 to 3 mm, the fat graft should be supported with one or two anchoring sutures (41).

If a leak is not seen intraoperatively but the signs and symptoms of a spinal fluid leak develop postoperatively, closed treatment consisting of complete bed rest with the head down at all times can be attempted. However, should this fail to stop the leak in 2 to 3 days and if imaging studies are consistent with a dural leak, surgical exploration of the wound with repair of the leak is indicated.

Unfortunately, CSF leaks exist that are not amenable to treatment or have failed attempted closure. In these circumstances and if the leak is above the L-2 level, a lumbar subarachnoid drain should be placed at the L-3, L-4, or L-5 level (32). The patient is kept on strict bed rest with continuous drainage, with a goal of 200 to 300 mL CSF drained every 24 hours (33), and prophylactic antibiotics should be started. After continuous drainage for 72 to 96 hours, the drain is clamped and the patient allowed to ambulate. The patient should be asked about symptoms of headaches, and careful examination of the wound for fluid accumulation is warranted. If any question about continued leak exists, the drain can be continued for a maximum of 7 days. At this point, the risk of catheter-induced infections begins to outweigh the benefit of the drain. One series revealed CSF fistula after spine surgery being cured by CSF drainage in 92% of cases with a 10% incidence of infection (60). Kitchell et al. (33) described using subarachnoid lumbar drains in cases of CSF fistula as a nonoperative alternative to surgical repair to be effective, with surgery reserved for those who have persistent leaks. The combined treatment protocol of an epidural blood patch and a 4-day course of spinal drainage was found to be highly effective, and with fewer complications than CSF diversion alone (42).

If leaks persist for longer than the 7 days for which a lumbar drain can be used, other forms of CSF diversion can be entertained. The placement of a temporary ventriculoperitoneal or lumboperitoneal shunt is a viable alternative that carries its own risks and sequelae.

COMPLICATIONS

Although dural tears may occasionally occur, it is the complications from such durotomies that are disconcerting. The trauma of unintended durotomy may lead to nerve root contusion, laceration, or even complete nerve section. In cases of surgically repaired durotomies without associated neural injury, the long-term outcomes show no increase in perioperative morbidity or compromise of final results and do not appear to increase the risk of postoperative infections, neural damage, or arachnoiditis (30,76). If dural tears are not repaired, the foremost risk of concern is the development of a chronic leaking fistula and increased risk of meningitis. Pseudomeningocele may form from the egress of CSF into the surrounding tissues, possibly involving nerve tissue and subsequent neurologic deficits.

Pseudomeningocele

Dural tears that go unrecognized or that are not properly treated can lead to the development of pseudomeningocele. The incidence of pseudomeningocele in lumbar spinal surgery has been estimated to be between 0.07% and 2.00% (22). Lumbar pseudomeningoceles are more common than cervical ones (57). Most pseudomeningoceles result as a complication from surgical treatment or spinal fractures (37,46–48,70); however, a report of traumatic pseudomeningocele formation occurring with spina bifida occulta has been described (29).

Although dural tears that leak relatively briskly are most likely to form CSF fistulae with wound breakdown, the leaks that occur slowly are likely to close spontaneously or form a pseudomeningocele. This false sac may subsequently entrap, in a ball-valve effect, either the spinal cord or the nerve roots, resulting in neurologic dysfunction or pain. In contrast to dural tears that lead to CSF fistulae, headache on standing is less common and less severe in pseudomeningocele. Rather, the patient may complain of recurrent back pain with or without radicular signs (78). The presence of persistent radiculopathy is a common complaint. A history of modest headache on standing, which is relieved by the recumbent position, and worsening or persistence of radiculopathy in a patient operated on for degenerative disease of the spine suggest the possibility of pseudomeningocele (40). The onset of symptoms ranges as a spectrum of insidious to acute deficits that present days to years after surgical intervention.

If the diagnosis of pseudomeningocele is suspected by history and physical examination, diagnosis is readily confirmed by MRI or CT (18,31,36) (Fig. 5). If the pseudomeningocele is diagnosed, surgical exploration with primary closure of the underlying dural defect is the treatment of choice. The repair techniques are similar to those previously described. Care must be taken to identify the nerve roots or nerve tissue involved in the pseudomeningocele and to locate

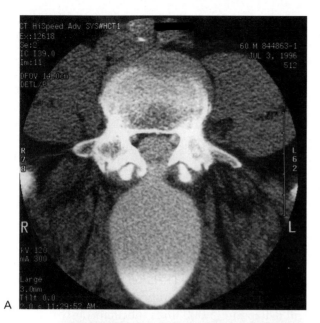

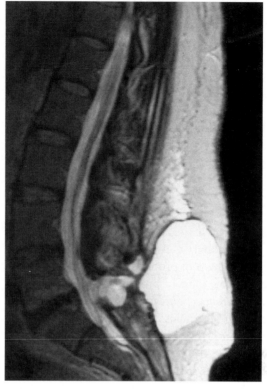

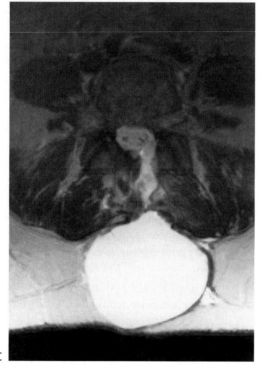

FIGURE 5. Examples of postoperative pseudomeningoceles. **A:** Contrast-enhanced computed tomography scan of a pseudomeningocele developed remotely following an L4-5 disk excision where a small incidental durotomy occurred. Despite satisfactory repair, pseudomeningocele developed. T2-weighted sagittal **(B)** and axial **(C)** magnetic resonance image (MRI) of pseudomeningocele 4 weeks postoperatively after uneventful L-5 to S-1 disk excision. This pseudomeningocele resolved spontaneously shortly after MRI was obtained. The patient remained asymptomatic during the entire postoperative course except for the presence of a fluctuant mass at the surgical site.

them properly within the dural sac. Reports using CSF drainage with or without blood patch have proven good results as a nonsurgical option (42,60). However, surgical repair should remain the primary treatment option, with CSF diversion being used for patients who are not surgical candidates.

Thromboembolic Disease

Incidence and Risk Factors

Well-accepted risk factors for the development of thromboembolic disease (TED) include advancing age, increased length of operation, presence of heart failure, history of a previous episode of TED, malignancy, and limb weakness (66). The presence of a family history of deep vein thrombosis (DVT) suggests the possibility of a hereditary hypercoagulable state such as antithrombin III deficiency or protein C or S deficiencies.

Although certain operations, such as hip arthroplasty, are known to be associated with a high risk of TED, the risk of this complication during elective spinal surgery without prophylaxis is less clear. Using radiolabeled iodine fibrinogen scanning to detect DVT, rates greater than 40% have been reported

(3,28,74). Interpretation of this is difficult because this method is unfortunately relatively nonspecific for distinguishing between deep and superficial thrombosis and may be insensitive for the detection of iliac thrombosis.

Patients with acute spinal cord injuries, however, are clearly a particularly high-risk group for the development of TED. Yelnik et al. (80), in a study of 127 spinal cord–injured patients, noted DVT by venography in 23%.

Prophylaxis

It has been estimated that the cost of diagnosis and treatment of pulmonary embolism (PE) is between 10 and 100 times the cost of prophylaxis (55), and, therefore, there is a clear logic to prophylaxis. The options for prophylaxis are mechanical methods, such as compression stockings, or the use of anticoagulants.

Mechanical prophylaxis has been shown to be effective in preventing DVT and has the advantage of being essentially risk free. The mechanism of action of mechanical devices probably involves prevention of venous stasis and promotion of thrombolysis (26). Ferree (16) studied 60 consecutive patients undergoing lumbar laminectomy with pre- and postoperative ultrasound examinations. The sole method of prophylaxis used was compression stockings. No PEs were present; calf vein thrombosis, which did not propagate proximally on serial ultrasound examinations, was detected in three patients (representing 5% of the total) (16). No patients, therefore, ultimately required anticoagulation. Similar results were noted by Smith et al. (63), who used compression stockings in combination with pneumatic compression stockings in a series of 317 patients undergoing a variety of complex spinal surgeries, with almost half the patients undergoing combined anterior and posterior procedures. A random group of 126 of these patients underwent ultrasound examination postoperatively, and no DVTs were noted; in one of these patients, a clinically evident DVT subsequently developed (63). Reasonable conclusions that can be drawn from these studies are that for the substantial majority of patients undergoing spinal surgery, including complex procedures, mechanical methods of prophylaxis are sufficient and that routine screening of postoperative patients is likely to have a low yield.

The use of anticoagulation should be considered in especially high-risk patient populations. Heparin is heterogeneous mucopolysaccharide isolated from bovine and porcine sources. It exerts its anticoagulant effect by binding to and accelerating the activity of antithrombin III, which, in turn, principally inhibits the action of clotting factor Xa. When used to prevent thrombus, heparin can be given in a fixed dose of 5,000 units subcutaneously twice a day or with a dose adjusted to increase the partial thromboplastin time (PTT) to 1.5 times the patient's baseline. A risk of bleeding is present, but heparin prophylaxis has been used safely for spinal surgery (4).

Low-molecular-weight heparins are produced by degradation of standard heparin. These agents also associate with antithrombin III to inhibit factor Xa and are effective prophylaxis for DVT. They exhibit less binding to plasma proteins than standard heparin and thus have a more predictable bioavailability and longer half-life. The administration of these agents does not alter the PTT. Among the agents available are enoxaparin (30 mg subcutaneously twice a day) and dalteparin (5,000 units subcutaneously per day).

As mentioned previously, patients with acute spinal cord injuries are an especially high-risk group for TED. Mechanical methods of prophylaxis alone do not appear to be adequate in this group of patients (21), although they can certainly be used to supplement other modalities. Low-dose standard heparin (5,000 units twice a day) also does not appear to provide adequate prophylaxis (45). Green et al. (20) used adjusted-dose standard heparin to prolong the PTT to 1.5 times control using an average of 13,200 units twice a day and found that this was effective, but bleeding complications developed in one-fourth of these patients. Low-molecular-weight heparin appears to be safe and effective in this group of individuals. Harris et al. (24) used enoxaparin, 30 mg every 12 hours, in a series of 105 patients with spinal injuries and noted no DVTs or PEs and a low rate of bleeding (24).

Prophylaxis can be stopped in those patients who regain sufficient strength to ambulate. The optimum duration of prophylaxis in patients who remain nonambulatory has not been clearly established, but 3 months is the usual recommendation (19).

Diagnosis

The diagnosis of DVT cannot be made by clinical examination alone. The classic signs and symptoms of leg pain, swelling, and Homan's sign have been shown to be remarkably unreliable for establishing or excluding the diagnosis (43), and confirmatory studies, therefore, are necessary.

The diagnosis can be reliably established with venography, and this was the mainstay of diagnosis for years. This invasive technique, however, involves the risk of exposure to radiation and contrast agents.

In recent years, the development of compression B-mode ultrasound has largely replaced venography. This technique uses pressure applied to the vessel wall during ultrasound examination; if clot is present, the vessel wall is prevented from collapse. It has been shown to have a sensitivity of greater than 90% and a specificity of 99% (3,10). Perhaps most significant is the study by Vaccaro et al. (73), which looked at patients whose ultrasound examination was negative and who were not treated and in whom PE did not develop. One can reasonably conclude that a normal compression B-mode ultrasound examination of good quality effectively excludes the diagnosis of DVT.

The diagnosis of PE remains one of the most vexing in clinical medicine. The potential consequences of missing the diagnosis are significant: The risk of death from recurrent PE in the absence of treatment may be as high as 25% (4). Unfortunately, the presenting symptoms are quite nonspecific, and there is no simple, safe, inexpensive confirmatory test. Autopsy studies have shown that between 60% and 80% of patients who die of PE were not suspected of having the condition (56), and yet in those patients suspected of having a PE, only one-third actually do (49,55).

The first steps in the evaluation of the patient suspected of having a PE are to obtain a chest radiograph, electrocardiogram, and arterial blood gas sample. The chest radiograph can exclude entities such as pneumonia, pneumothorax, or pleural effusion. The electrocardiogram can identify myocardial ischemia and may show evidence of right heart strain. The arterial blood gas is usually abnormal in the presence of PE: If the alveolar-arterial gradient of oxygen is normal and the carbon dioxide pressure is greater than 36 torr, the likelihood of PE is remote (11).

Pulmonary angiography can establish or exclude the diagnosis of PE with a high degree of reliability. This expensive and invasive procedure, however, carries the small but definite risk of arrhythmia, adverse reaction to contrast dye, and renal failure. The mortality from this procedure is approximately 0.3%, with a nonfatal complication rate of about 6% (64). Because of this and the fact that such a minority of patients who are suspected of having had a PE actually have had one, pulmonary angiography is generally not used as the first confirmatory test. If, however, clinical suspicion of PE remains after other tests, pulmonary angiography should be obtained.

Because most PEs originate from DVTs in the lower extremities, one strategy is to perform ultrasound examination of the lower extremities. If a DVT is detected, the treatment is the same as for PE. Unfor-

tunately, in greater than one-fourth of patients with documented PE, there is no evidence of DVT in the lower extremities (27). In most cases, this presumably reflects embolization of the entire clot. A negative lower-extremity ultrasound examination does not, therefore, exclude the diagnosis of PE.

Ventilation/perfusion ($\dot{V}/\dot{Q}$) scans are widely used for the diagnosis of PE but can be a source of confusion. These studies are reported as high probability, intermediate probability, low probability, and normal. The Prospective Investigation of Pulmonary Embolism Diagnosis (PIOPED) study (49) was a prospective study of more than 900 patients suspected of having sustained a PE that correlated clinical suspicion with subsequent imaging studies. The prior probability of PE was estimated on clinical grounds as high (>80%), intermediate (20–79%), and low (<20%). The patients then underwent $\dot{V}/\dot{Q}$ scanning and pulmonary angiography. The results are displayed in Table 1. A normal scan usually excludes the diagnosis. A high-probability scan, in the presence of high or intermediate clinical suspicion, is usually diagnostic of PE. If the clinical suspicion is low and the scan is low probability, it is unlikely that the patient has had a PE. An intermediate-probability scan with any level of suspicion or a low-probability scan associated with high or intermediate clinical suspicion does not exclude the diagnosis, and pulmonary angiography should be considered.

In recent years, there has been interest in spiral-CT for the diagnosis of PE. This has shown promise in identification of emboli located up to the level of the segmental pulmonary arteries (52). Identification of emboli in the subsegmental branches has been less reliable (35,75), and the place of this technique in the overall diagnostic algorithm for PE is uncertain. With refinement in technique and additional experi-

TABLE 1. LIKELIHOOD OF ANGIOGRAPHY-PROVEN PULMONARY EMBOLISM BASED ON CLINICAL SUSPICION AND VENTILATION/PERFUSION ($\dot{V}/\dot{Q}$) SCAN RESULTS

$\dot{V}/\dot{Q}$ scan interpretation category	Clinical suspicion of pulmonary embolism		
	High	Intermediate	Low
High	96%	88%	56%
Intermediate	66%	28%	16%
Low	40%	16%	4%
Normal	0	6%	2%

From The PIOPED Investigators. Value of the ventilation/perfusion scan in acute pulmonary embolism: results of the Prospective Investigation of Pulmonary Embolism Diagnosis (PIOPED). *JAMA* 1990;263:2753–2759, with permission.

ence, it may be an alternate to $\dot{V}/\dot{Q}$ scanning in many situations.

Treatment

The goal of treatment of TED is to prevent PE. The risk of untreated DVT progressing to PE in the absence of treatment has been reported to be as high as 75% (67). DVT above the calf should be treated with anticoagulation. Heparin, followed by oral warfarin, is effective at preventing death from PE (5). The usual practice is to start heparin with a bolus injection of 5,000 units followed by 1,000 units per hour over the next 24 hours (69). The dose is adjusted to keep the PTT 1.5 to 2.5 times the patient's baseline level. Oral warfarin can be started at the same time and continued for a minimum of 3 months (34). When the international normalized ratio is between 2.0 and 3.0, the heparin can be stopped. This usually requires about 5 days of intravenous heparin. The principal complications of heparin are bleeding and thrombocytopenia. The period of time following spinal surgery that anticoagulation can be safely begun must be determined on an individual basis. Because heparin has a short half-life of approximately 1 hour, minor bleeding can be handled by stopping the infusion. In situations of life-threatening hemorrhage, reversal of heparin activity can be accomplished with protamine sulfate. The development of thrombocytopenia occurs in up to 15% of patients who receive heparin and is due to the development of antibodies that bind to platelets. This becomes apparent by falling platelet counts, usually between 3 and 15 days of treatment, and, therefore, monitoring platelet counts is important during the initiation of therapy. It is usually reversible by stopping the heparin.

Low-molecular-weight heparin (enoxaparin, 1 mg/kg subcutaneously twice a day) has been used instead of standard heparin for the initial treatment of TED and appears to be safe and effective (34,38). The advantages of this are that it does not require monitoring of the PTT, there is less risk of thrombocytopenia, and treatment can potentially be done on an outpatient basis. One drawback is that protamine sulfate is less effective at reversing life-threatening hemorrhage when low-molecular-weight heparins are used. For patients who cannot tolerate anticoagulation or have a serious complication or contraindication to anticoagulation, vena caval interruption devices, such as the Greenfield filter, are an alternative for prevention of fatal PE.

Delirium

Delirium, an acute deterioration in global cognitive function, is surprisingly common in hospitalized elderly patients. Studies have identified it to occur in 15% to 40% of hospitalized patients older than 65 years of age (50,77). It is, however, often underrecognized (53). Identified risk factors for the development of this syndrome include increasing age, preexisting cognitive deficits, and a history of alcohol abuse (39,50,77).

The diagnostic criteria for this condition are delineated in the *Diagnostic and Statistical Manual of Mental Disorders, Fourth Edition* (*DSM-IV*) (13), and these are listed in Table 2. The symptoms often first become apparent at night and clear during the daytime, and there is a consequent disturbance in the sleep-wake cycle. The patient is usually confused and disoriented and often has some degree of agitation and impulsiveness.

The syndrome is potentially reversible, but it is an ominous development. Studies have demonstrated that patients who experience delirium have longer length of stay, higher in-hospital and 1-month mortality, and higher rates of nursing home placement when compared to patients without this complication (9,50). A metaanalysis demonstrated that only approximately half of patients had returned to their cognitive baseline at 1 month (9).

Treatment

As part of the diagnostic evaluation, a careful physical examination is warranted. The presence of any new lateralizing neurologic signs should raise the question of stroke, and a CT scan of the head should

---

TABLE 2. DIAGNOSTIC CRITERIA FOR DELIRIUM

Disturbance of consciousness (i.e., reduced clarity of awareness of the environment) with reduced ability to focus, sustain, or shift attention

A change in cognition (such as memory deficit, disorientation, language disturbance) or the development of a perceptual disturbance that is not better accounted for by a preexisting, established, or evolving dementia

The disturbance develops over a short period of time (usually hours to days) and tends to fluctuate during the course of the day

Evidence is shown from the history, physical examination, or laboratory findings that the disturbance is caused by the direct physiologic consequences of a general medical condition

From *Diagnostic and Statistical Manual of Mental Disorders, 4th ed. (DSM-IV)*. Washington, DC: American Psychiatric Association, 1994.

be obtained. Infection can precipitate delirium, and common sources of potential nosocomial infection should be excluded, such as the wound, urinary tract, and respiratory system. Meningitis should be considered in patients who have had a CSF leak or undergone intradural procedures.

Laboratory studies can be helpful and should include a complete blood count, urinalysis, electrolytes, glucose, blood urea nitrogen, and creatinine. Arterial blood gas analysis to exclude hypoxia should be done; pulse oximetry is a noninvasive alternative. Medications that are administered should be reviewed and consideration given to discontinuation of any agents that are nonessential, especially those with anticholinergic properties (39).

Once infectious or other clearly organic causes have been excluded, treatment is largely supportive. Careful nursing care with frequent reorientation can be invaluable (71). The goal in treating agitation should be to prevent the patient from injury; this is usually best accomplished with careful use of haloperidol (39).

REFERENCES

1. Agrillo U, Simonetti G, Martino V. Postoperative cerebrospinal fluid problems after lumbar surgery. *J Neurosurg Science* 1991;35:93–95.
2. Anderson PA, Bohlman HH. Anterior decompression and arthrodesis of the cervical spine: long-term motor impingement. *J Bone Joint Surg Am* 1992;74:683–691.
3. Appelman PT, Dejong TE, Lampmann LE. Deep venous thrombosis of the leg: US findings. *Radiology* 1987;163:743–746.
4. Barnett HG, Clifford JR, Lewellyan RC. Safety of mini-dose heparin administration for neurosurgical patients. *J Neurosurg* 1977;47:27–30.
5. Barritt DW, Jordan SC. Anticoagulant drugs in the treatment of pulmonary embolism: a controlled clinical trial. *Lancet* 1960;1:1309–1312.
6. Reference deleted.
7. Cain JE, Dryer RF, Barton BR. Evaluation of dural closure technique: suture methods, fibrin adhesive sealant, and cyanoacrylate polymer. *Spine* 1988;13:720–724.
8. Cammisa FP, Eismont FJ, Green BA. Dural laceration occurring with burst fractures and associated laminar fractures. *J Bone Joint Surg Am* 1989;71:1044–1051.
9. Cole MG, Primeau FJ. Prognosis of delirium in elderly hospital patients. *Can Med Assoc J* 1993;149:41–46.
10. Cronan JJ, Dorfman GS. Lower extremity deep venous thrombosis: further experience with and refinement of US assessment. *Radiology* 1988;168:101–107.
11. Cvitanic O, Marion PL. Improved use of arterial blood gas analysis in suspected pulmonary embolism. *Chest* 1989;95:48–51.
12. Deyo RA, Cherkin DC, Loeser JD, et al. Morbidity and mortality in association with operations on the lumbar spine. The influence of age, diagnosis, and procedure. *J Bone Joint Surg Am* 1992;74:536–543.
13. *Diagnostic and Statistical Manual of Mental Disorders, 4th ed. (DSM-IV)*. Washington, DC: American Psychiatric Association, 1994.
14. Eismont FJ, Wiesel SW, Rothman RH. Treatment of dural tears associated with spinal surgery. *J Bone Joint Surg Am* 1981;63:1132–1136.
15. Epstein NE, Epstein JE. Lumbar decompression for spinal stenosis. Surgical indications and techniques with and without fusion. In: Frymoyer JW, ed. *The adult spine: principles and practice.* Philadelphia: Lippincott–Raven Publishers, 1997:2082.
16. Ferree BA. Deep venous thrombosis following lumbar laminotomy and laminectomy. *Orthopedics* 1994;17:35–38.
17. Goldberg EJ, Andersson GBJ. Dural tears in lumbar spine surgery. In: Andersson GBJ, McNeill TW. *Lumbar spinal stenosis.* Chicago: Mosby–Year Book, 1992:415.
18. Graham JJ. Complications of cervical spine surgery. *Spine* 1989;14:1046–1050.
19. Green D, Hull RD, Mammen EF, et al. Deep vein thrombosis in spinal cord injury. *Chest* 1992;102:633S–635S.
20. Green D, Lee MY, Ito VY, et al. Fixed VS adjusted dose heparin with the prophylaxis of thromboembolism in spinal cord injury. *JAMA* 1988;260:1255–1258.
21. Green D, Rossi EC, Yao JST, et al. Deep venous thrombosis in spinal cord injury: effect of prophylaxis with calf compression, aspirin and dipyridamole. *Paraplegia* 1982;20:227–234.
22. Hadani FG, Knoler N, Tadmor R. Entrapped lumbar nerve root in pseudomeningocele after laminectomy: report of three cases. *Neurosurgery* 1986;19:405–407.
23. Hardaker WT Jr, Cook WA Jr, Friedman AH, et al. Bilateral transpedicular decompression and Harrington rod stabilization in the management of severe thoracolumbar burst fractures. *Spine* 1992;17:167–171.
24. Harris S, Chen D, Green D. Enoxaparin for thromboembolism prophylaxis in spinal injury: preliminary report on experience with 105 patients. *Am J Phys Med Rehabil* 1996;75:326–327.
25. Reference deleted.
26. Hull RD. Venous thromboembolism in spinal cord injury patients. *Chest* 1992;102:658S–663S.
27. Hull RD, Hirsh J, Carter CJ, et al. Pulmonary angiography, ventilation scanning and venography for clinically suspected pulmonary embolism with abnormal perfusion lung scan. *Ann Intern Med* 1983;98:891–899.
28. Joffe SN. Incidence of postoperative deep venous

thrombosis in neurosurgical patients. *J Neurosurg* 1975; 42:201–203.

29. Johnson JP, Lane JM. Traumatic lumbar pseudomeningocele occurring with spina bifida occulta. *J Spinal Disord* 1998;11:80–83.

30. Jones AM, Stambough JL, Balderston RA, et al. Long term results of lumbar spine surgery complicated with unintended incidental durotomy. *Spine* 1989;14:443–446.

31. Keenen TL, Antony J, Benson DR. Dural tears associated with lumbar burst fractures. *J Orthop Trauma* 1990;4:243–245.

32. Keiper G, Stambough JL. Complications of cervical spine surgery: dural tears and cerebrospinal fluid leaks. In: Clark CR, ed. *The cervical spine.* Philadelphia: Lippincott–Raven Publishers, 1998:899–901.

33. Kitchell SH, Eismont FJ, Green BA. Closed subarachnoid drainage for the management of cerebrospinal fluid leakage after an operation on the spine. *J Bone Joint Surg Am* 1989;71:984–987.

34. Koopman MMW, Buller HR. Low molecular-weight heparins in the treatment of venous thromboembolism. *Ann Intern Med* 1998;128:1037–1039.

35. Kuzo RS, Goodman LR. CT evaluation of pulmonary embolism: technique and interpretation. *AJR Am J Roentgenol* 1997;109:959–965.

36. Laffey PA, Kricun ME. Sonographic recognition of postoperative meningocele. *AJR Am J Roentgenol* 1984; 143:177–178.

37. Lee KS, Hardy IM. Post laminectomy lumbar pseudomeningocele: report of four cases. *Neurosurgery* 1992; 30:111–114.

38. Levine MN, Gent M, Hirsh J, et al. A comparison of low-molecular-weight heparin administered primarily at home with unfractionated heparin administered in the hospital for proximal deep-vein thrombosis. *N Engl J Med* 1996;334:677–681.

39. Lipowski ZJ. Update on delirium. *Psychiatr Clin North Am* 1992;15:335–346.

40. Marshall LF. Cerebrospinal fluid leaks: etiology and repair. In: Rothman RH, Simeone FA, eds. *The spine.* Philadelphia: WB Saunders, 1992;1892–1899.

41. Mayfield FH, Korakawa K. Watertight closure of spinal dura mater. Technical note. *J Neurosurg* 1975;143:639–640.

42. McCormack BM, Wassmann H, Polinski C. Pseudomeningocele/CSF fistula in a patient with lumbar spinal implants treated with epidural blood patch and a brief course of closed subarachnoid drainage. A case report. *Spine* 1996;21:2273–2276.

43. McLachlin J, Richards T, Paterson. An evaluation of clinical signs in the diagnosis of venous thrombosis. *Arch Surg* 1962;85:738–744.

44. McNeill TW, Andersson GBJ. Complications of degenerative lumbar spine surgery. In: Bridwell KH, DeWald RL, eds. *The textbook of spinal surgery.* Philadelphia: Lippincott–Raven Publishers, 1997:1672.

45. Merli GJ, Herbison GJ, Ditunno JF, et al. Deep vein thrombosis: prophylaxis in acute spinal cord injured patients. *Arch Phys Med Rehabil* 1988;69:661–664.

46. Miller PR, Elder FW Jr. Meningeal pseudocysts (meningocele spurious) following laminectomy. *J Bone Joint Surg* 1968;50A:268–276.

47. Nairus JG, Richman JD, Douglas RA. Retroperitoneal pseudomeningocele complicated by meningitis following a lumbar burst fracture. A case report. *Spine* 1996; 21:1090–1093.

48. O'Connor D, Maskery N, Griffiths WE. Pseudomeningocele nerve root entrapment after lumbar discectomy. *Spine* 1998;23:1501–1502.

49. The PIOPED Investigators. Value of the ventilation/perfusion scan in acute pulmonary embolism: results of the Prospective Investigation of Pulmonary Embolism Diagnosis (PIOPED). *JAMA* 1990;263:2753–2759.

50. Pompei P, Foreman M, Rudberg MA, et al. Delirium in hospitalized older persons: outcomes and predictors. *J Am Geriatr Soc* 1994;42:809–815.

51. Ramirez LF, Thisted R. Complications and demographic characteristics of patients undergoing lumbar discectomy in community hospitals. *Neurosurgery* 1989;25:226–230; discussion, 230–231.

52. Remy-Jardin M, Remy J, Deschilde F, et al. Diagnosis of pulmonary embolism with spiral CT: comparison with pulmonary angiography and scintigraphy. *Radiology* 1996;200:699–706.

53. Rockwood K, Cosway S, Stolee P, et al. Increasing the recognition of delirium in elderly patients. *J Am Geriatr Soc* 1994;42252–42256.

54. Romano PS, Campa DR, Rainwater JA. Elective cervical discectomy in California: postoperative in-hospital complications and their risk factors. *Spine* 1997;22:2677–2692.

55. Rosenow EC. Venous and pulmonary thromboembolism: an algorithmic approach to diagnosis and management. *Mayo Clin Proc* 1995;70:45–49.

56. Ryu JH, Olson EJ, Pellikka PA. Clinical recognition of pulmonary embolism: problem of unrecognized and asymptomatic cases. *Mayo Clin Proc* 1998;73:873–879.

57. Schumacher HW, Wassmann H, Polinski C. Pseudomeningocele of the lumbar spine. *Surg Neurol* 1988;29:77–78.

58. Schwab FJ, Nazarian DG, Mahmud F, et al. Effects of spinal instrumentation on fusion of the lumbosacral spine. *Spine* 1995;20:2023–2028.

59. Shaffrey CI, Spotnitz WD, Shaffrey ME, et al. Neurosurgical applications of fibrin glue: augmentation of dural closure in 134 patients. *Neurosurgery* 1990;26:207–210.

60. Shapiro SA, Scully T. Closed continuous drainage of cerebrospinal fluid via a lumbar subarachnoid catheter for treatment or prevention of cranial/spinal cerebrospinal fluid fistula. *Neurosurgery* 1992;30:241–245.

61. Shapiro SA, Snyder W. Spinal instrumentation with a low complication rate. *Surg Neurol* 1997;48:566–574.

62. Smith MD, Bolesta MJ, Leventhal M, et al. Postoperative cerebrospinal fluid fistula associated with erosion of the dura. *J Bone Joint Surg Am* 1992;74:270–277.

63. Smith MD, Bressler EL, Lonstein JE, et al. Deep venous

thrombosis and pulmonary embolism after major reconstructive operations on the spine: a prospective analysis of three hundred and seventeen patients. *J Bone Joint Surg* 1994;76-A:980–985.

64. Sostman HD, Newman GE. Evaluation of the patient with suspected pulmonary embolism. In: Strandness DE, van Breda A, eds. *Vascular diseases.* New York: Churchill Livingstone, 1994.

65. Spangfort EV. The lumbar disc herniation. A computer-aided analysis of 2,504 operations. *Acta Orthop Scand* 1972;142[Suppl]:1–95.

66. Swann KW, Black PM. Deep venous thrombosis and pulmonary embolism in neurosurgical patients: a review. *J Neurosurg* 1984;61:1055–1062.

67. Swann KW, Black PM, Baker MF. Management of symptomatic deep venous thrombosis and pulmonary embolism on a neurosurgical service. *J Neurosurg* 1986; 64:563–567.

68. Takayama S, Hatsuda N, Matsumura K, et al. Creutzfeldt-Jakob disease transmitted by cadaveric dural graft: a case report. *Neurol Surg* 1993;21:167–170.

69. Taylor DC, Nantel SH. Anticoagulant therapy for acute deep venous thrombosis and pulmonary embolism. In: Strandness DE, Van Breda A, eds. *Vascular diseases.* New York: Churchill Livingstone, 1994.

70. Toppich HG, Feldmann H, Sandvoss G, et al. Intervertebral space nerve root entrapment after lumbar disc surgery. *Spine* 1994;19:249–250.

71. Trockman G. Caring for the confused or delirious patient. *Am J Nursing* 1978;78:1495–1499.

72. Turner JA, Jersek M, Herron L, et al. Surgery for lumbar stenosis: an attempted meta-analysis of the literature. *Spine* 1992;17:1–8.

73. Vaccaro JP, Cronan JJ, Dorfman GS. Outcome analysis of patients with normal compression US examinations. *Radiology* 1990;175:645–649.

74. Valladares J, Hankinson J. Incidence of lower extremity deep venous thrombosis in neurosurgical patients. *Neurosurgery* 1980;6:138–141.

75. Van Russum AB, Pattynama PMT, Ton ERTA, et al. Pulmonary embolism: validation of spiral CT angiography in 149 patients. *Radiology* 1996;210:467–470.

76. Wang JC, Riew DK, Bohlman HH. Dural tears secondary to operations on the lumbar spine. Management and results after a two-year-minimum follow-up of eighty-eight patients. *J Bone Joint Surg Am* 1998;80:1728–1732.

77. Williams-Russo P, Urquhart BL, Sharrock NE, et al. Post-operative delirium: predictors and prognosis in elderly orthopedic patients. *J Am Geriatr Soc* 1992;40: 759–767.

78. Wood GW II. Low back pain and disorders of the intervertebral disc. In: Crenshaw AH, ed. *Campbell's operative orthopaedics.* St. Louis: Mosby–Year Book, 1992:3764.

79. Yamada S, Aiba T, Endo Y, et al. Creutzfeldt-Jakob disease transmitted by a cadaveric dura mater graft. *Neurosurgery* 1994;34:740–744.

80. Yelnik A, Dizien O, Bussel B, et al. Systematic lower limb phlebography in acute spinal cord injury in 147 patients. *Paraplegia* 1991;29:253–260.

81. Zeidman SM, Ducker TB. Posterior cervical laminoforaminotomy for radiculopathy: review of 172 cases. *Neurosurgery* 1993;33:356–362.

82. Zeidman SM, Ducker TB, Raycroft J. Trends and complications in cervical spine surgery. *J Spine Disord* 1997;10:523–526.

INDEX

Note: Page numbers followed by *f* indicate figures; numbers followed by *t* indicate tables.